We lovingly dedicate this book

to our families:

especially Phil, Ken, and Jim

Preface

Introduction to Basic Cardiac Dysrhythmias was written to help the beginning learner unravel the mysteries of those squiggly lines seen on the monitor and rhythm strip. Our intent is to explain what happens inside the heart when a dysrhythmia is seen, as well as how the dysrhythmia appears on a monitor or rhythm strip.

Although the text is designed for students without a medical background, the learner with limited cardiac knowledge should also find it helpful.

The term **dysrhythmia** is used in the title and throughout the text because we believe it is an accurate description of the information presented. We have used simple medical terminology whenever feasible; numerous illustrations are also included to make learning as easy as possible.

The hearts found in the illustrations are not drawn to scale; the atria, atrioventricular junction, and septum are drawn larger than normal, to show the conduction pathway of the heart clearly. A sequential approach is used, following the normal electrical conduction pathway of the heart.

All rhythm strips are from a Lead II placement and reflect examples of cardiac rhythms found in the adult patient.

- **Chapter 1** covers the basic anatomy and physiology of the cardiac, pulmonary, and vascular systems, with corresponding illustrations for additional clarification. Medical terms are introduced with simple explanations or definitions.

- **Chapter 2** explains the equipment and supplies used in telemetry, the components of a cardiac complex, and information for interpreting rhythm strips.

- **Chapters 3 to 7** explain basic cardiac dysrhythmias, following the normal, sequential conduction pathway of the heart (i.e., atrial, junctional, and ventricular dysrhythias), as well as heart blocks, aberrant and escape beats, followed by pacemaker rhythms.

- **Chapter 8** offers a concise review of all dysrhythmias discussed in the book, providing sample rhythm strips and brief explanations of the parameters involved in identifying each dysrhythmia.

- **Chapter 9** focuses on the treatment of basic dysrhythmias and follows current American Heart Association standards.

- **Chapter 10** includes at least one example of each dysrhythmia shown in the book, as well as space for the reader to write in the measurements of each component and the name of the dysrhythmia.

- **Chapter 11** provides various case studies for additional review of dysrhythmias and treatment.

Review questions and practice strips can be found at the end of each chapter to assist readers in measuring their progress in learning. A section of flash cards, as well as a glossary and index, can be found at the end of the book.

We gratefully acknowledge the efforts of others who were so instrumental in the completion of this text. Many thanks to all of our nursing friends and colleagues for their encouragement and constant "eagle eyes" for varied rhythm strips and to all the nurses and monitor technicians who attended our courses and provided such valuable feedback about our original study guide.

Last, but certainly not least, our loving thanks to our families for their patience, understanding, and encouragement.

Introduction to Basic Cardiac Dysrhythmias

Introduction to Basic Cardiac Dysrhythmias

Second Edition

Sandra Atwood, RN, BA

Cheryl Stanton, RN, CEN

Jenny Storey, RN, BSN

Original illustrations by Jenny Storey, RN, BSN
Modified versions by Mark Wieber

with 484 illustrations

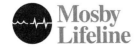

St. Louis Baltimore Boston Carlsbad Chicago Naples New York Philadelphia Portland
London Madrid Mexico City Singapore Sydney Tokyo Toronto Wiesbaden

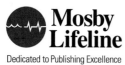

A Times Mirror
Company

Publisher: David Dusthimer
Executive Editor: Claire Merrick
Developmental Editor: Nancy Peterson
Editor: Julie Scardiglia
Assistant Editor: Lisa Esposito
Project Manager: Chris Baumle
Production Editor: Susie Coladonato
Design Manager: Nancy McDonald
Cover Design: Ellen Dawsen
Manufacturing Supervisor: Andrew Christensen

Second Edition

Copyright 1996 by Mosby-Year Book, Inc.
A Mosby Lifeline Imprint of Mosby-Year Book, Inc.

Previous edition copyrighted 1990

Printed in the United States of America
Composition by Graphic World
Printing/binding by Quebecor Printing

Mosby-Year Book, Inc.
11830 Westline Industrial Drive
St. Louis, Missouri 63146

Library of Congress Cataloging-in-Publication Data

Atwood, Sandra
Introduction to basic cardiac dysrhythmias, second edition/ Sandra Atwood, Cheryl Stanton,
Jenny Storey; illustrations by Jenny Storey.
    p. cm.
  ISBN 0-8016-0258-0
  1. Electrocardiography. 2. Arrhythmia—Diagnosis. I. Stanton, Cheryl,
II. Storey, Jenny. III. Title.
  (DNLM: 1. Arrhythmia. WG 330 A887i)
RC683.5E5A78 1990
616.1'28—-dc20
DNLM/DLC
for Library of Congress   89-13340
                                        CIP

Introduction to the Second Edition

We have made some significant changes in the second edition of *Introduction to Basic Cardiac Dysrythmias*. The most important difference is the addition of a new chapter, Chapter 11, "Case Studies." We added this chapter so students could apply their new knowledge in a practical manner. Other changes include the addition of 90 rhythm strips to Chapter 10 and the addition of a medication review in Chapter 9, which is based on the latest ACLS guidelines of the American Heart Association.

Other additions include the following new information:
- Explanation and examples of cardiac output, including the formula for the calculation of cardiac output
- Basic description and explanation of the effects of the autonomic nervous system on cardiac rate
- Definition, common symptoms, and basic treatment of myocardial infarction
- Use of calipers for determining the regularity of a rhythm
- Updated illustrations and materials
- Information about, and an illustration, of an AICD unit
- Flashcards for an additional means of dysrhythmia identification practice

NOTE TO THE READER
While the authors and the publisher have made every attempt to check the accuracy of this text, the possibility of error can never be eliminated. The information presented here represents accepted practices in the United States, but is not offered as a standard of care. It is the reader's responsibility to learn and follow the protocols of their locality, and to follow the direction of a licensed physician. It is also the reader's responsibility to stay informed of procedural changes and new drugs used in emergency care.

Contents

3 SINUS AND ATRIAL DYSRHYTHMIAS — 41

4 JUNCTIONAL DYSRHYTHMIAS — 65

Anatomy and Physiology

Chapter One

Objectives

On completion of this chapter, the reader should be able to:

1. List the two main organs of the cardiovascular system.
2. Identify the four heart chambers, three cardiac muscle layers, and four main heart valves.
3. Explain the basic function of the lungs.
4. Describe the three main types of blood vessels.
5. Describe the flow of a drop of blood from the vena cava through the heart and lungs to the aorta.
6. Explain how to measure cardiac output.
7. Explain the four common characteristics of all cardiac cells.
8. Define the following terms: polarization, depolarization, and repolarization.
9. Describe the movement of an electrical impulse, following the normal cardiac conduction pathways.
10. Explain the actions of the sympathetic and parasympathetic nervous systems on the heart rate.

Outline

ANATOMY

The main organs of the cardiovascular system are the heart and lungs. These organs work together to circulate oxygenated blood through blood vessels to all body cells.

Heart

The adult heart is a hollow, muscular organ that is located in the chest cavity, between the sternum (breastbone) and the spinal column. The normal adult heart weighs about one pound (0.45 kilogram) and is approximately the size of an adult fist.

The heart functions as a double pump. The pumping action occurs when the muscular walls of each heart chamber contract (squeeze), causing blood to be forced out of the chambers.

Heart Chambers

The heart has four chambers: right atrium, left atrium, right ventricle, and left ventricle (Fig. 1-1). The *atria* (plural for atrium) are thin-walled, upper chambers that function as reservoirs, or holding areas, for blood. *Ventricles* are the lower chambers of the heart. The right ventricle has a thin muscular wall, while the muscle of the left ventricular wall is much thicker. The atria contract at the same time, followed by the ventricles contracting at the same time. These contractions usually occur in a rhythmic beat, making a, "lub, dub; lub, dub" sound.

The heart is further divided by a muscular wall called the *septum.* The septum separates the atria and ventricles into right and left sides (Fig. 1-2). The right side of the heart pumps blood to the lungs, while the left side of the heart pumps blood throughout the body.

The pumping action of the left ventricle produces a pulse, or wave of pressure, which can be counted. This pulse is called the ventricular rate and is usually defined as heart beats per minute.

> NOTE: The hearts are drawn for simplicity and ease of illustration. They are **not** drawn to scale.

Heart Muscle

The heart is made of specialized muscle tissue that is not found anywhere else in the body. This specialized tissue forms the cardiac wall and has three main layers. The first layer of the cardiac wall is called the *endocardium* and lines the chambers of the heart and covers the valves.

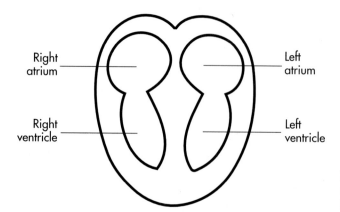

Right atrium

Left atrium

Right ventricle

Left ventricle

Fig. 1-1 The four chambers of the heart.

The second layer of the cardiac wall is the *myocardium.* This layer is the heart muscle and provides the pumping action needed to circulate blood. The *epicardium* is the third layer of the cardiac muscle and is a thin, protective membrane that covers the outside of the heart.

The heart is contained in a loose-fitting sac called the *pericardium* or *pericardial* sac (Fig. 1-3). A small amount of fluid can be found in the space between the epicardium and pericardium. This fluid *(pericardial fluid)* acts as a lubricant, allowing the heart to move within the sac as it beats.

The myocardium and pericardium are further divided into sublayers, which are discussed in 12 Lead electrocardiogram courses.

Heart Valves

The heart has four valves that are covered with endocardial tissue. These four valves are located in the following areas of the heart:

> *Tricuspid valve*—Between the right atrium and the right ventricle
> *Pulmonic valve*—Between the right ventricle and the pulmonary artery
> *Mitral valve*—Between the left atrium and the left ventricle
> *Aortic valve*—Between the left ventricle and the aorta (Fig. 1-4)

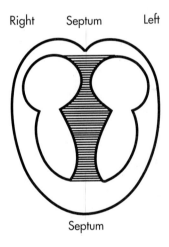

Right   Septum   Left

Septum

Fig. 1-2 Septum that divides the right and left sides of the heart.

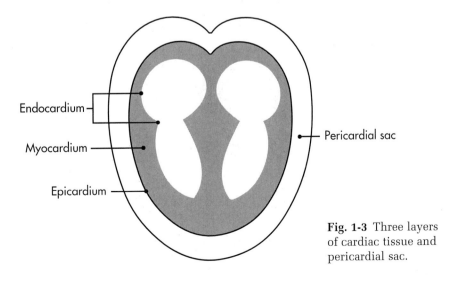

Endocardium

Myocardium

Epicardium

Pericardial sac

Fig. 1-3 Three layers of cardiac tissue and pericardial sac.

These valves are flaplike structures that open and close in response to the pumping action of the heart. The opening and closing of the heart valves permit the flow of blood in a forward direction and prevent blood from flowing backward.

For example, in the left side of the heart, as the blood enters the empty left atrium, the blood causes increased pressure against the atrial walls. When the atrial pressure becomes greater than the ventricular pressure, the mitral valve opens, allowing most of the blood to flow into the left ventricle. The atrium then gives a mild contraction (atrial kick), emptying the remaining blood into the left ventricle.

As the left ventricle contracts, the mitral valve closes and the aortic valve opens. The closed mitral valve prevents the flow of blood back into the left atrium. The open aortic valve allows the blood to be pumped from the heart and then carried to all body cells.

The noises caused by the normal closing of the valves are known as *heart sounds*. In an adult, a *murmur* is an abnormal sound made by blood flowing through a valve that is not functioning correctly. This sound can be heard when listening to the heart with a stethoscope. Heart murmurs frequently are caused by an improperly functioning mitral valve.

Lungs

The lungs are two large organs that are located within the chest cavity. The main function of the lungs is to remove carbon dioxide from the blood and to replace it with oxygen (Fig. 1-5).

The exchange of carbon dioxide for oxygen takes place in the lungs, inside millions of tiny sacs called *alveoli*. The alveoli are tiny, grapelike clusters of tissue that are surrounded by very small blood vessels called *capillaries*. Because the walls of both the alveoli and the capillaries are only one-cell thick, the exchange of oxygen and carbon dioxide occurs easily.

Blood Vessels

Blood vessels are located throughout the body, and their primary purpose is transportation. They carry oxygenated blood to all body cells and then transport blood with carbon dioxide from the body cells to the lungs.

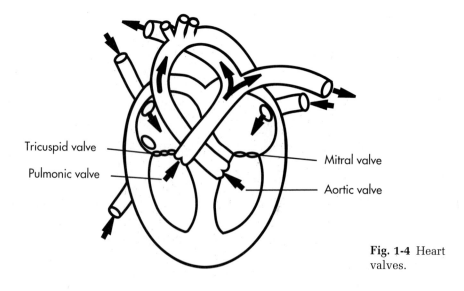

Tricuspid valve

Pulmonic valve

Mitral valve

Aortic valve

Fig. 1-4 Heart valves.

The three main types of blood vessels are *arteries, veins,* and *capillaries* (Fig. 1-6). Arteries carry blood away from the heart, while veins carry blood to the heart. The exchange of nutrients and waste products for the body cells takes place in the capillaries.

Arteries

Arteries are blood vessels that carry oxygenated blood away from the heart to all parts of the body. Arteries have the thickest walls of all blood vessels because they must withstand the pumping pressure of the heart. The *aorta* is the largest artery in the body.

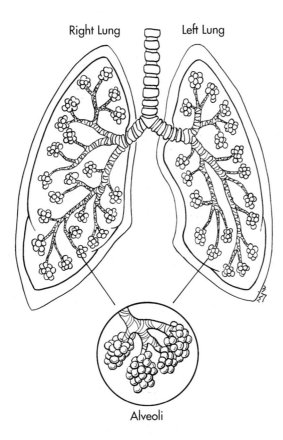

Fig. 1-5 Lungs and alveoli.

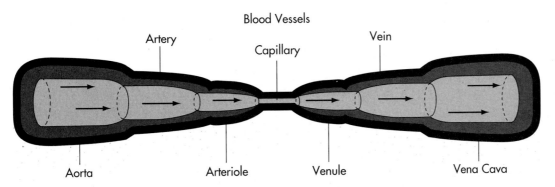

Fig. 1-6 Gradual change in the size of blood vessels and vessel walls.

The arteries divide into *arterioles,* which are smaller blood vessels with thinner walls. The arterioles connect arteries to capillaries.

Veins

Veins are vessels that carry blood with carbon dioxide from the body cells back to the heart. The venous walls are thinner than the arterial walls and contain tiny valves (similar to cardiac valves) that prevent the backward flow of blood. The *vena cava* is the largest vein in the body. The smallest veins are called *venules,* which connect veins to capillaries.

> NOTE: The one exception to the definition of arteries and veins is found in the heart/lung circulation. The pulmonary arteries carry blood with carbon dioxide to the lungs, and the pulmonary veins carry blood with oxygen to the heart.

Capillaries

Capillaries, the smallest blood vessels in the body, also have the thinnest walls of any blood vessel. The exchange of oxygen and waste products between the blood and the body cells takes place through the capillary walls.

Coronary Arteries

The heart muscle receives its blood supply from *coronary arteries.* These special arteries branch off the aorta and supply oxygenated blood to each portion of the heart muscle.

For example, the right coronary artery divides into the posterior descending artery and the marginal artery, both of which again divide into smaller arteries (Fig. 1-7). Therefore, the right coronary artery and its branches are able to provide oxygenated blood to the muscle tissue of the right atrium, the left ventricle, and the right ventricle. The left coronary artery also branches (divides) into smaller arteries, which provide oxygenated blood to the muscle tissue of the left atrium, the left ventricle, and the right ventricle. Most of this oxygenated blood flows to the cardiac muscle between heart beats (contractions) while the myocardium is resting.

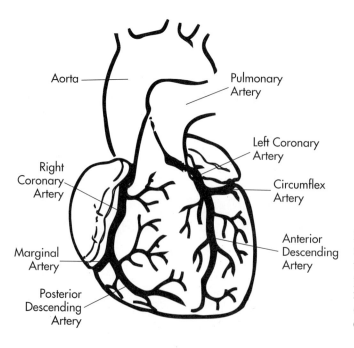

Aorta

Pulmonary Artery

Left Coronary Artery

Right Coronary Artery

Circumflex Artery

Marginal Artery

Anterior Descending Artery

Posterior Descending Artery

Fig. 1-7 Coronary vessels: arteries that supply oxygen and nutrients to cardiac muscle cells.

Myocardial Infarction

A coronary artery may become partially or completely blocked by blood clots or a build-up of cholesterol on the inside of the artery wall. When a blockage occurs, the cardiac muscle usually nourished by that artery does not receive enough oxygen.

The decreased supply of oxygen to tissue is called *ischemia.* Ischemia that is not diagnosed and treated usually leads to *myocardial infarction* (death of cardiac tissue). The death of cardiac tissue usually lessens the ability of the cardiac muscle to contract and pump blood efficiently.

A myocardial infarction (MI, heart attack, or coronary) can affect any area of the heart.

The location of the myocardial infarction may cause an interruption in the cardiac electrical conduction pathways. This interruption may cause dysrhythmias (abnormal cardiac rhythms), which will be discussed in Chapters 3 through 7.

Symptoms of an MI may include chest pain or pressure that is described as a heavy feeling, a dull ache, a feeling of being squeezed, or a discomfort similar to indigestion. The pain or pressure may radiate (move) down the left arm or into the neck, jaw, back, or shoulders. Other signs include nausea; vomiting; difficulty breathing; and pale, cool, sweating skin. Confusion or loss of consciousness may also be present.

MECHANICAL PHYSIOLOGY

Heart/Lung Circulation

The right side of the heart receives blood from the vena cava and sends this blood to the lungs. The lungs filter carbon dioxide from the blood and exchange it for oxygen. The oxygenated blood then flows to the left side of the heart, which pumps the blood into the aorta. Blood is circulated through the heart and lungs in the following order:

vena cava → right atrium → tricuspid valve → right ventricle → pulmonic valve → pulmonary arteries → lungs → pulmonary veins → left atrium → mitral valve → left ventricle → aortic valve → aorta → rest of the body, including the heart (Fig. 1-8).

Cardiac Output

One method of measuring how efficiently the heart is pumping and circulating blood to the body cells is by determining the *cardiac output.* Cardiac output is the amount of blood pumped by the left ventricle in 1 minute.

Cardiac output (CO) is measured by multiplying the ventricular rate (VR) by the stroke volume (SV), which is the amount of blood pumped by the left ventricle with each beat. The formula is: $CO = SV \times VR$.

CO—cardiac output is the amount of blood pumped by the left ventricle in 1 minute. The normal amount is usually 5000 to 6000 cc.

SV—stroke volume is the amount of blood pumped by the left ventricle with each contraction or beat, approximately 70 cc.

VR—ventricular rate is the number of times the left ventricle contracts in 1 minute; the normal rate is 60 to 100.

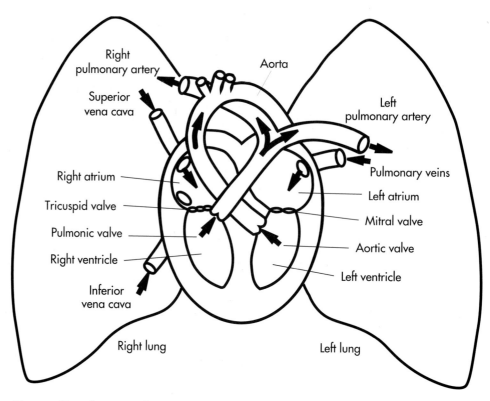

Right
pulmonary artery

Aorta

Superior
vena cava

Left
pulmonary artery

Right atrium

Pulmonary veins

Tricuspid valve

Left atrium

Pulmonic valve

Mitral valve

Right ventricle

Aortic valve

Inferior
vena cava

Left ventricle

Right lung

Left lung

Fig. 1-8 Heart/lung circulation.

Example: CO = SV × VR; the stroke volume is 70 cc, and the ventricular rate is
80; CO = 70 × 80 = 5600 = normal cardiac output.

When the cardiac output is abnormal, the heart will try to balance it by
changing either the stroke volume or the ventricular rate. For example, if a person exercises and becomes physically fit, the stroke volume usually increases,
because the heart muscle is stronger and pumps more blood with each beat.
The ventricular rate then decreases to keep the cardiac output within the normal range.

Example: CO = SV × VR; with an increased stroke volume of 90 cc and a decreased ventricular rate of 60: CO = 90 × 60 = 5400 = normal cardiac
output.

The opposite is also true. When the heart cannot pump the usual amount of
blood, due to injury or disease, the stroke volume decreases. The ventricular
rate will then increase to maintain a normal cardiac output.

Example: CO = SV × VR; with a decreased stroke volume of 50 cc and an increased ventricular rate of 110: CO = 50 × 110 = 5500 = normal cardiac output.

If the heart is unable to increase the stroke volume or the ventricular rate,
the cardiac output will decrease.

Example: CO = SV × VR; with a decreased stroke volume of 50 cc and a ventricular rate of 60: CO = 50 × 60 = 3000 = decreased cardiac output.

A decreased (poor) cardiac output may cause damage to major organs such as the heart and brain. This damage occurs because there is not enough blood being circulated to carry oxygen to the body cells.

Any combination of signs and symptoms, such as pale, cool and clammy skin; shortness of breath; confusion; dizziness; decreased blood pressure; and/or chest pains, may indicate poor cardiac output.

ELECTROPHYSIOLOGY

All muscle tissue contracts in response to an electrical stimulus or impulse. For example, skeletal muscle will contract after receiving stimulation from a nerve. However, *cardiac muscle* is unique; not only can it respond to an electrical impulse, cardiac muscle also has pacemaker cells that can generate electrical impulses.

The following definitions explain four common characteristics of cardiac cells:

Automaticity—the ability of cardiac pacemaker cells to generate their own electrical impulses

Excitability—irritability; the ability of cardiac cells to respond to an electrical stimulus; when a cardiac cell is highly irritable, less stimulus is required to cause a contraction

Conductivity—the ability of cardiac cells to receive an electrical stimulus and then transmit it to other cardiac cells

Contractility—the ability of cardiac cells to shorten, causing cardiac muscle contraction in response to an electrical stimulus

Contractility is a mechanical function of the heart. Automaticity, excitability, and conductivity are electrical functions.

Depolarization and Repolarization

The following terms explain the phases of the normal electrical activity of the heart:

Polarization—the phase of readiness; the muscle is relaxed and the cardiac cells are ready to receive an electrical impulse

Depolarization—the phase of contraction; the cardiac cells have transmitted an electrical impulse, causing the cardiac muscle to contract

Repolarization—the recovery phase; the muscle has contracted and the cells are returning to a ready state

All tissue, including cardiac muscle, is made of many single cells that contain chemicals such as potassium and sodium. The cells normally have *potassium* (K) on the inside of the cell and *sodium* (Na) on the outside. These cells are *polarized,* or in the ready state (Fig. 1-9A).

When a pacemaker cell generates an electrical impulse to a polarized cardiac cell, most of the potassium moves to the outside of the cell and most of the sodium moves to the inside of the cell. This movement of the potassium and sodium through the cell wall causes a "spark" of electricity. The electrical spark is then conducted to the remaining cells in that part of the heart, causing *depolarization* (Fig. 1-9B). While in this state, the cardiac cells contract. They cannot respond to any further electrical impulses until they have repolarized.

After the electrical impulse has passed through the cells, the potassium reenters the cells and the sodium leaves, causing *repolarization* (Fig. 1-9C). However, all cells do not repolarize at the same time. Therefore, some cardiac cells are able to conduct an additional electrical impulse sooner than others.

Electrical Conduction Pathway

Although any cardiac pacemaker cell is capable of initiating an electrical impulse, the normal pacemaker is the *sinoatrial node*. The normal electrical conduction pathway of the heart occurs in the following order:

> sinoatrial node → internodal and intra-atrial pathways → atrioventricular node → bundle of His → bundle branches → Purkinje's fibers → ventricular muscle (Fig. 1-10).

Sinoatrial node (SA node)   The sinoatrial node is located in the upper portion of the right atrium and is called the *pacemaker of the heart.* The SA node initiates an electrical impulse that

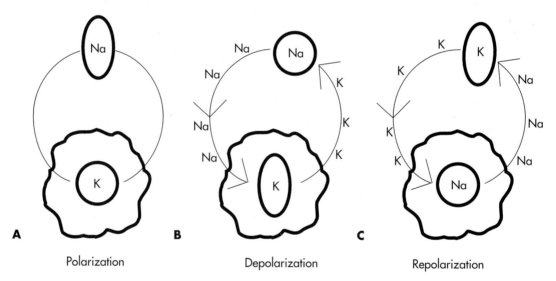

A	B	C
Polarization	Depolarization	Repolarization

Fig. 1-9, A-C. Electrical conduction within cardiac cells showing exchange of sodium and potassium.

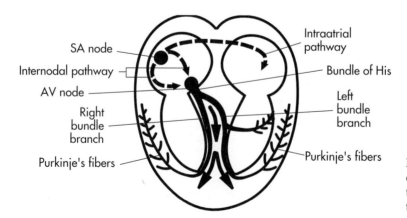

Fig. 1-10 Normal electrical conduction pathway of the heart.

travels downward, throughout the muscle of both atria. This impulse travels through the atrial muscles by way of the *intraatrial conduction pathways,* causing depolarization of the atrium. The same impulse is also transmitted from the SA node to the atrioventricular node through the *internodal conduction pathways.* The SA node usually generates 60 to 100 electrical impulses per minute.

Atrioventricular node (AV node)	The atrioventricular node is located in the general area of the lower right atrium near the septum. The AV node continues transmitting the impulse from the atria to the bundle of His. If the SA node fails to function, pacemaker cells between the atria and the AV node *(AV junction)* are capable of functioning as a *secondary pacemaker.* This area of the electrical conduction system usually generates 40 to 60 electrical impulses per minute.
Bundle of His	The bundle of His, located below the AV node, continues transmitting the electrical impulse to the bundle branches.
3 – Bundle branches (BB)	The lower portion of the bundle of His divides into a *right bundle branch* (leading into the right ventricle) and a *left bundle branch* (leading into the left ventricle). The bundle branches continue transmitting the electrical impulse to the Purkinje's fibers.
Purkinje's fibers	Extending from the bundle branches into the muscular walls of the ventricles, the Purkinje's fibers conduct the electrical impulse from the bundle branches to cells of the ventricular muscle.
Ventricular muscle	The cells of the ventricular muscle receive an electrical stimulus from the Purkinje's fibers and contract. If the SA node **and** the AV junction do not initiate an electrical impulse, an impulse can be generated from any pacemaker cell in the ventricles including the Purkinje's fibers or the bundle branches. These impulses are usually generated at a rate of 20 to 40 impulses per minute.

Autonomic Nervous System

The electrical conduction system of the heart is affected by the *autonomic nervous system.* The function of the autonomic nervous system is to maintain the body in a normal state by controlling several organs, including the heart as well as the blood vessels. This control is done automatically, without a person being aware it is happening.

The autonomic nervous system is divided into two parts: the *sympathetic* and the *parasympathetic* systems.

The sympathetic nervous system prepares the body to react in times of stress or emergencies, increasing cardiac output by increasing the heart rate, blood pressure, and force of cardiac contractions. This is known as the "fight or flight response." The sympathetic nerves can be stimulated by anger, pain, fright, caffeine, and some drugs.

The parasympathetic nervous system affects the heart in the opposite way by decreasing the rate of cardiac contractions. This reaction usually occurs after the stress or emergency is over, allowing the body to restore energy. The parasympathetic nerves can be stimulated by straining to have a bowel movement, a urinary bladder that is too full, vomiting, and some drugs.

Medications are available to reverse the effects of the sympathetic and parasympathetic nervous systems on the heart, when necessary. For example, when the parasympathetic nerves have been stimulated and decrease the heart rate too much, drugs such as atropine block the parasympathetic nerves and allow the heart rate to increase.

Chapter 1: Review

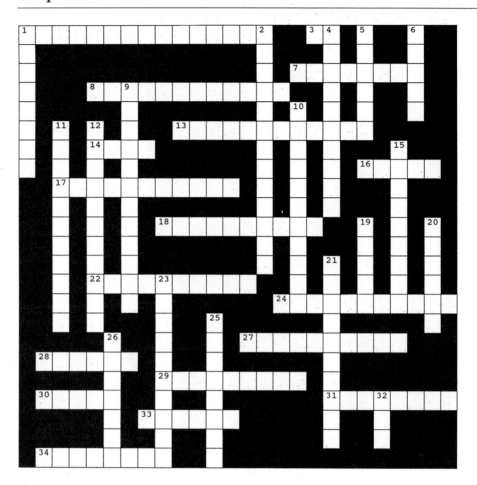

ACROSS

1. Part of autonomic nervous system that decreases heart rate.

3. The _____ node transmits electrical impulses between the SA node and the bundle of His.

7. Atrioventricular area known as the secondary pacemaker of the heart.

8. Ability of cardiac cells to respond to electrical impulses.

13. Ability of cardiac cells to generate electrical impulses.

14. SA _____ is the primary pacemaker of the heart.

16. Largest artery in the body.

17. Tissue forming the sac that surrounds the heart.

18. The SA node initiates _____ impulses.

22. Conduction pathway between the SA node and the AV junction.

24. First or inner layer of heart wall.

27. Cardiac cells _____ after they have transmitted an electrical impulse.

28. Bundle of His conducts electrical impulses to the _____ branches.

29. The _____ nervous system maintains the body in a normal state.

30. Wave of pressure that can be counted; heartbeats per minute.

31. Lack of oxygen to tissue.

33. Valve between the left atrium and left ventricle.

34. The ventricular muscle cells receive electrical impulses from the

       _____'s fibers.

DOWN

1. Valve between the right ventricle and artery leading to lungs.

2. Ability of cardiac muscle to shorten in response to an electrical impulse.

4. Lower chambers of the heart.

5. Blood vessel that carries oxygenated blood to body tissues.

6. Organs that exchange oxygen for carbon dioxide.

9. Ability of cardiac cells to transmit electrical impulses.

10. Heart/lung _____ describes the way blood travels between the heart and the lungs.

11. Part of the autonomic nervous system that increases heart rate.

12. Conduction pathway between the right and left atrium.

15. Valve between the right atria and the right ventricle.

19. Upper chambers of the heart.

20. Abnormal sound made by blood passing through damaged valves.

21. Muscle layer of the heart.

23. When the cardiac cells _____, they are able to conduct an electrical impulse again.

25. Arteries that supply the heart muscle with oxygen; also another name for a myocardial infarction.

26. Small grape-like structures in the lungs where the exchange of carbon dioxide and oxygen occurs.

32. The AV node transmits electrical impulses to the bundle of _____.

The solution to this crossword puzzle is in the answer section.

Monitoring and Telemetry

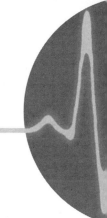

Telemetry refers to the process of monitoring cardiac electrical activity. This process includes a machine, graph paper, the identification of complex components, and the interpretation of rhythm strips.

MONITORS AND TELEMETRY UNITS

The movement of electrical impulses through the heart can be seen by using a machine that is called an *electrocardiograph* or *monitor*. The monitor shows the electrical impulses as a pattern of waves on the monitor screen (Fig. 2-1).

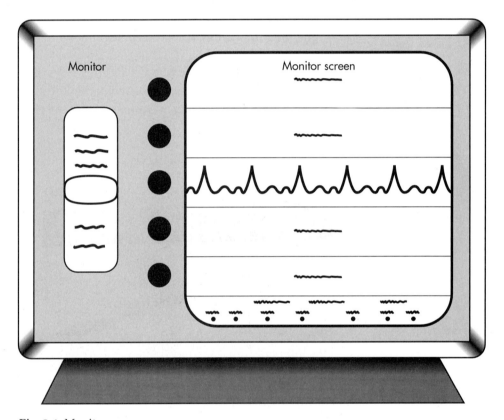

Fig. 2-1 Monitor screen.

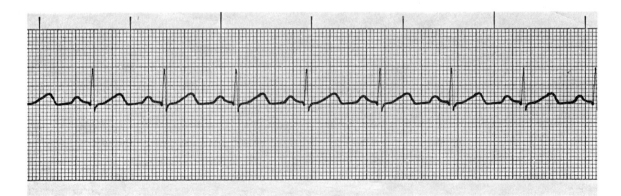

Fig. 2-2 Rhythm strip.

These wave patterns can also be transferred to graph paper for a printed record of the electrical impulses as they travel through the heart. This printed record is called a *rhythm strip* (Fig. 2-2).

Many monitors feature a *freeze mode* to stop the action on the screen. A *delay mode* may also be available to print a specific part of the wave pattern that has already been seen. These special features allow the observer to study the wave pattern more closely.

Remember: the monitor does **not** show the actual **contraction** of the cardiac muscle, only the conduction of the electrical impulses through the heart. Cardiac contractions can only be confirmed by the presence of a pulse.

Electrodes and Leads

The monitor receives electrical impulses from the patient's heart through a system of electrodes placed on the body. *Electrodes* are adhesive pads that contain a conductive gel and are attached to the patient's skin.

Electrodes are connected to the monitor by clearly marked wires called *leads* (Fig. 2-3). A positive, a negative, and a ground lead must be used for the monitor to receive a clear picture of the cardiac electrical impulses.

The leads from the electrodes may be connected either directly to a monitor or to a telemetry unit. The *telemetry unit* is a small, battery-operated box that resembles a transistor radio. It transmits the electrical impulses to a monitor at a nursing station or other central location (Fig. 2-4).

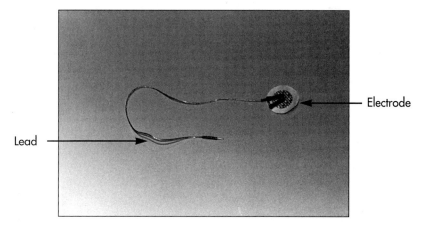

Fig. 2-3 Monitor lead and electrode.

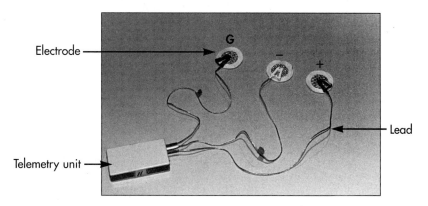

Fig. 2-4 Telemetry unit with leads and electrodes.

Lead Placement

The placement of the electrodes on the patient's body determines the angle at which the electrical impulses are received and therefore, the part of the heart being observed. The 12-Lead *electrocardiogram* (EKG, ECG) "looks" at the heart from 12 different viewing angles. However, most patients are monitored using only one or two "viewing angles." The patterns of the electrodes on the patient are called *Leads*.

> NOTE: The term *leads* is used in two different ways:
> 1. The wires leading from electrodes to the monitor. The word "leads" is not capitalized in this definition.
> 2. The different types of electrode placements. In this definition, the word "Leads" is capitalized.

The standard EKG Leads are I, II, III, aVR, aVL, aVF, V1, V2, V3, V4, V5, and V6. Leads I, II, III, aVR, aVL and aVF are known as *limb* or *peripheral* Leads. Leads V1, V2, V3, V4, V5, and V6 are known as *chest* or *precordial* Leads. In limb Leads, electrodes are placed on the arms and legs or outer areas of the chest. In chest Leads, electrodes are attached to very specific areas of the chest.

The placement of electrodes for the chest Leads is sometimes changed slightly to "see" a specific area of the heart more clearly. The chest Leads (V1 through V6) are then referred to as *modified chest Leads* (MCL) and become MCL I through MCL VI.

Patients are usually monitored in Lead II or MCL I. Lead II shows the movement of the electrical impulse (depolarization) through the ventricles most clearly, while MCL I shows the depolarization of the atria.

In Lead II, the negative electrode is placed on the patient's right upper chest and the positive electrode on the left lower chest. The ground electrode is usually positioned on the left upper chest; however, the ground lead may be placed anywhere on the body, because its purpose is to reduce static (Fig. 2-5).

In the MCL I Lead, the positive electrode is placed on the patient's midchest to the right of the sternum and the negative electrode on the left upper chest. The ground electrode may be applied anywhere on the body, but is usually positioned on the left lower chest (Fig. 2-6).

> NOTE: All rhythms included in this book are described as they appear in Lead II on an adult patient.

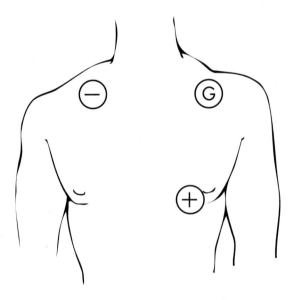

Fig. 2-5 Placement of electrodes for Lead II monitoring.

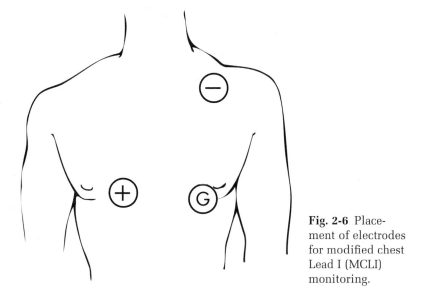

Fig. 2-6 Placement of electrodes for modified chest Lead I (MCLI) monitoring.

Graph Paper

The rhythm strip provides a printed record of cardiac electrical activity and is printed on ruled *graph paper.* Graph paper is divided into small squares that are 1 mm in height and width. The paper is further divided by darker lines every fifth square, both vertically (top to bottom) and horizontally (side to side). Each large square is 5 mm high and 5 mm wide.

Graph paper measures both time and amplitude. *Time* is measured on the horizontal line. Each small square is equal to **0.04 second** and each large square (5 small squares) is **0.20 second**. These squares measure the length of time it takes an electrical impulse to pass through a specific part of the heart (Fig. 2-7).

The force of the electrical impulse is measured by *amplitude.* Amplitude is measured on the vertical line. Each small square on the graph paper is equal to **0.1 millivolt** (mV), and each large square (5 small squares) is **0.5 mV**.

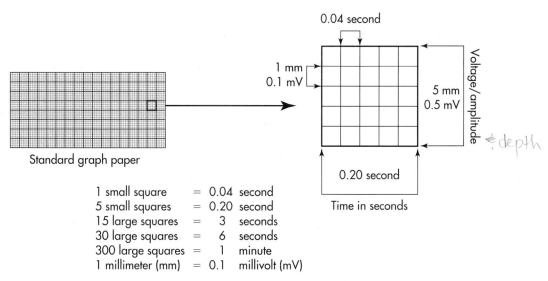

Standard graph paper

1 small square	=	0.04	second
5 small squares	=	0.20	second
15 large squares	=	3	seconds
30 large squares	=	6	seconds
300 large squares	=	1	minute
1 millimeter (mm)	=	0.1	millivolt (mV)

Fig. 2-7 Standard monitoring graph paper illustrating time and amplitude measurements.

COMPLEX COMPONENTS

Each *wave* seen on the graph paper or monitor screen represents an electrical impulse in a specific part of the heart. (All wave components used in this book are described as they appear in Lead II.)

Baseline

The *baseline*, or *isoelectric line*, is the straight line, without any waves, that can be seen on either the monitor or the graph paper. It represents the absence of electrical activity in the cardiac tissue. All waves begin and end at the baseline. A *deflection* (wave) above the baseline is positive (+) and indicates electrical flow **toward** a positive electrode. A deflection below the baseline is negative (-) and indicates an electrical flow **away from** a positive electrode (Fig. 2-8).

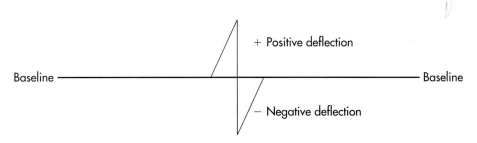

Fig. 2-8 Baseline (isoelectric line) with positive and negative deflections.

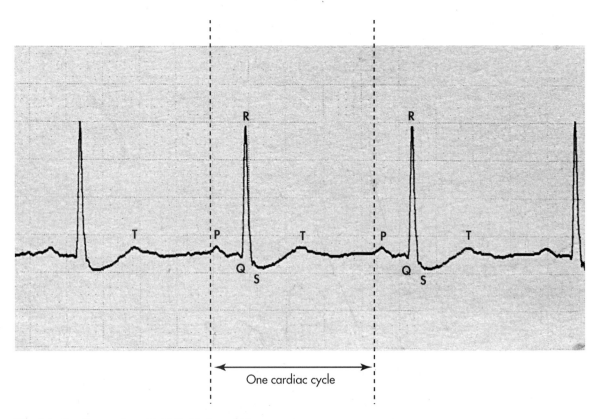

Fig. 2-9 Cardiac cycle with P, Q, R, S, and T waves.

The conduction of an electrical impulse for a single heart beat normally contains five major waves: P, Q, R, S, and T. The combination of these five waves represents a single heartbeat, or one *cardiac cycle* (Fig. 2-9).

P Wave

The *P wave* is the first positive (upward) deflection before the QRS complex. The P wave represents the depolarization of both the right and the left atria (Fig. 2-10). The repolarization of the atria is not usually seen on the rhythm strip because the wave that shows the recovery of the atrial cells is buried in the QRS complex.

PR Interval

The *PR interval* (PRI) represents the time it takes an electrical impulse to be conducted through the atria and the atrioventricular node until the impulse begins to cause ventricular depolarization. The PR interval is measured from the beginning of the P wave to the beginning of the next deflection of the baseline. The normal PR interval is **0.12 to 0.20 second,** or three to five small squares on the graph paper (Fig. 2-11).

QRS Complex

The *QRS complex* usually contains three waves: the Q, R, and S. The *Q wave* is the first negative (downward) deflection following the PR interval. The *R wave* is the first positive deflection after the P wave. The *S wave* is the first negative deflection that follows the R wave (Fig. 2-12). Although the Q wave may not be present in all Leads, this combination of waves is still called a **QRS complex.**

The QRS complex represents ventricular depolarization, or the conduction of an electrical impulse from the bundle of His through the ventricular muscle.

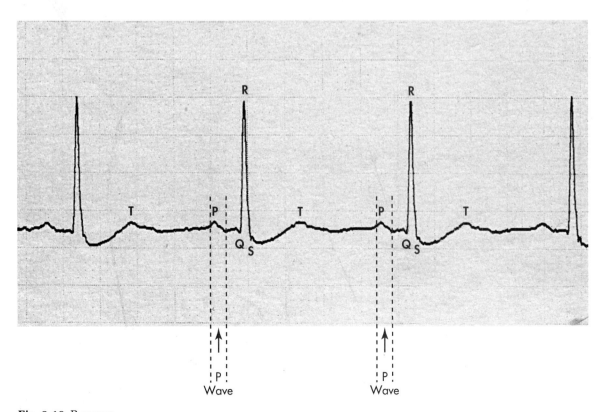

Fig. 2-10 P waves.

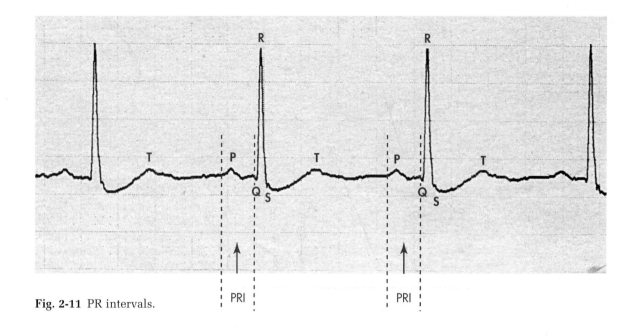

Fig. 2-11 PR intervals.

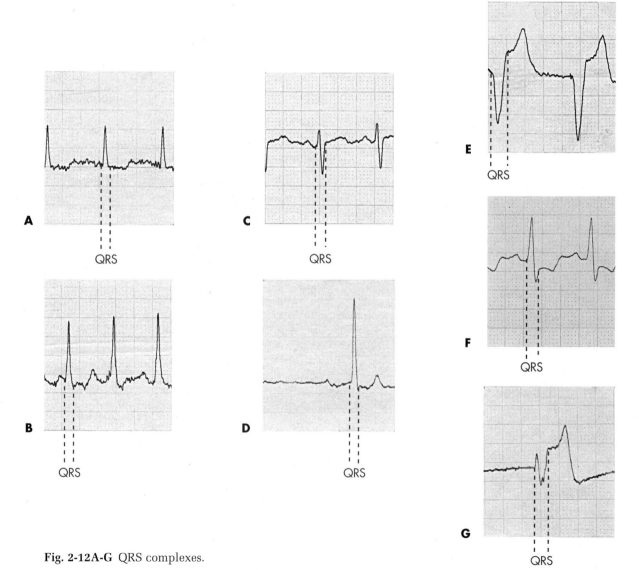

Fig. 2-12A-G QRS complexes.

The measurement of the QRS complex starts at the beginning of the Q wave (or the R wave if the Q wave is not present). The QRS measurement ends where the S wave meets the baseline, or where the S wave would meet the baseline if it did not curve into the ST segment.

The QRS complex normally measures less than **0.12 second**, or less than three small squares on the graph paper (Fig. 2-12).

ST Segment

The portion of the line that leads from the end of the S wave to the beginning of the T wave is the *ST segment* (Fig. 2-13A). The ST segment may be normal (flat), elevated (above the baseline), or depressed (below the baseline) (Fig. 2-13B and C). The beginning of the T wave may be difficult to determine in elevated ST segments. Changes in the ST segment can be used to diagnose a cardiac problem only when seen in a 12-Lead ECG.

T Wave

The *T wave* follows the ST segment and indicates the repolarization of the ventricular myocardial cells (Fig. 2-14A). The T wave may be either above or below the isoelectric line.

A T wave greater than half the height of the QRS complex is *elevated* and may indicate new ischemia (lack of oxygen) of the cardiac muscle (Fig. 2-14B). A *depressed* (inverted) T wave follows an upright QRS complex, is below the isoelectric line, and looks upside down (Fig. 2-14C). An inverted T wave is frequently an indication of previous cardiac ischemia.

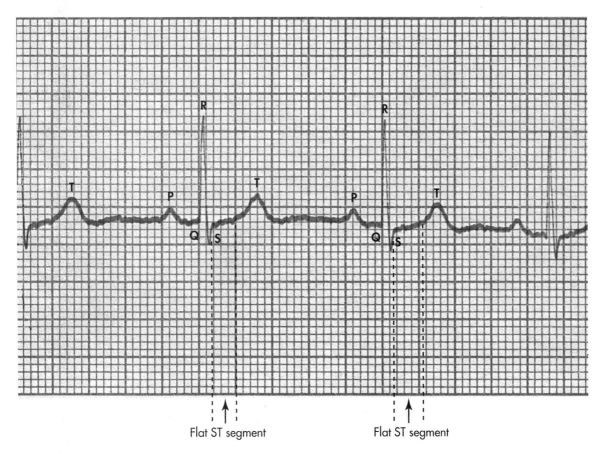

Flat ST segment   Flat ST segment

Fig. 2-13A Normal ST segments.

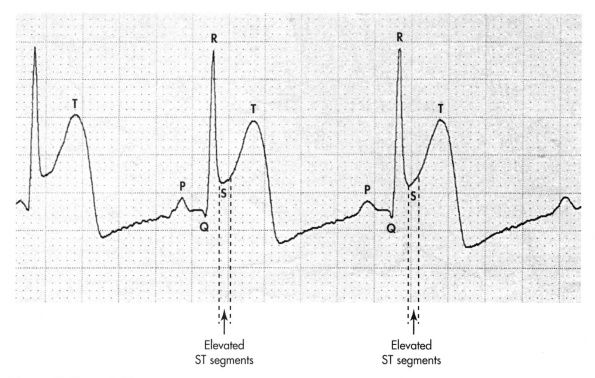

Fig. 2-13B Elevated ST segments.

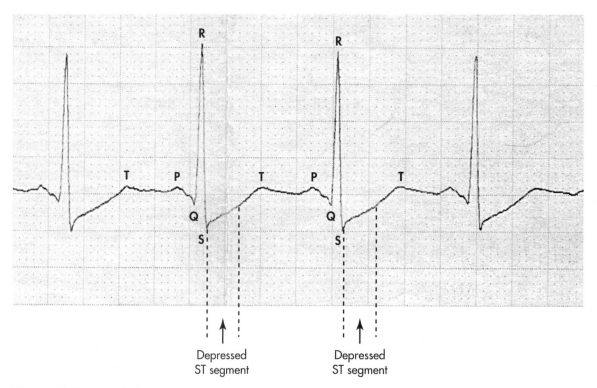

Fig. 2-13C Depressed ST segments.

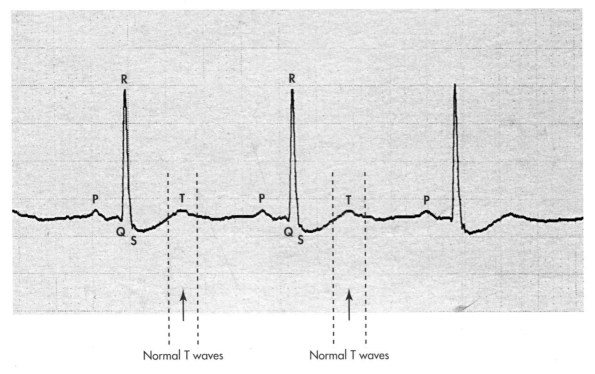

Fig. 2-14A Normal T waves.

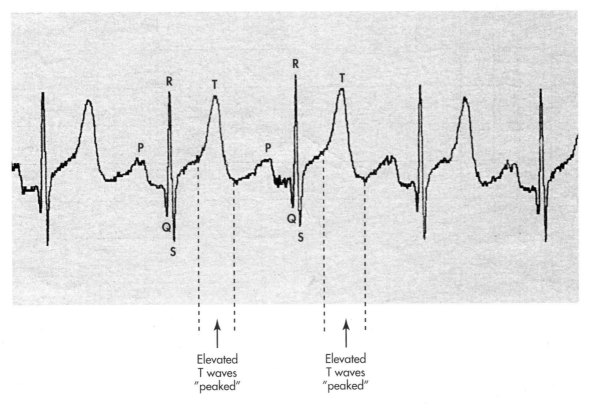

Fig. 2-14B Elevated T waves.

Bundle Branch Block

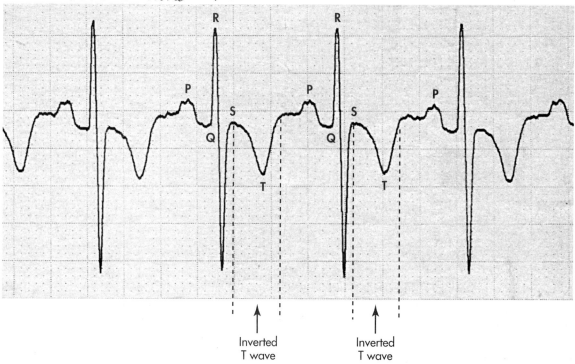

Fig. 2-14C Depressed "inverted" T waves.

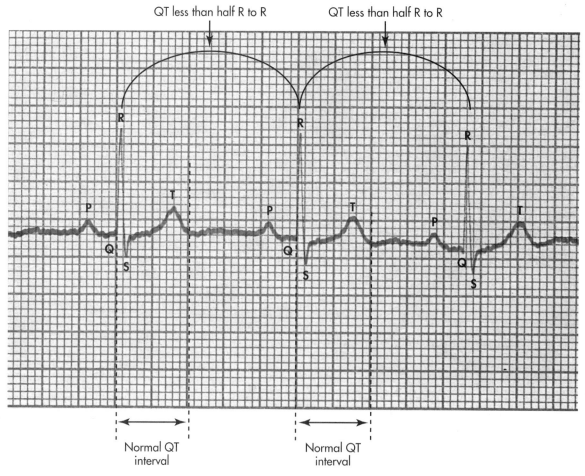

Fig. 2-15A Normal QT intervals.

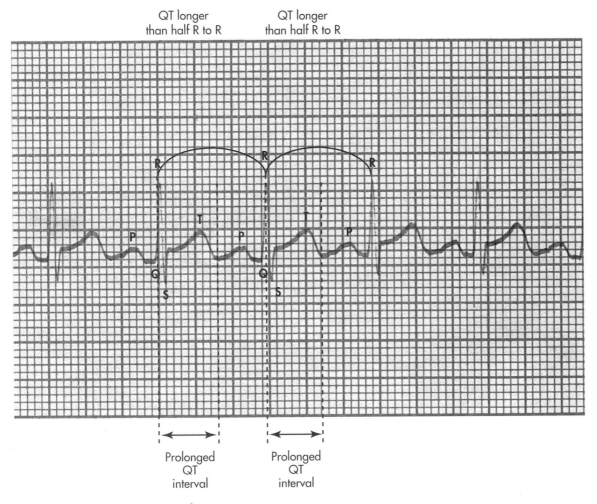

Fig. 2-15B Prolonged QT intervals.

QT Interval

The depolarization and repolarization of the ventricles are shown by the *QT interval*. The QT interval is measured from the beginning of the QRS complex to the end of the T wave.

QT intervals are either normal or prolonged. A normal QT interval is equal to, or less than, one half the R to R interval of that complex (Fig. 2-15A). A QT interval that is greater than one half the R to R interval of that complex is *prolonged* (Fig. 2-15B).

> NOTE: The rhythm strip represents **only** the conduction of electrical impulses through the myocardial cells. Normally, it also represents the contraction of the heart muscle. However, this is not always true, so **you must treat the patient** and any symptoms that are present, **not the monitor.**

REFRACTORY PERIODS

In addition to identifying wave and complex formations, it will be helpful to understand refractory periods.

The *refractory period* is the time between depolarization and the return of the cardiac cells to the ready or polarized state. While the cells are recovering, the atria and ventricles are refilling with blood, preparing to contract again. The refractory period is divided into two phases:

1. *Absolute refractory period*—the cardiac cells have not completed repolarization and **cannot** be stimulated to conduct an electrical impulse and contract again (depolarize). This period is measured from the beginning of the QRS complex through approximately the first third of the T wave.

2. *Relative refractory period*—the cardiac cells have repolarized to the point that **some** cells can again be stimulated to depolarize, if the stimulus is strong enough. However, if these cells are stimulated during this period, they will probably conduct the electrical impulse in a slow, abnormal pattern. This period is measured from the end of the absolute refractory period to the end of the T wave. The relative refractory period is also known as the *vulnerable period of repolarization* (Fig. 2-16).

This information allows more accurate interpretation of dysrhythmias, particularly those involving premature ventricular contractions (*see* Chapter 6, "Ventricular Dysrhythmias").

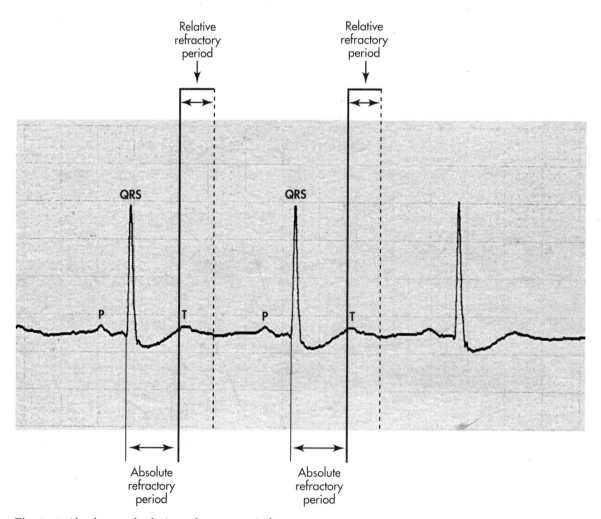

Fig. 2-16 Absolute and relative refractory periods.

INTERPRETING A RHYTHM STRIP

A *rhythm strip* is a tool that assists the observer in the interpretation of a patient's cardiac rhythm. It also is useful to monitor changes in the cardiac cycle. However, a 12-Lead ECG is necessary to diagnose a cardiac problem.

To interpret a cardiac rhythm accurately, you must evaluate P waves (including the ratio of P waves to QRS complexes), PR intervals, QRS complexes, rhythm (regularity), and rate.

These components may be evaluated in any order, however, they must all be evaluated on every rhythm strip. Rhythm interpretation is easier if each component is examined in the same order with each strip.

First, look at the general appearance of the entire rhythm strip, then examine each individual component.

Complex Formation

The **appearance** of the P, Q, R, S, and T waves, and the **ratio** of P waves to QRS complexes should be evaluated. Examine each cardiac cycle from the beginning to its end.

1. *P waves*—examine each P wave.
   a. Are P waves present?
   b. Are they all upright?
   c. Do all P waves look alike?
   d. Is there a P wave before every QRS complex?
   e. Are the P to P intervals equal?
2. *PR intervals*—measure each PR interval.
   a. Are PR intervals present?
   b. Are all PR intervals equal?
   c. Are all PR intervals within the normal range of 0.12 to 0.20 second?
3. *QRS complexes*—examine and measure each QRS complex.
   a. Are QRS complexes present?
   b. Do all QRS complexes look alike?
   c. Is there a QRS complex after every P wave?
   d. Are the R to R intervals equal?
   e. Are all QRS complexes within the normal range of less than 0.12 second?

ST segments, T waves, and QT intervals are not required for the interpretation of cardiac rhythms. However, they can be important as indicators of changes in a patient's cardiac condition, such as new ischemia. Therefore, any change in the ST segment, T wave, or QT interval should be included in the interpretation of a cardiac rhythm strip.

Rhythm

The term *rhythm* is used to describe how regularly the complexes occur. To determine if the complexes occur regularly, measure the R to R intervals and the P to P intervals (if P waves are present). If the R to R intervals are equal, the rhythm is regular (Fig. 2-17). If the P to P and/or the R to R intervals vary by less than 0.06 second (1.5 small squares), the rhythm can be considered regular. If the intervals vary by more than 0.06 second, the rhythm is irregular. The P to P intervals are also measured to determine if the atrial rhythm is regular.

Calipers provide the most accurate method of measuring rhythm. Place the point of one caliper leg on the top of an R wave (Fig. 2-18A). Adjust the caliper so the point of the second caliper leg is on the top of the next R wave. Then move the caliper so that the point of the first leg is on the second R wave. If the rhythm is regular, the second caliper point will be on the top of the third R

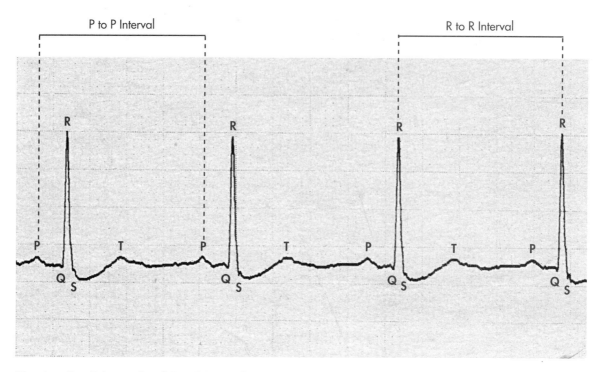

Fig. 2-17 P to P interval and R to R interval.

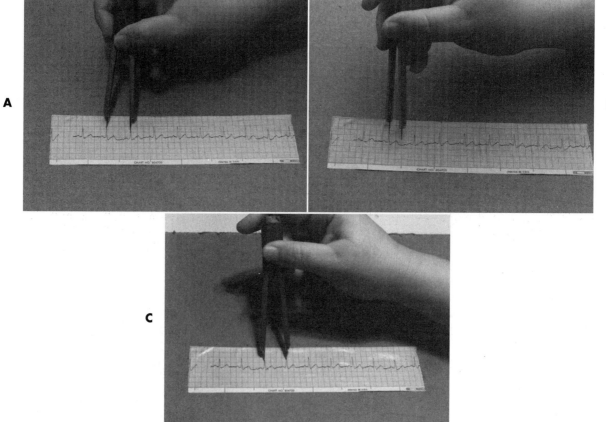

Fig. 2-18 Measuring rhythm with calipers, using R to R intervals: **(A)** mark two R waves **(B)** move caliper to next R wave **(C)** continue checking remaining R waves for regularity.

wave (Fig. 2-18B). Continue moving the calipers across the rhythm strip, measuring the distance between each two R waves, to check the regularity of the R waves (Fig. 2-18C). The rhythm is irregular if the measurement differs by more than 0.06 second. The P to P rhythm can be checked in the same way using P waves instead of R waves.

When calipers are not available, an acceptable alternative involves the use of a blank piece of paper and a pencil. Place the paper over the rhythm strip so only the tips of the R waves are showing. Mark small dots on the paper where the first two R waves occur. Then move the paper so the first dot is now on the second R wave. If the rhythm is regular, the second dot will fall on the next R wave. Continue moving the paper across the rhythm strip in this manner to check the regularity of each R wave. The P to P rhythm can be checked in the same way (Fig. 2-19).

Rate

Rate is the number of electrical impulses conducted through the myocardium in 1 minute. **Atrial rate** is determined by the number of P waves seen, while **ventricular rate** is determined by the number of R waves. The ventricular rate should be the same as the patient's pulse, if the myocardium is contracting with each QRS complex and if the cardiac output is within normal limits.

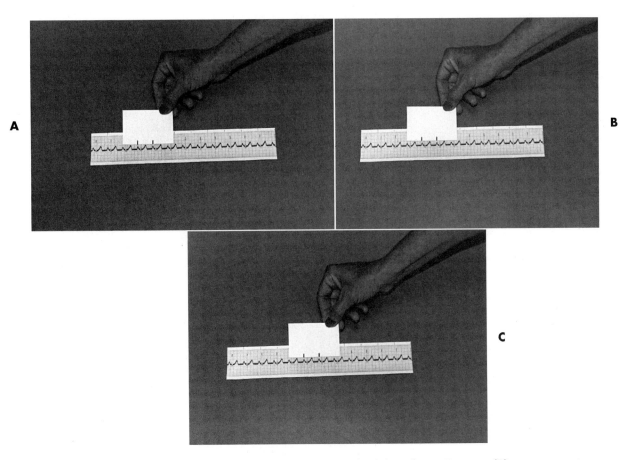

Fig. 2-19 Measuring rhythm with paper, using P to P intervals: **(A)** mark two P waves **(B)** move paper to next P wave **(C)** continue checking remaining P waves for regularity.

Many methods of calculating rate exist, but the following are the methods used most frequently:

1. *Calculation by a 6-second rhythm strip.* The graph paper may have small indicator lines (vertical lines) in the top margin of the paper that measure 1-second intervals. Every 3 seconds the indicator line is longer or darker. The space between three *long* lines equals 6 seconds. To calculate heart rate, count the number of R waves in a 6-second rhythm strip and multiply by 10. If a QRS complex falls directly under the beginning or ending indicator line, it is included in the total number of R waves counted. If the graph paper does not have 1- or 3-second indicator lines, count the number of R waves in 30 large squares and multiply by 10. (Thirty large squares equal 6 seconds). This calculation gives an *approximate* heart rate per minute (Fig. 2-20).

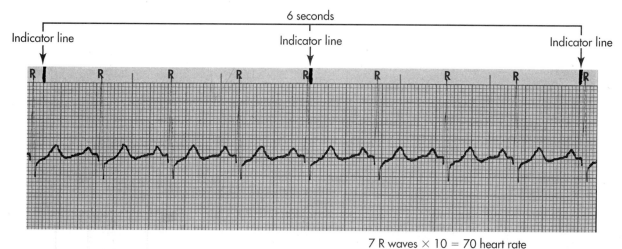

7 R waves × 10 = 70 heart rate
30 large squares (30 × 0.20 sec) = 6 seconds
10 × 6 seconds = 60 seconds or 1 minute

Fig. 2-20 Six-second rhythm strip method of calculating heart rate.

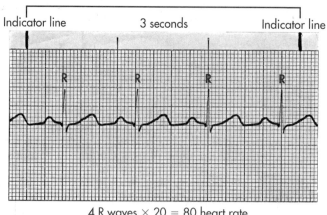

4 R waves × 20 = 80 heart rate
15 large squares (15 × 0.20 sec) = 3 seconds
20 × 3 seconds = 60 seconds or 1 minute

Fig. 2-21 Three-second rhythm strip method of calculating heart rate.

2. *Calculation by a 3-second rhythm strip.* The space between two long indicator lines equals 3 seconds. Count the number of R waves between the two long lines and multiply by 20, or count the number of R waves in 15 large squares and multiply by 20. This calculation gives an *approximate* heart rate per minute (Fig. 2-21).

3. *Calculation by division.* This method is more precise than the first two methods; however, **it should only be used when the rhythm is regular**. To use this method, count the number of large squares between two R waves and divide 300 by this number to determine the heart rate. For example, 300 divided by 3 (number of large squares between two R waves) equals 100. The heart rate is 100.

   When counting the number of large squares between two R waves, if part of a large square is included, count each small square as 0.2. Add the number of large and small squares and then divide 300 by that number. For example, 4 large and 4 small squares equal 4.8 squares; 300 divided by 4.8 equals 62.5. The heart rate is approximately 63 (Fig. 2-22).

   An additional method using calculation by division involves counting the number of small squares between two R waves. Then divide 1500 by that number to determine the rate. For example, in Figure 2-22, 24 small squares are between the two R waves. 1500 divided by 24 equals 62.5, or a heart rate of approximately 63.

4. *Calculation by a 1-minute rhythm strip.* This method is the most accurate for calculating rate. Count the number of R waves in a 1-minute rhythm strip. This method is rarely used because it requires a relatively long period of time to perform.

All heart rates in this book have been calculated by the 6-second rhythm strip method unless stated otherwise and are only approximate rates.

Take time to practice identifying the various components of many rhythm strips. These components are the *basic building blocks* needed for future identification of rhythms and dysrhythmias. The more you practice, the easier it will become to identify each component.

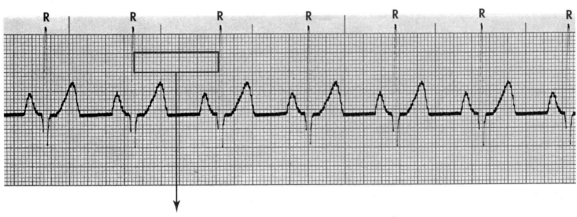

Steps:
1. 4 large and 4 small squares between R waves
2. 4 small squares × 0.2 = 0.8
3. 300 ÷ 4.8 = 63
   Approximate heart rate = 63

Steps:
1. 24 small squares between R waves
2. 1500 ÷ 24 = 62.5
3. Approximate heart rate = 63

Fig. 2-22 Division methods of calculating heart rate.

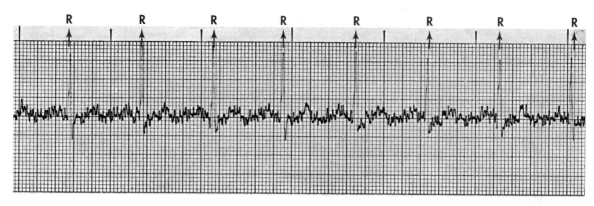

Fig. 2-23 60 cycle interference

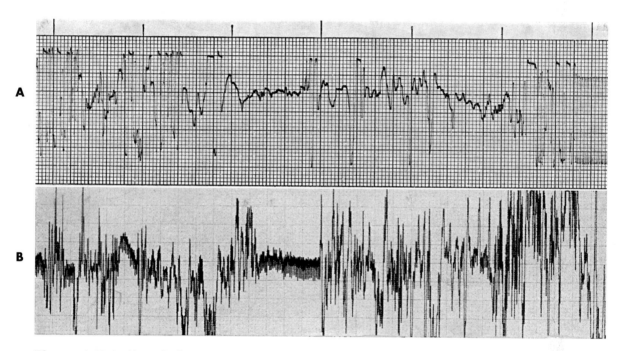

Fig. 2-24A, B Artifact; rhythm not visible.

ARTIFACT

Artifact is interference or static seen on the monitor screen or rhythm strip. This interference may be caused by the electrode losing contact with the patient's skin, patient movement or shivering, a broken cable or lead wire, or improper grounding.

One type of artifact is *60-cycle interference*, which appears as a fuzziness of the baseline. The P wave may not be seen because of this interference, but the QRS is usually visible (Fig. 2-23).

The 60-cycle interference is usually seen when the electrodes have lost contact with the patient's skin. This situation may result from excessive chest hair, sweaty skin, or the loss of conductive gel.

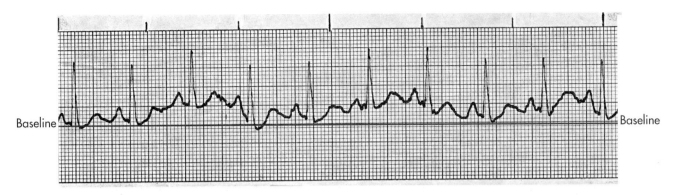

Baseline   Baseline

Fig. 2-25 Wandering baseline.

NOTE: The conductive gel of the electrodes may dry out with prolonged use or improper storage. Be sure that the conductive gel is still moist and the electrodes are firmly attached to the patient's skin.

The 60-cycle interference also may be caused by either the patient or the lead cable touching a metal object, such as a bed rail. A blanket between the metal object and the patient or lead wire should correct the interference.

Artifact that completely hides both the P wave and the QRS complex may be caused by either a loose lead or patient movement (Fig. 2-24). Patient assessment is very important because this artifact can mimic a lethal dysrhythmia on the monitor or rhythm strip.

Patient movement or deep, rapid breathing also may cause an artifact in which the baseline moves up and down rapidly on the monitor screen or rhythm strip. This type of artifact is called a *wandering baseline* and is usually corrected when the patient lies still or when the electrode placement is changed (Fig. 2-25).

Review Questions

1. True or false? The monitor only shows the conduction of the electrical impulses through the heart, not the actual contraction of the heart muscle.

2. True or false? Leads are color-coded wires that connect the telemetry unit to the patient's cardiac muscle.

3. True or false? Lead II and MCL I are the two Leads most often used to monitor patients.

4. True or false? When interpreting a rhythm strip, it is important to check complex formation, rhythm, and rate.

5. The P wave represents the depolarization of both the right and left _____.

6. The normal PR interval measures _____ to _____ second.

7. The QRS complex is measured from the beginning of the _____ to the end of the _____ wave.

8. What does a normal T wave represent on the rhythm strip? _____

   _____

9. A normal QT interval measures _____

   _____.

10. Explain how to calculate heart rate using the 6-second rhythm strip method. _____

    _____

    _____

11. Calculate the heart rate using both division methods when the distance between two R waves is:

    a. Three large squares _____

       _____

       _____

    b. Seven large squares and two and a half small squares _____

       _____

       _____

12. List two facts about PR intervals that are important to measure when interpreting a rhythm strip.

    a. _____

    b. _____

13. List four facts about QRS complexes that are important to evaluate when interpreting a rhythm strip.

    a. _____

    b. _____

    c. _____

    d. _____

14. What are three common causes of artifact?

a. _____

b. _____

c. _____

15. Explain the difference between relative and absolute refractory periods.

_____

_____

_____

_____

Rhythm Strip Review

Example:

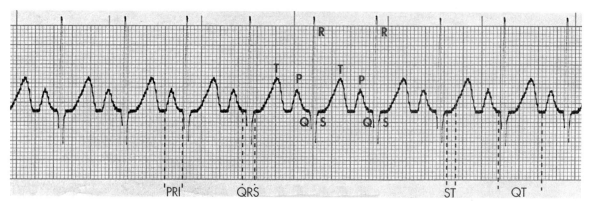

IDENTIFY: P wave, QRS complex, ST segment, T wave, and QT interval.

MEASURE: PR interval <u>0.20</u>   Rhythm <u>Regular</u>

QRS complex <u>0.06 - 0.08</u>   Heart rate <u>90</u>

QT interval <u>Prolonged</u>

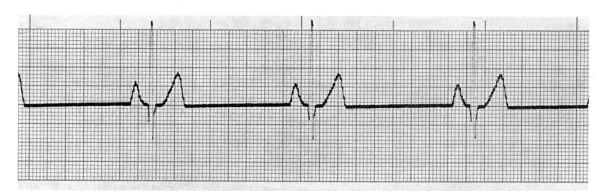

1. IDENTIFY: P wave, QRS complex, ST segment, T wave, and QT segment.

   MEASURE: PR interval <u>.20</u>   Rhythm <u>Reg</u>

   QRS complex <u>.08</u>   Heart rate <u>30</u>

   QT interval <u>Normal</u>

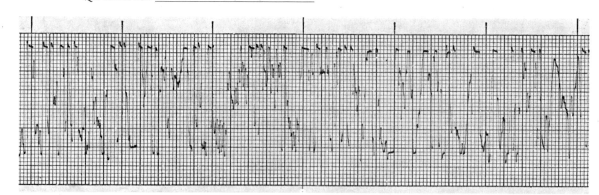

2. IDENTIFY: P wave, QRS complex, ST segment, T wave, and QT segment.

   MEASURE: PR interval <u>unmeasurable</u>   Rhythm _____

   QRS complex _____   Heart rate _____

   QT interval _____

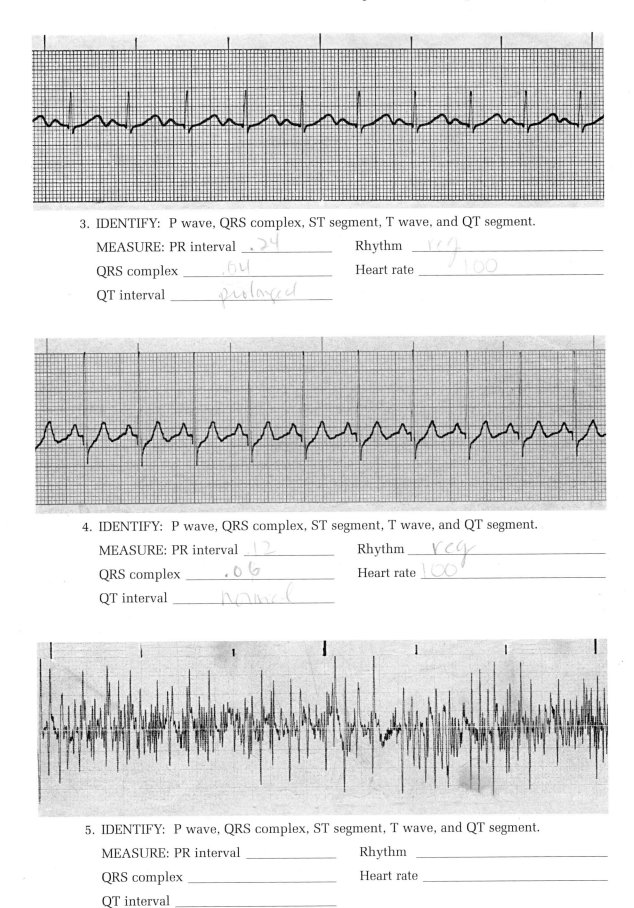

3. IDENTIFY: P wave, QRS complex, ST segment, T wave, and QT segment.

   MEASURE: PR interval _.24_   Rhythm _reg_

   QRS complex _.04_   Heart rate _100_

   QT interval _prolonged_

4. IDENTIFY: P wave, QRS complex, ST segment, T wave, and QT segment.

   MEASURE: PR interval _.12_   Rhythm _reg_

   QRS complex _.06_   Heart rate _100_

   QT interval _normal_

5. IDENTIFY: P wave, QRS complex, ST segment, T wave, and QT segment.

   MEASURE: PR interval _____   Rhythm _____

   QRS complex _____   Heart rate _____

   QT interval _____

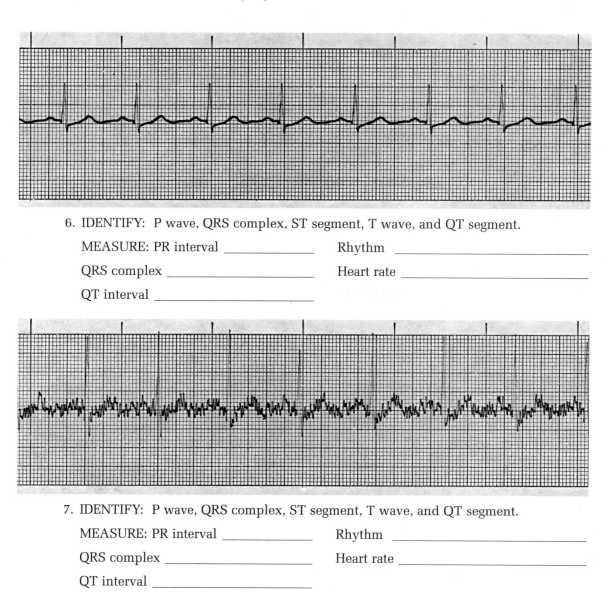

6. IDENTIFY: P wave, QRS complex, ST segment, T wave, and QT segment.

MEASURE: PR interval _____   Rhythm _____

QRS complex _____   Heart rate _____

QT interval _____

7. IDENTIFY: P wave, QRS complex, ST segment, T wave, and QT segment.

MEASURE: PR interval _____   Rhythm _____

QRS complex _____   Heart rate _____

QT interval _____

Sinus and Atrial Dysrhythmias

Chapter Three

Objectives

On completion of this chapter, the reader should be able to:

1. Describe the conduction of a normal electrical impulse from the sinoatrial node to the Purkinje's fibers.
2. Describe a normal sinus rhythm, including measurements of the components.
3. Identify sinus bradycardia, sinus tachycardia, and sinus arrhythmia.
4. Explain the differences between a sinus exit block and a sinus arrest, including measurements of the components.
5. Describe the appearance of a premature atrial contraction, including measurements of the components.
6. Explain the primary difference between paroxysmal atrial tachycardia and supraventricular tachycardia.
7. Describe the appearance of a wandering atrial pacemaker dysrhythmia, including measurements of the components.
8. Describe the appearance of an atrial flutter, including measurements of the components and types of blocks.
9. Describe atrial fibrillation, including measurements of the components.

Outline

Sinus and Atrial Dysrhythmias

A. Sinus Rhythms
1. Normal Sinus Rhythm
2. Sinus Bradycardia
3. Sinus Tachycardia
4. Sinus Arrhythmia
5. Sinus Exit Block and Sinus Arrest

B. Atrial Dysrhythmias
1. Premature Atrial Contraction
2. Paroxysmal Atrial Tachycardia
3. Supraventricular Tachycardia
4. Wandering Atrial Pacemaker
5. Atrial Flutter
6. Atrial Fibrillation

C. Review Questions

D. Rhythm Strip Review

SINUS RHYTHMS

The sinoatrial (SA) node is located in the upper portion of the right atrium and is referred to as the *pacemaker of the heart* (*see* Chapter 1, "Anatomy and Physiology"). The SA node normally initiates the electrical impulse that travels throughout the heart, leading to depolarization of the atria and ventricles (Fig. 3-1). If the SA node fails to generate an electrical impulse, any other pacemaker cell within the atria is capable of initiating an impulse.

The SA node, as well as other pacemaker cells in the atria, normally generates 60 to 100 electrical impulses per minute. This is known as the *inherent* heart rate of the atria. In sinus rhythms, the electrical impulse travels from the SA node, through the atria to the atrioventricular (AV) node, continuing through the bundle of His and bundle branches, to the Purkinje's fibers, and ending in the ventricular muscle.

Because the electrical impulse follows this normal pathway throughout the heart, an upright P wave is present, representing atrial depolarization. The PR

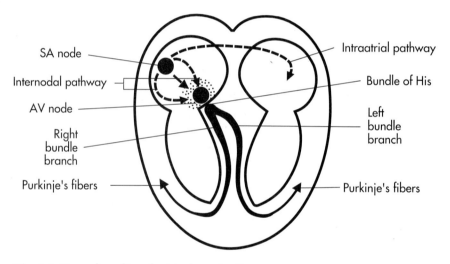

Fig. 3-1 Normal cardiac electrical conduction.

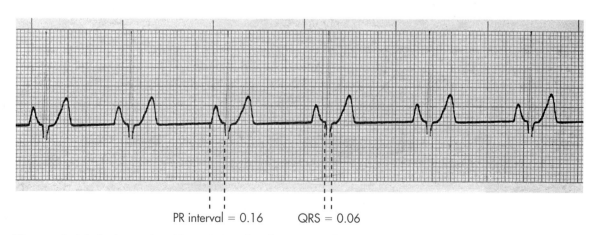

PR interval = 0.16   QRS = 0.06

Fig. 3-2 Atrial rhythm strip with PR interval and QRS complex.

interval is within the normal limits of 0.12 to 0.20 second. The QRS complex, representing ventricular depolarization, measures less than 0.12 second (Fig. 3-2). However, in some sinus rhythms, the size and shape of the P waves and the length of PR intervals may vary.

Rhythms originating from the SA node are *sinus rhythms* or *sinus dysrhythmias* (abnormal rhythms), while rhythms originating from other atrial sites are *atrial dysrhythmias*. The term *dysrhythmia* is used with all cardiac rhythms except normal sinus rhythm.

Sinus dysrhythmias are usually not serious. However, as with any rhythm, **patient assessment** is essential to determine their tolerance of the dysrhythmia.

> **NOTE:** The patient is considered symptomatic (medically unstable) if any of the following occur: chest pain, weakness, faintness, sudden change in blood pressure, confusion, or unresponsiveness.

Normal Sinus Rhythm

Normal sinus rhythm (NSR) is the ONLY rhythm considered "normal." In this rhythm the SA node initiates all the electrical impulses that are transmitted throughout the heart. The SA node generates an impulse that travels downward, throughout both the right and the left atria causing atrial depolarization. The impulse is then transmitted through the AV node, the bundle of His, and both bundle branches to the Purkinje's fibers and ends in the ventricular muscle, where it causes ventricular depolarization (Fig. 3-3).

Because the electrical impulse follows the normal conduction pathway, an upright P wave precedes every QRS complex. All PR intervals range from 0.12 to 0.20 second, and the QRS complex is less than 0.12 second. All P waves look alike, and all QRS complexes are the same size and shape.

In normal sinus rhythm, both the atria and the ventricles depolarize at regular intervals. Therefore, the P to P intervals and R to R intervals are regular. In addition, the P to P intervals are the same length as the R to R intervals. Normal sinus rhythm is very regular, and the rate is 60 to 100 electrical impulses per minute (Fig. 3-4).

> **NOTE:** All rhythms included in this book are described as they appear in Lead II on an adult patient.

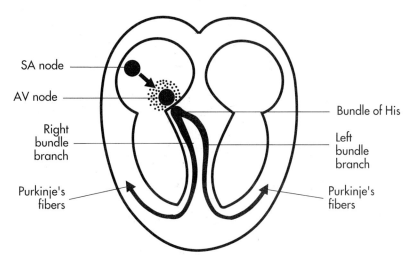

Fig. 3-3 Normal conduction pathway.

Sinus Bradycardia

Sinus bradycardia (sinus brady) is a dysrhythmia that occurs when all the electrical impulses originate from the SA node and follow the normal cardiac conduction pathway. However, the rate is slower than 60 impulses per minute (Fig. 3-3).

An upright P wave occurs before every QRS complex. The PR intervals remain within the normal range of 0.12 to 0.20 second, and the QRS complexes are less than 0.12 second. All P waves look alike, and QRS complexes are the same size and shape. Because the P to P intervals and the R to R intervals are regular and equal in length, the rhythm is regular. The rate can vary, but it must be slower than 60 electrical impulses per minute in sinus bradycardia (Fig. 3-5).

Sinus bradycardia may be normal for sleeping individuals as well as for athletes. However, it may become a dangerous dysrhythmia if the rate falls significantly or the patient becomes symptomatic, showing signs of poor cardiac output. These symptoms include pale, cool, clammy skin; shortness of breath; decreased blood pressure; confusion; dizziness; and/or chest pain.

Some common causes of sinus bradycardia are vomiting and/or drugs such as digitalis, morphine, and sedatives.

Sinus Tachycardia

Sinus tachycardia (sinus tach) occurs when all the electrical impulses originate from the SA node at a rate between 101 to 150 per minute (Fig. 3-3).

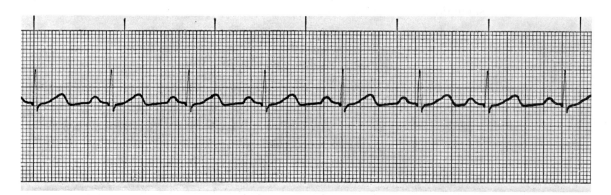

Fig. 3-4 Normal sinus rhythm; heart rate, 80.

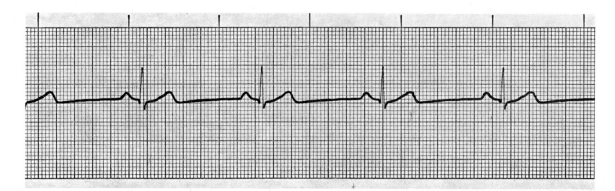

Fig. 3-5 Sinus bradycardia; heart rate 40.

Because the impulse follows the normal conduction pathway, an upright P wave occurs before every QRS complex. PR intervals remain within the normal range of 0.12 to 0.20 second, and QRS complexes are less than 0.12 second (Fig. 3-6A). All P waves look alike, and all QRS complexes are the same size and shape.

As the rate of the tachycardia increases, the P waves are frequently hidden in the T wave of the preceding QRS complex, causing a slight change in the appearance of the T wave (Fig. 3-6B).

Because the P to P intervals and R to R intervals are usually regular and equal in length, the rhythm usually is regular. The rate can vary, but it usually falls between 101 and 150 electrical impulses per minute.

Sinus tachycardia may become a serious dysrhythmia if the patient becomes symptomatic.

The most common causes of sinus tachycardia are pain, fever, acute anemia, hemorrhage, exercise, fear, sudden excitement, anxiety, or the effects of drugs such as atropine, nicotine, caffeine, or amphetamines.

Sinus Arrhythmia

Sinus arrhythmia occurs when the SA node initiates all the electrical impulses, but at irregular intervals. The P to P intervals and the R to R intervals change with respirations, producing an irregular rhythm (Fig. 3-3).

Since the impulses are all generated by the SA node and follow the normal conduction pathway, an upright P wave still occurs before every QRS complex. The PR intervals remain within 0.12 to 0.20 second, and the QRS complexes are less than 0.12 second. All P waves look alike, and the QRS complexes are the same in size and shape.

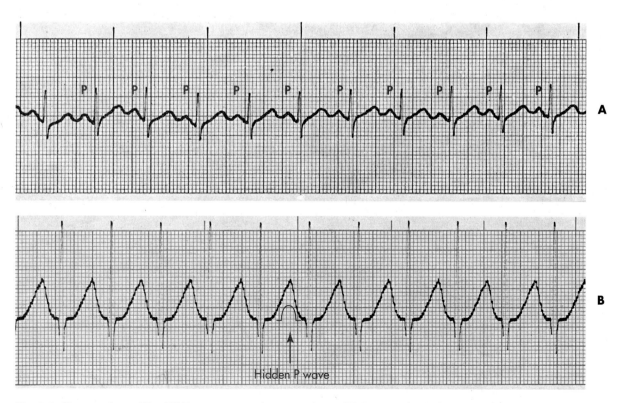

Fig. 3-6 Sinus tachycardia. **(A)** P waves seen; heart rate, 110 **(B)** P waves buried in preceding T waves; heart rate, 110.

Because the heart rate increases as the patient inhales and decreases as the patient exhales, the 6-second rhythm strip is a more reliable method of determining heart rate. However, the overall heart rate will usually be 60 to 100 electrical impulses per minute. P to P and R to R intervals are irregular, causing the rhythm to be irregular. The longest R to R interval will be **less** than twice the length of any of the remaining R to R intervals (Fig. 3-7).

Although sinus arrhythmia is normal for infants and young children, it may a warning of a diseased SA node or coronary artery disease in the adult patient. Sinus arrhythmia is usually not serious unless the patient's cardiac output decreases and the patient becomes medically unstable (symptomatic).

As with any rhythm, **patient assessment** is essential to determine the patient's tolerance of the dysrhythmia.

> NOTE: Normal sinus rhythm, sinus bradycardia, sinus tachycardia, and sinus arrhythmia all follow the normal conduction pathway of the heart, only the rate or rhythm varies.

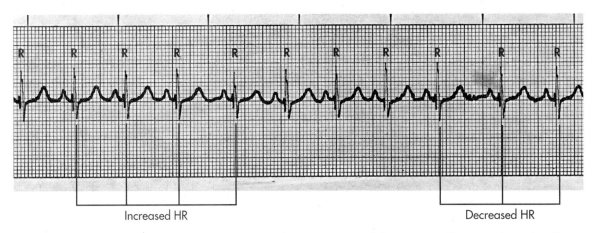

Increased HR   Decreased HR

Fig. 3-7 Sinus arrhythmia. Heart rate increases with inspiration and decreases with expiration; overall heart rate, 100.

Sinus Exit Block and Sinus Arrest

Sinus exit block (sinus block) occurs when the SA node initiates an electrical impulse that is blocked and not conducted to the atria. The atria do not depolarize, and a P wave will not be seen.

Sinus arrest occurs when the SA node does **not** initiate an electrical impulse. Because an impulse is not generated, the atria do not depolarize and a P wave will not be seen.

Both dysrhythmias appear similar on the monitor screen or rhythm strip. P waves are absent and QRS complexes are not seen because an impulse is not conducted to the ventricles to cause depolarization. The lack of a P wave and QRS complex forms a *pause* on the monitor and rhythm strip.

The length of the pause may help to determine whether the dysrhythmia is a sinus exit block or a sinus arrest. The pause of a sinus exit block is equal to exactly two or more cardiac cycles of the underlying rhythm. For example, the P to P interval of the underlying rhythm will fit into the pause of a sinus exit block exactly two times, or exactly three times, and so forth (Fig. 3-8). The SA node continues to fire at its normal rate, so the rhythm will usually be regular except where the pause occurs.

The pause of a sinus arrest is not equal to exactly two or more cardiac cycles of the underlying rhythm. It may be less than or more than two times the cardiac cycle of the underlying rhythm. For example, the P to P interval of the underlying rhythm will not fit into the pause of a sinus arrest exactly two times, or exactly three times, and so forth. Because the SA node is not firing, any pacemaker cell in the heart can begin to initiate electrical impulses. Therefore, the complex that ends the sinus arrest may be either atrial, junctional, or ventricular (Fig. 3-9). The rhythm after the sinus arrest may be different than the rhythm before the pause.

Both dysrhythmias may be caused by myocardial infarction, hypoxia (lack of oxygen), or drugs such as digitalis or quinidine.

As with any rhythm, **patient assessment** is essential to determine the patient's tolerance of the dysrhythmia. Treatment should be started if the patient is medically unstable e.g., if the patient has pale, sweaty skin; low blood pressure; chest pain; weakness; or any other symptoms of poor cardiac output (*see* Chapter 9, "Medication Review and Adult Treatment Guidelines").

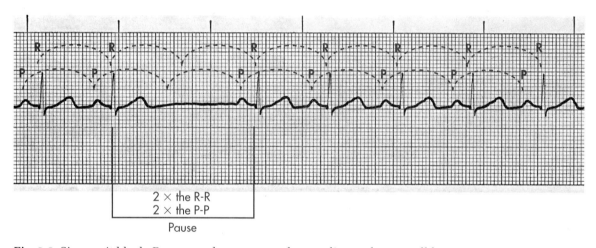

Fig. 3-8 Sinus exit block. Pause equal to two complete cardiac cycles; overall heart rate, 70.

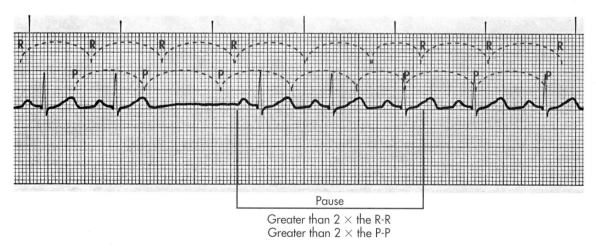

Fig. 3-9 Sinus arrest. P to P and R to R intervals regular, except during pause; overall heart rate, 60.

ATRIAL DYSRHYTHMIAS

When the SA node fails to generate an electrical impulse, any other pacemaker site within the atria is capable of initiating the impulse. Cardiac rhythms originating from atrial sites are *atrial dysrhythmias.*

In atrial rhythms, the electrical impulse travels through the atria to the AV node, continuing through the bundle of His and bundle branches, to the Purkinje's fibers, ending in the ventricular muscle. The depolarization of the atria varies depending on the atrial rhythm, while the ventricles usually depolarize in a normal manner.

Most atrial dysrhythmias are usually not *lethal* (death producing). However, as with any rhythm, **patient assessment** is essential to determine the patient's tolerance of the dysrhythmia.

Premature Atrial Contraction

A *premature atrial contraction* (PAC) is an individual complex that occurs earlier than the next expected complex of the underlying rhythm. It originates from any atrial site outside the SA node (Fig. 3-10). PACs usually occur in an underlying sinus rhythm, which may be regular except for the PAC.

> NOTE: Although the term **contraction** is used with a PAC, remember this complex represents electrical activity of cardiac muscle and may **not** reflect an actual contraction.

A PAC usually has the same characteristics as other atrial complexes. However , the P wave may appear different in size or shape than the P waves of the underlying rhythm, or it may be hidden in the T wave of the preceding complex.

The PAC is followed by a pause before the underlying rhythm returns. Two different types of pauses follow a premature complex: noncompensatory or compensatory. To determine the type of pause on the rhythm strip, measure the R to R intervals before and after the PAC in the following manner:

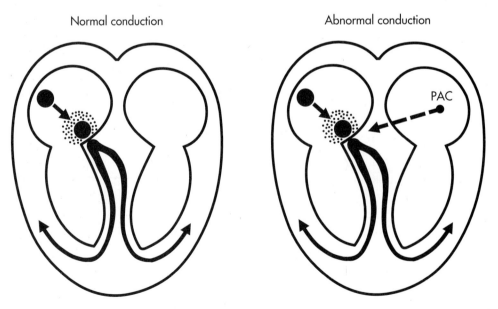

Normal conduction   Abnormal conduction

PAC

Fig. 3-10 Left heart shows normal electrical conduction pathway. Right heart shows conduction pathway of a premature atrial contraction (PAC).

1. *Noncompensatory pause.* Measure from the R wave of the complex before the PAC to the R wave of the complex after the PAC. This measurement will be less than two times the R to R interval of the underlying rhythm. This type of pause may also be called an *incomplete* compensatory pause.
2. *Compensatory pause.* Measure from the R wave of the complex before the PAC to the R wave of the complex after the PAC. This measurement will be two times the R to R interval of the underlying rhythm. This type of pause may also be called a *complete* compensatory pause.

A PAC is usually followed by a noncompensatory pause.

The underlying rhythm **must** also be identified when interpreting rhythm strips containing a PAC. Although a premature atrial contraction may occur in any rhythm, it is easier to identify in a sinus rhythm or any rhythm with a bradycardia rate (Fig. 3-11A, B). When determining the rate of a rhythm containing a PAC, the R wave of the PAC is included in the total count of R waves.

A PAC represents increased irritability of the atria. Increased irritability indicates that the cardiac cells are able to respond to even a mild electrical stimulus and may depolarize in an unpredictable rate or manner. PACs may be caused by pain, fever, fear, anxiety, sudden excitement, exercise, or the effects of drugs such as digitalis, atropine, nicotine, caffeine, and amphetamines.

A PAC by itself is not a serious dysrhythmia. However, PACs are frequently monitored, since they may lead to a more serious dysrhythmia, such as paroxysmal atrial tachycardia.

Although a PAC is **not** a true atrial dysrhythmia but an individual complex, it is included in this chapter because it originates from the atria.

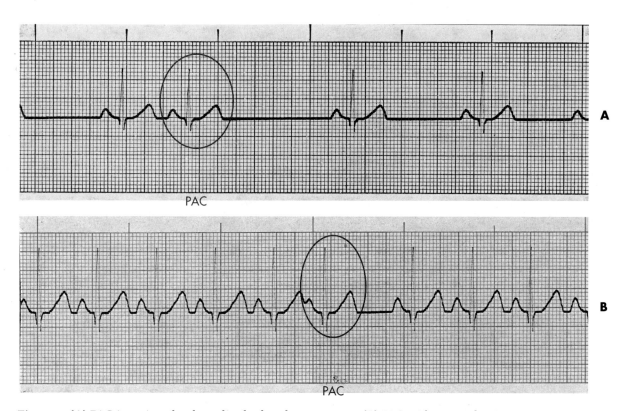

Fig. 3-11 (A) PAC in a sinus bradycardic rhythm; heart rate, 40. **(B)** PAC with a complete compensatory pause in a sinus rhythm; heart rate, 90.

Paroxysmal Atrial Tachycardia

Paroxysmal atrial tachycardia (PAT) is the sudden onset of a tachycardia with a rate greater than 151 electrical impulses per minute. PAT is frequently triggered by a PAC.

Because PAT is usually initiated by an irritable site in the atria, a P wave occurs before every QRS complex (Fig. 3-12). However, because of the rapid rate of PAT, the P wave may be hidden in the T wave of the preceding complex. If P waves are seen, the PR intervals range from 0.12 to 0.20 second and the QRS complexes are usually less than 0.12 second.

Since the P to P intervals and R to R intervals are regular and equal in length, the rhythm is regular. The rate may vary from 151 to 250, or more, electrical impulses per minute. Because the rate is so rapid, the ventricles do not have time to fill completely before each contraction, causing a decrease in cardiac output.

Because most of the blood flow through the coronary arteries occurs between heartbeats, the rapid heart rate of a PAT may also decrease the amount of oxygenated blood circulated to the heart muscle (myocardium).

The patient may complain of symptoms such as weakness, dizziness, palpitations, or a feeling that the heart is doing "flip-flops." PAT may stop as suddenly as it starts, or it may require medical treatment if the patient becomes medically unstable.

A paroxysmal atrial tachycardia is not a lethal dysrhythmia but should be monitored closely, since this rapid rate cannot be tolerated for long periods of time.

To interpret a PAT, the **beginning** of the PAT **must** be seen and the underlying rhythm that precedes the PAT must be identified (Fig. 3-13). If the onset of the PAT is not seen, the dysrhythmia is called *supraventricular tachycardia*, providing it fits the other characteristics of PAT.

A PAT may be caused by stimulants such as caffeine, nicotine, or amphetamines.

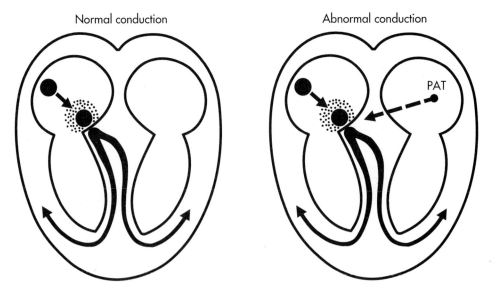

Fig. 3-12 Left heart shows normal electrical conduction pathway. Right heart shows conduction pathway of paroxysmal atrial tachycardia (PAT).

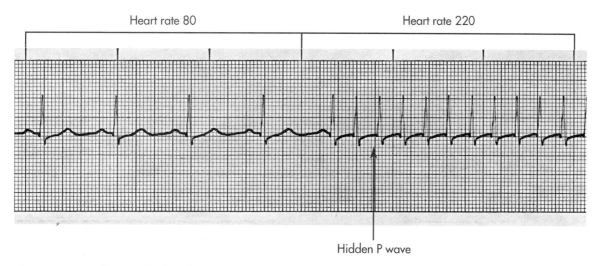

Fig. 3-13 Normal sinus rhythm; heart rate, 80, progressing to PAT; heart rate, 220.

Supraventricular Tachycardia

Supraventricular tachycardia (SVT) is the term used when a dysrhythmia fits all the characteristics of a PAT, but the beginning of the dysrhythmia is not seen. SVT is a general term that refers to **any** dysrhythmia that cannot be identified by other means, originates from an irritable site **above the bundle of His** and has a rate greater than 151 (Fig. 3-14).

A P wave usually occurs before every QRS complex. However, the P wave may be hidden in the T wave of the preceding complex because of the rapid rate of the SVT. If P waves are seen, the PR intervals usually range from 0.12 to 0.20 second and the QRS complexes usually measure less than 0.12 second.

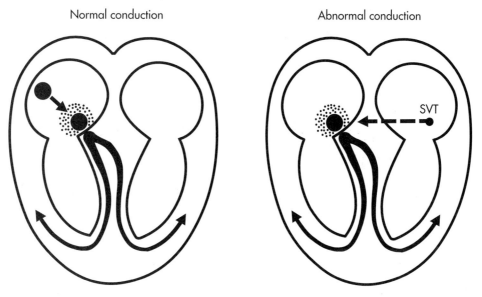

Fig. 3-14 Left heart shows normal electrical conduction pathway. Right heart shows conduction pathway of supraventricular tachycardia (SVT).

Any P waves that can be seen usually look alike, and the QRS complexes are usually the same size and shape. The P to P intervals and R to R intervals are regular and equal in length, and the rhythm is regular (Fig. 3-15).

The rate of the SVT varies from 151 to 250, or more, electrical impulses per minute. A rhythm resembling SVT but with a heart rate less than 151 is called *sinus tachycardia*.

SVT is usually triggered by an irritable site within the atria. This irritability can be caused by stimulants such as caffeine, nicotine, or amphetamines.

SVT is treated if the patient becomes medically unstable. This dysrhythmia is usually not lethal, but the patient should be assessed frequently because the rapid rate can not be tolerated for long periods of time.

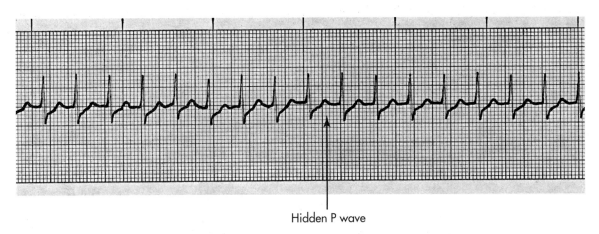

Hidden P wave

Fig. 3-15 SVT. P waves hidden in preceding T waves, onset not seen; heart rate, 170.

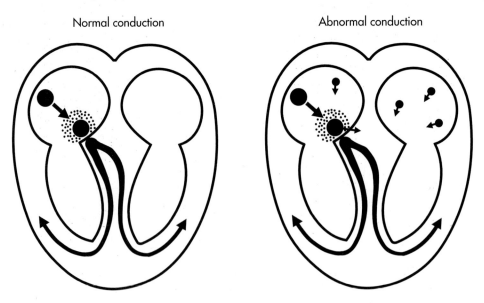

Normal conduction   Abnormal conduction

Fig. 3-16 Left heart shows normal electrical conduction pathway. Right heart shows conduction pathway of wandering atrial pacemaker.

Wandering Atrial Pacemaker

A *wandering atrial pacemaker dysrhythmia* originates from at least **three** different sites above the bundle of His. These sites may include any pacemaker site in the atria, including the SA node, the AV junction, or a combination of these areas (Fig. 3-16).

The size and shape of each individual complex is determined by the site of origin for that complex. If the site is from the atria, a P wave occurs, followed by a QRS complex less than 0.12 second. The PR interval is usually 0.12 to 0.20 second, but may vary because the atrial point of origin varies.

If the complex is from the AV junctional area, the P waves may be inverted, may be hidden, or may follow the QRS complex. Therefore, P waves may not be seen before every QRS complex, and PR intervals may vary or be absent.

The P to P intervals (if present) and R to R intervals vary, producing an irregular rhythm. The rate may also vary, but usually remains between 60 and 100 electrical impulses per minute (Fig. 3-17).

A wandering pacemaker dysrhythmia may be caused by heart disease, myocardial infarction, or drug toxicity.

This dysrhythmia is usually not lethal. However, it is frequently treated because it indicates increased irritability within the cardiac muscle. This increased irritability may cause the dysrhythmia to progress to a more serious dysrhythmia.

The patient's symptoms vary depending on the rate of the wandering atrial pacemaker and the patient's tolerance of the dysrhythmia.

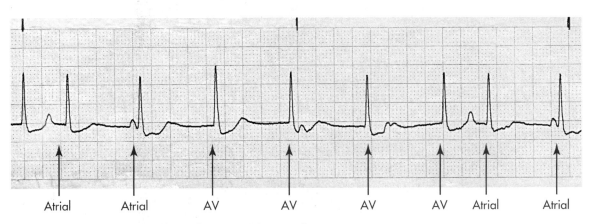

| Atrial | Atrial | AV | AV | AV | AV | Atrial | Atrial |

Fig. 3-17 Wandering atrial pacemaker. Sites of origin; heart rate, 90.

Atrial Flutter

Atrial flutter occurs when a single irritable site in the atria initiates many electrical impulses at a rapid rate (Fig. 3-18). The electrical impulses are conducted throughout the atria so rapidly that normal P waves are not produced. Instead of P waves, *flutter waves* (F waves) are formed.

Flutter waves have a typical "saw-toothed" or jagged appearance on the rhythm strip. They may not all look exactly the same, since some F waves may be buried in the QRS complex, ST segment, or T wave.

The negative (downward) stroke of the F wave represents atrial depolarization conducted by an abnormal pathway. The positive (upward) stroke of the F wave indicates atrial repolarization.

During atrial flutter, the atria usually depolarize more rapidly than normal, while the ventricles usually depolarize at a normal rate. Therefore, every atrial impulse cannot be conducted to the ventricles, and a QRS complex is not present for every F wave.

The ventricles usually depolarize and repolarize at regular intervals, allowing them to respond to the atrial impulse at a regular rate, which may result in a regular ventricular rhythm.

The QRS complexes typically measure less than 0.12 second and usually occur at regular intervals. The ventricular rate, as measured by the number of QRS complexes, is usually 60 to 100 electrical impulses per minute. However, the atrial rate (F waves) usually ranges from 250 to 350 impulses per minute (Fig. 3-19).

When an atrial flutter has a ventricular rate of less than 60 impulses per minute, it is called *atrial flutter with a slow ventricular response*. When the ventricular rate is 100 to 150 impulses per minute, it is called *atrial flutter with a rapid ventricular response*.

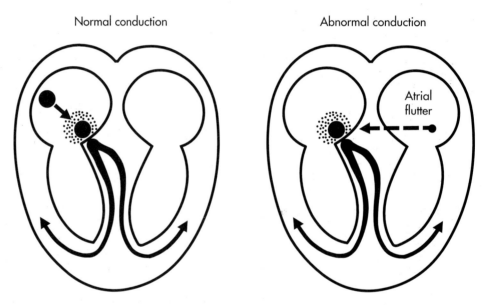

Fig. 3-18 Left heart shows normal electrical conduction pathway. Right heart shows conduction pathway of atrial flutter.

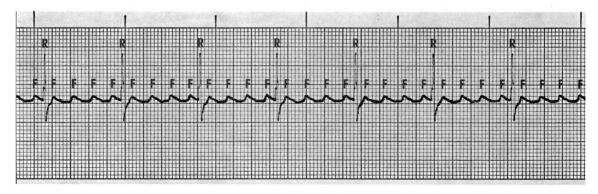

Fig. 3-19 Atrial flutter. Atrial heart rate, 290; ventricular heart rate, 70.

Since the ratio of flutter waves to each QRS complex further describes the dysrhythmia, it is important to determine the number of flutter waves for every QRS complex (Fig. 3-20).

Example: Two F waves with one QRS complex = 2:1 block
Three F waves with one QRS complex = 3:1 block
Four F waves with one QRS complex = 4:1 block
Five F waves with one QRS complex = 5:1 block

If the number of flutter waves is the same before every QRS complex, the R to R intervals are equal throughout, and the rhythm is regular. When the number of F waves before each QRS complex varies, the R to R interval is irregular and the rhythm is called *atrial flutter with variable ventricular response* (Fig. 3-21).

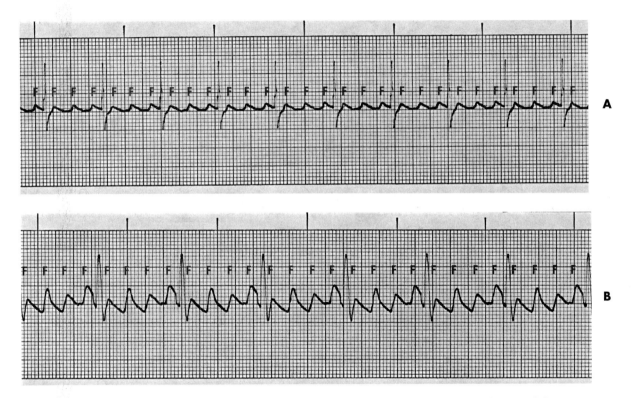

Fig. 3-20 (A) Atrial flutter, 3:1 block. Atrial heart rate, 280; ventricular heart rate, 100. **(B)** Atrial flutter, 4:1 block. Atrial heart rate, 260; ventricular heart rate, 60.

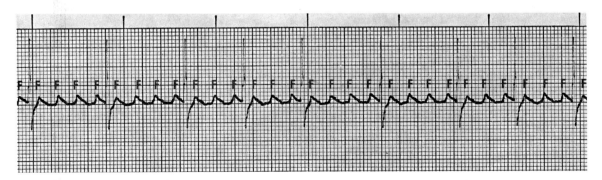

Fig. 3-21 Atrial flutter with variable block. Atrial heart rate, 280; ventricular heart rate, 90.

Atrial flutter may be caused by heart disease, myocardial infarction, or drug toxicity. This dysrhythmia is usually not lethal. However, it is frequently treated because it indicates increased irritability within the atria. This increased irritability may cause the dysrhythmia to progress to a more serious dysrhythmia.

The patient's symptoms vary depending on the cause of the atrial flutter, the ventricular response, and the patient's tolerance of the dysrhythmia.

Atrial Fibrillation

In *atrial fibrillation* (A Fib) an increased irritability of all the cardiac cells in the atria exists. Because of this increased atrial irritability, many sites within the atria attempt to initiate electrical impulses (Fig. 3-22).

Since so many electrical impulses are initiated, most of the impulses are not conducted; therefore, the atria is not completely depolarized with each impulse. The atrial muscle does not contract forcefully, only a quivering movement (*fibrillatory waves*) occurs. These fibrillatory waves (fib. waves) appear on the rhythm strip or monitor screen as a wavy line between each QRS complex. No true P waves or PR intervals exist.

At irregular intervals, one electrical impulse **is** conducted through the AV junction and ventricles, resulting in ventricular depolarization and a QRS complex. QRS complexes usually remain within the normal range of less than 0.12 second, and the R to R intervals are irregular throughout the rhythm strip. Frequently, one of the first clues that a dysrhythmia might be atrial fibrillation is seeing R to R intervals that are irregularly irregular (with no pattern to the irregularity).

Although the atrial heart rate is usually 350 to 500, or more, electrical impulses per minute, the ventricular heart rate is usually within the normal limits of 60 to 100 impulses per minute. This dysrhythmia is known as *controlled atrial fibrillation* (Fig. 3-23).

Atrial fibrillation with a ventricular rate of less than 60 impulses per minute is called *atrial fibrillation with a slow ventricular response*. When this dysrhythmia has a ventricular rate of 101 to 150 impulses per minute, it is called

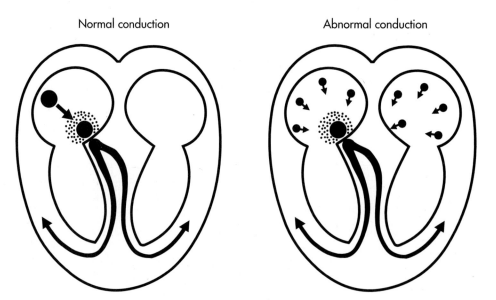

Normal conduction   Abnormal conduction

Fig. 3-22 Left heart shows normal electrical conduction pathway. Right heart shows conduction pathway of atrial fibrillation.

atrial fibrillation with rapid ventricular response (Fig. 3-24). Atrial fibrillation with a ventricular rate greater than 150 impulses per minute is called *uncontrolled atrial fibrillation.*

This dysrhythmia is not usually considered lethal and may be normal in elderly patients. However, a new occurrence of atrial fibrillation is frequently treated, because it indicates an increased irritability within the atria and may progress to a more serious dysrhythmia.

Treatment will depend on the patient's tolerance of the dysrhythmia and the patient's symptoms. For example, a patient with atrial fibrillation and a ventricular response of 50 impulses per minute, with stable vital signs, may not require treatment. However, a patient with atrial fibrillation with a ventricular response of 50, who is medically unstable, requires treatment immediately.

Medically unstable symptoms include those of poor cardiac output:

1. pale or cyanotic; cool, clammy skin
2. shortness of breath
3. weakness or dizziness
4. chest pain
5. unresponsiveness

Symptoms vary depending on the cause of the atrial fibrillation, the ventricular response, cardiac output, and the patient's tolerance of the dysrhythmia.

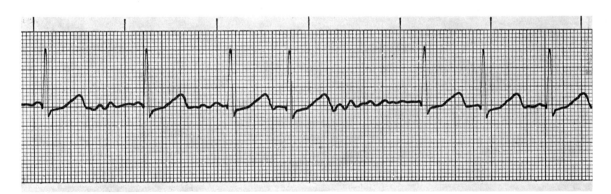

Fig. 3-23 Controlled atrial fibrillation. Ventricular heart rate, 70.

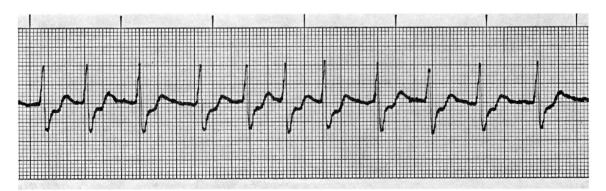

Fig. 3-24 Atrial fibrillation with a rapid ventricular response. No distinguishable P waves. Ventricular heart rate, 110.

Atrial fibrillation may be caused by severe heart disease or myocardial infarction. It may also occur with excessive use of alcohol or caffeine.

NOTE: Atrial fibrillation is usually not a lethal dysrhythmia; however, it **must not** be confused with *ventricular fibrillation*, which **is** a lethal dysrhythmia (*see* Chapter 6, "Ventricular Dysrhythmias").

Review Questions

1. True or false? The SA node normally generates 60 to 100 electrical impulses per minute.

2. True or false? Sinus bradycardia may become a lethal dysrhythmia if the heart rate falls significantly or the patient becomes symptomatic.

3. True or false? The complex that ends a sinus arrest can only be initiated from the atria.

4. True or false? A PAC is an atrial contraction that occurs later than the next expected complex of the underlying rhythm.

5. True or false? In sinus arrhythmia, the heart rate increases with inspirations and decreases with expirations.

6. The number of electrical impulses for sinus tachycardia is between _____ and _____ per minute.

7. In atrial fibrillation, the QRS complexes usually measure less than _____ second.

8. Sinus exit block occurs when the SA node fails to initiate an electrical impulse for a length of time equal to _____ complete cardiac cycles.

9. If the onset of PAT is not seen, the dysrhythmia is called:

   a. premature atrial tachycardia

   b. supraventricular tachycardia

   c. sinus tachycardia

   d. atrial flutter

10. SVT is a dysrhythmia that originates from an irritable site located:

    a. above the bundle of His

    b. within the ventricles

    c. within the bundle branches

    d. below the bundle branches

11. List three possible causes of a wandering atrial pacemaker dysrhythmia.

    a. _____

    b. _____

    c. _____

12. Explain the meaning of "variable ventricular response" in atrial flutter.

    _____

    _____

Rhythm Strip Review

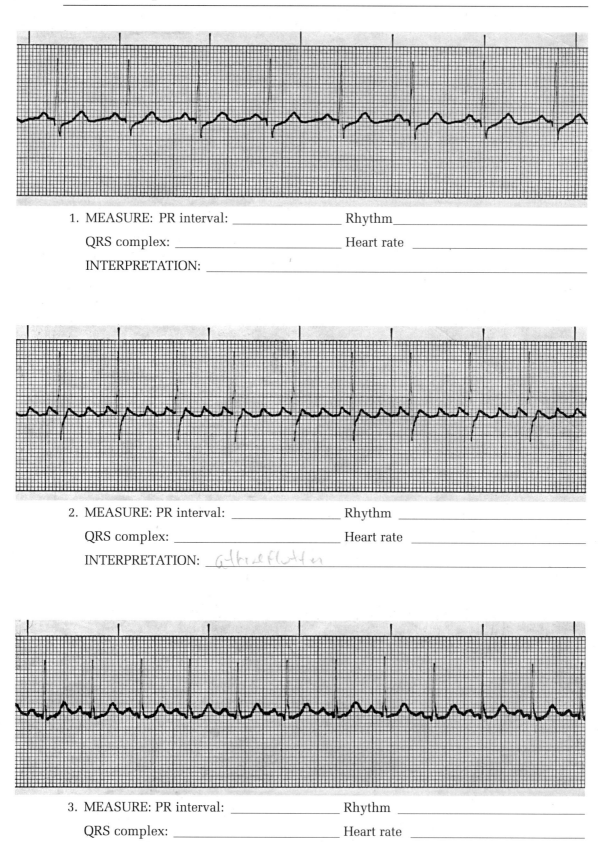

1. MEASURE: PR interval: _____ Rhythm _____

   QRS complex: _____ Heart rate _____

   INTERPRETATION: _____

2. MEASURE: PR interval: _____ Rhythm _____

   QRS complex: _____ Heart rate _____

   INTERPRETATION: _Atrial flutter_ _____

3. MEASURE: PR interval: _____ Rhythm _____

   QRS complex: _____ Heart rate _____

   INTERPRETATION: _____

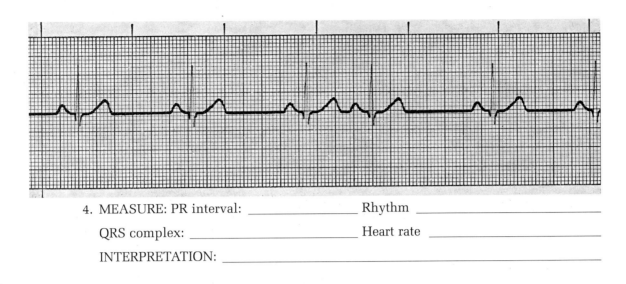

4. MEASURE: PR interval: _____ Rhythm _____

   QRS complex: _____ Heart rate _____

   INTERPRETATION: _____

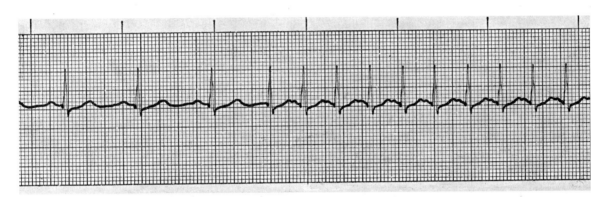

5. MEASURE: PR interval: _____ Rhythm _____

   QRS complex: _____ Heart rate _____

   INTERPRETATION: _____

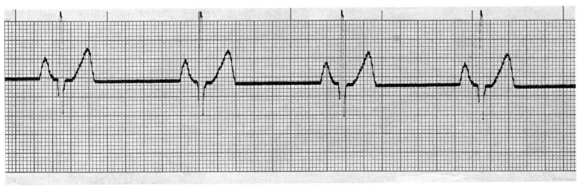

6. MEASURE: PR interval: _____ Rhythm _____

   QRS complex: _____ Heart rate _____

   INTERPRETATION: _____

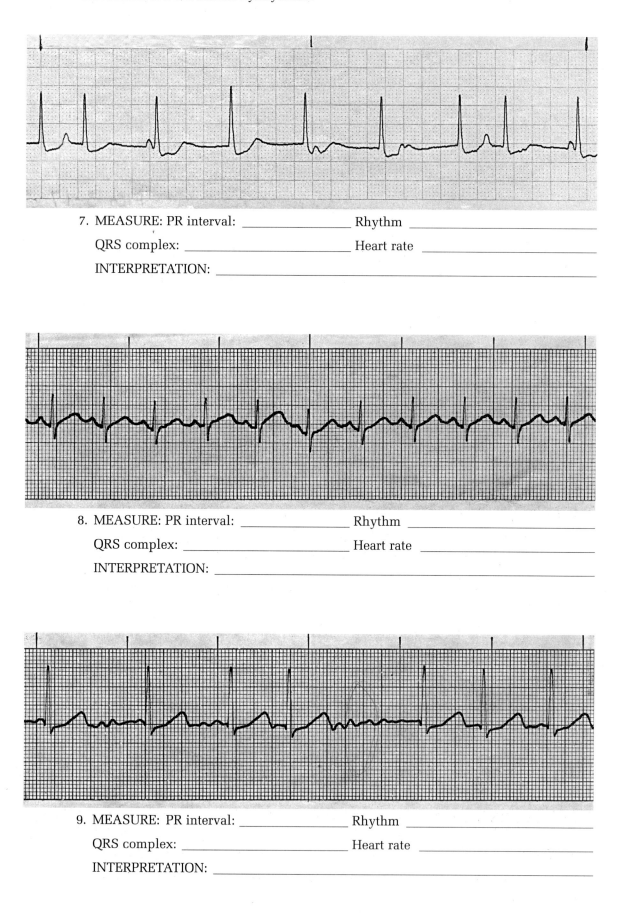

7. MEASURE: PR interval: _____ Rhythm _____

    QRS complex: _____ Heart rate _____

    INTERPRETATION: _____

8. MEASURE: PR interval: _____ Rhythm _____

    QRS complex: _____ Heart rate _____

    INTERPRETATION: _____

9. MEASURE: PR interval: _____ Rhythm _____

    QRS complex: _____ Heart rate _____

    INTERPRETATION: _____

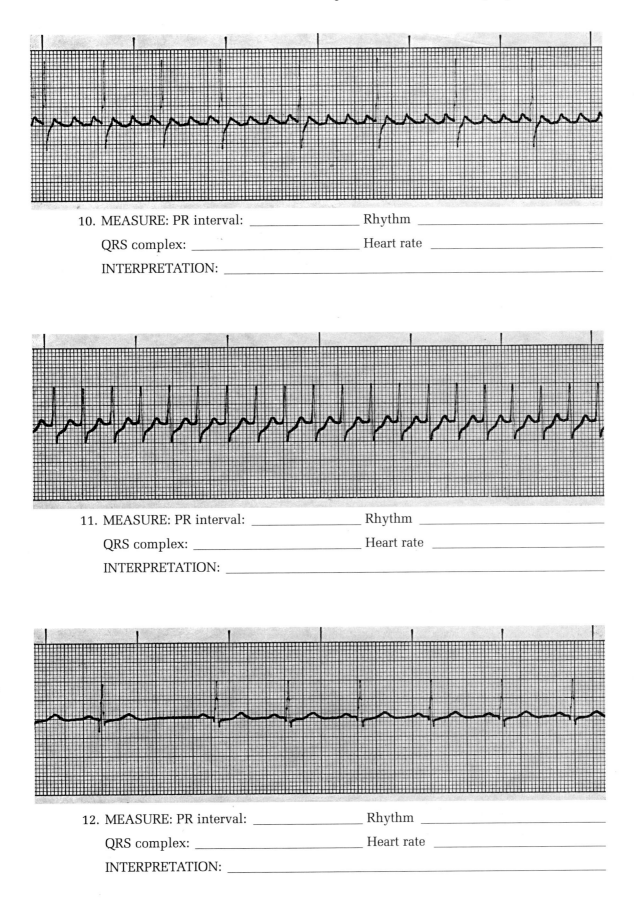

10. MEASURE: PR interval: _____ Rhythm _____

    QRS complex: _____ Heart rate _____

    INTERPRETATION: _____

11. MEASURE: PR interval: _____ Rhythm _____

    QRS complex: _____ Heart rate _____

    INTERPRETATION: _____

12. MEASURE: PR interval: _____ Rhythm _____

    QRS complex: _____ Heart rate _____

    INTERPRETATION: _____

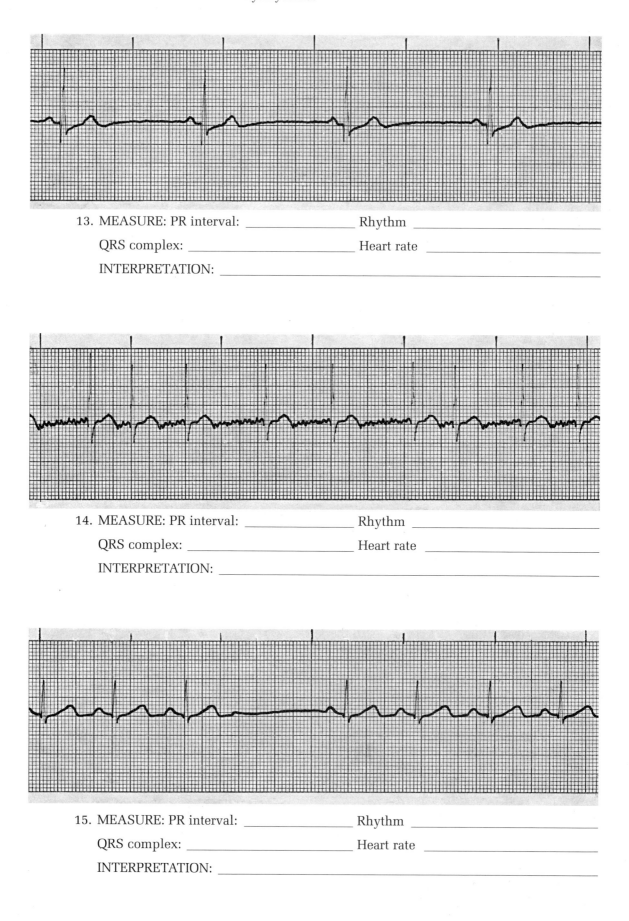

13. MEASURE: PR interval: _____ Rhythm _____

    QRS complex: _____ Heart rate _____

    INTERPRETATION: _____

14. MEASURE: PR interval: _____ Rhythm _____

    QRS complex: _____ Heart rate _____

    INTERPRETATION: _____

15. MEASURE: PR interval: _____ Rhythm _____

    QRS complex: _____ Heart rate _____

    INTERPRETATION: _____

Junctional Dysrhythmias

Chapter Four

JUNCTIONAL RHYTHMS

As discussed in Chapter 3, "Sinus and Atrial Dysrhythmias," the sinoatrial (SA) node and the atria may fail to generate the electrical impulses needed to begin depolarization for many reasons, such as drug toxicity, myocardial infarction, or heart disease. When this failure occurs, the atrioventricular (AV) node may assume its role of the secondary cardiac pacemaker of the heart (*see* Chapter 1, "Anatomy and Physiology").

The AV node is located in the general area of the lower right atrium, near the septum. It is an indistinct area and difficult to pinpoint exactly (Fig. 4-1). The cardiac tissue immediately surrounding the AV node is usually called the *AV junction* and is also capable of initiating electrical impulses (Fig. 4-1).

Rhythms that start in either the AV node or the AV junctional area are called *junctional rhythms* or nodal rhythms. The term *nodal* is rarely used today, since junctional is more accurate.

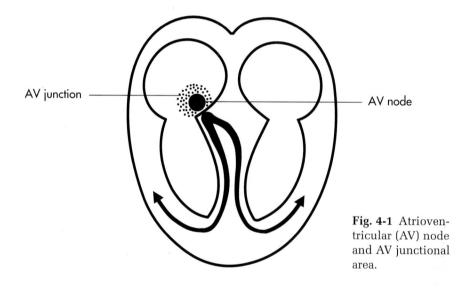

Fig. 4-1 Atrioventricular (AV) node and AV junctional area.

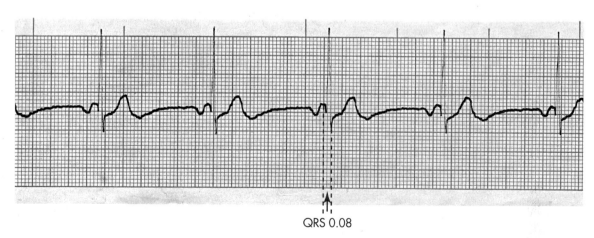

QRS 0.08

Fig. 4-2 Heart shows junctional/ventricular conduction pathway. Rhythm strip shows ventricular response.

Because the AV junction is not the primary pacemaker of the heart, it is not as efficient as the SA node and has a slower rate. The AV junctional rate is 40 to 60 electrical impulses per minute. This rate is also known as the inherent heart rate of the AV junctional area.

A junctional rhythm is not usually a lethal dysrhythmia. However, as with any rhythm, **patient assessment** is essential to determine the patient's tolerance of the dysrhythmia.

In a junctional rhythm, the electrical impulse travels in a normal pathway from the AV junction, through the bundle of His and bundle branches, to the Purkinje's fibers, and ending in the ventricular muscle.

Since the electrical impulse follows the normal pathway through the ventricles, the QRS complex usually measures less than 0.12 second (Fig. 4-2).

However, the impulse that depolarizes the atria must travel in a backwards, or *retrograde*, motion from the AV junction up through the atria (Fig. 4-3). This retrograde motion accounts for all three characteristic changes in the P wave, which identify an AV junctional dysrhythmia: *inverted, buried (hidden),* or *retrograde* (Fig. 4-4).

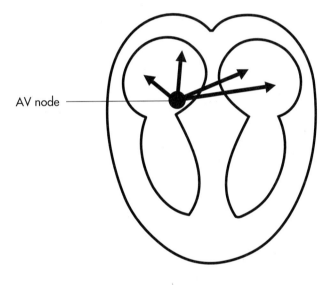

AV node

Fig. 4-3 Retrograde electrical conduction pathway from AV node to atria.

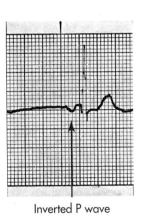

Inverted P wave

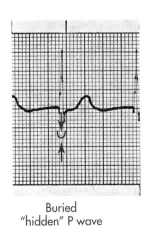

Buried "hidden" P wave

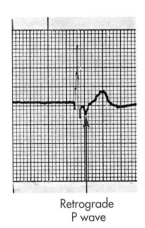

Retrograde P wave

Fig. 4-4 Inverted, buried, and retrograde P waves.

Inverted P Wave

If the electrical impulse originates high in the AV junctional area, the atria are depolarized quickly, although in a retrograde manner (Fig. 4-5). This retrograde depolarization causes the P wave to be inverted, or upside down (Fig. 4-6).

Since the electrical impulse originates in the AV junction, the distance the impulse must travel to depolarize the ventricles is shorter than normal. The depolarization of the ventricles, reflected by the QRS complex, occurs quickly and may cause a shortened PR interval of less than 0.12 second.

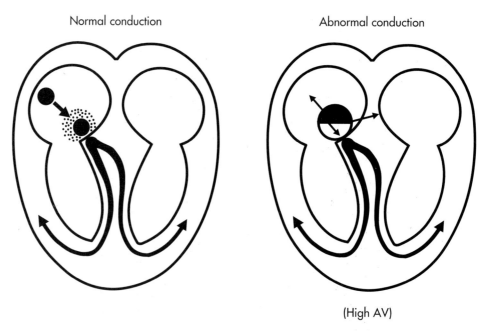

Normal conduction   Abnormal conduction

(High AV)

Fig. 4-5 Left heart shows normal electrical conduction pathway. Right heart shows conduction pathway of high AV junctional area.

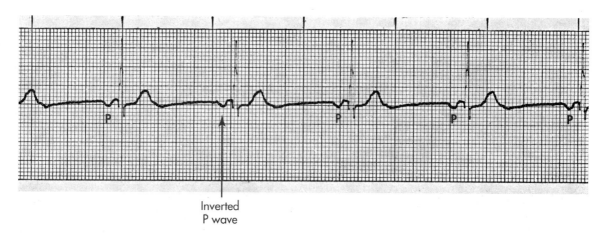

Inverted
P wave

Fig. 4-6 Junctional rhythm with inverted P waves.

Buried P Wave

When the electrical impulse originates in the mid AV junctional area, the distance the impulse must travel up through the atria (retrograde) and down through the ventricles is almost the same. This similar distance causes the atria and the ventricles to depolarize at almost the same time (Fig. 4-7).

Because the force of the atrial depolarization is less than the force of the ventricular depolarization, the P wave is hidden by the QRS. This P wave is described as buried, or hidden, and consequently a PR interval is not seen (Fig. 4-8).

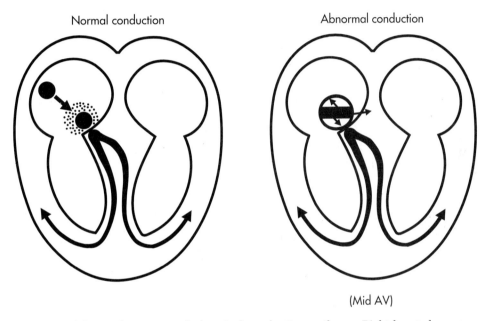

Normal conduction   Abnormal conduction

(Mid AV)

Fig. 4-7 Left heart shows normal electrical conduction pathway. Right heart shows conduction pathway of mid AV junctional area.

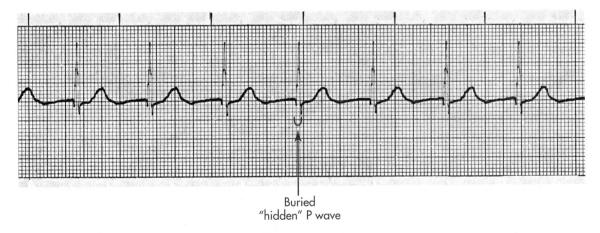

Buried
"hidden" P wave

Fig. 4-8 Junctional rhythm with buried, or hidden, P waves.

Retrograde P Wave

When the electrical impulse originates in the lower part of the AV junctional area, the distance the impulse must travel to the atria is greater than the distance to the ventricles (Fig. 4-9). Therefore, the atria depolarize slightly later than the ventricles, producing a retrograde P wave after the QRS.

The P wave is said to be retrograde because it appears after the QRS complex; no measurable PR interval is present. The P wave is inverted because the atria are depolarized in a retrograde manner (Fig. 4-10).

> NOTE: The term retrograde is used in two different ways:
> 1. To appear behind or after
> 2. To occur in a backward or reverse motion

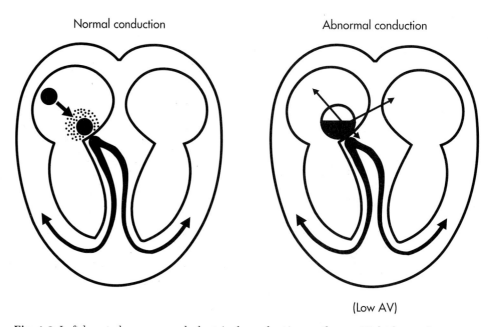

Normal conduction   Abnormal conduction

(Low AV)

Fig. 4-9 Left heart shows normal electrical conduction pathway. Right heart shows conduction pathway of lower AV junctional area.

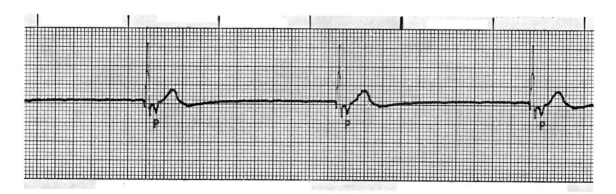

Fig. 4-10 Junctional rhythm with retrograde P waves.

JUNCTIONAL BRADYCARDIA

Junctional bradycardia occurs when all the electrical impulses originate from a single site within the AV junctional area, at a rate less than 40 impulses per minute.

The P wave is either inverted, buried, or retrograde. The PR interval, if present, is usually less than 0.12 second. However, the QRS complex usually remains less than 0.12 second. Because the P to P intervals, if seen, and the R to R intervals are regular and equal in length, the rhythm is regular. The rate can vary, but it must be less than 40 electrical impulses per minute (Fig. 4-11).

Junctional bradycardia may be caused by heart disease or drugs such as digitalis, quinidine, or sedatives.

A junctional bradycardia may become a serious dysrhythmia if the rate falls significantly or the patient becomes symptomatic.

Remember: any patient with a heart rate of less than 60 electrical impulses per minute has a bradycardic rate. This is known as an *absolute bradycardia*. However, because the inherent rate of the AV junction is 40 to 60 electrical impulses per minute, only a junctional rhythm with a rate below 40 impulses per minute can be called a junctional bradycardia.

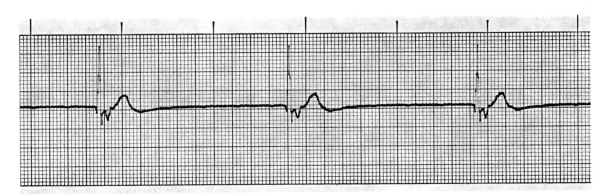

Fig. 4-11 Junctional bradycardia with retrograde P waves; heart rate, 30.

ACCELERATED JUNCTIONAL RHYTHM

Accelerated junctional rhythm occurs when all the electrical impulses originate from a single site within the AV junctional area, at a rate between 61 and 100 impulses per minute.

The P wave is either inverted, buried, or retrograde. The PR interval, if present, is usually less than 0.12 second. Since the electrical impulse follows the normal conduction pathway through the ventricles, the QRS complex usually remains normal, measuring less than 0.12 second.

Because the P to P intervals, if seen, and the R to R intervals are regular and equal in length, the rhythm is regular. The rate can vary, but it must be between 61 and 100 electrical impulses per minute (Fig. 4-12).

Any patient with a heart rate greater than 100 electrical impulses per minute has a tachycardic rate. However, only those rhythms that are junctional and have a rate between 61 and 100 impulses per minute can be called accelerated

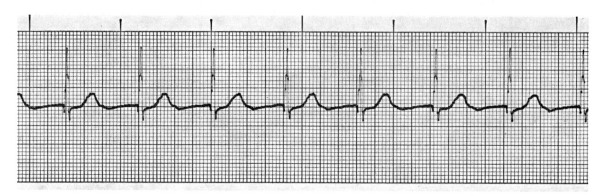

Fig. 4-12 Accelerated junctional rhythm with hidden P waves; heart rate, 70.

junctional rhythms. A junctional rhythm with a rate between 101 and 150 impulses per minute is called *junctional tachycardia*.

Both accelerated junctional rhythm and junctional tachycardia may be caused by heart disease or drugs such as atropine, caffeine, or amphetamines. It also may result from pain, fever, or acute anemia. Exercise or street drugs also can cause these dysrhythmias if heart disease is present.

Either accelerated junctional rhythm or junctional tachycardia may become a serious dysrhythmia, if the rate increases significantly or the patient becomes symptomatic. Assessment is required to determine the appropriate treatment as well as the patient's tolerance to the dysrhythmia.

PREMATURE JUNCTIONAL CONTRACTION

A *premature junctional contraction* (PJC) is an individual complex that originates from a single site in the AV junctional area and occurs earlier than the next expected complex of the underlying rhythm (Fig. 4-13). PJCs are common and can occur in any rhythm.

Although PJCs are **individual** complexes and **not** true rhythms, they are included in this chapter because they originate from the AV junctional area.

A PJC has the same characteristics as other junctional complexes. The P wave is either inverted, buried, or retrograde. The PR interval, if seen, may be less than 0.12 second, but the QRS complex is usually normal; less than 0.12 second.

The P to P and the R to R intervals of the underlying rhythm vary, depending on that rhythm. The occurrence of a PJC, in even the most regular rhythm, causes the P to P and the R to R intervals to be irregular.

The PJC may be followed by a complete compensatory pause, which allows the underlying rhythm to depolarize at its normal rate, as though the PJC had never occurred. The R to R interval from the complex before the PJC to the complex after the PJC, is at least two times the R to R interval of the underlying rhythm.

Although a PJC may occur in any rhythm, it is easier to identify within a sinus or bradycardic rhythm. When determining the rate of any rhythm containing a PJC, the R wave of the PJC is included in the total count of the R waves.

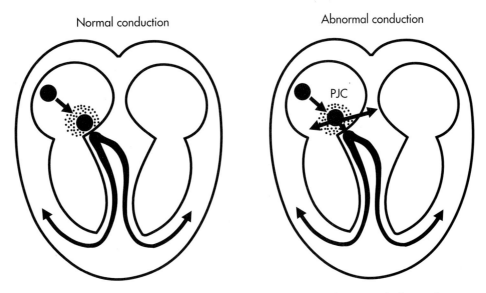

Fig. 4-13 Left heart shows normal electrical conduction pathway. Right heart shows conduction pathway of a premature junctional contraction (PJC).

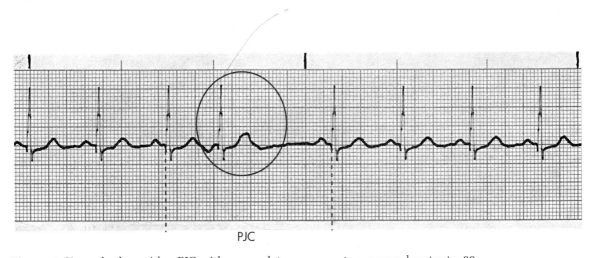

PJC

Fig. 4-14 Sinus rhythm with a PJC with a complete compensatory pause; heart rate, 80.

The underlying rhythm must be identified when interpreting a rhythm strip containing a PJC. For example, the underlying rhythm might be a sinus rhythm or a junctional rhythm with a PJC (Fig. 4-14).

Premature junctional contractions may be caused by pain, fever, fear, anxiety, sudden excitement, exercise, or the effects of drugs such as digitalis, atropine, nicotine, caffeine, and amphetamines. PJCs also may be caused by an increased irritability of the myocardium. This increased irritability indicates that the cardiac cells are able to respond to even a mild electrical stimulus and may depolarize in an unpredictable rate or manner

A PJC, by itself, is not a lethal dysrhythmia. However, it should be monitored closely, since it may trigger a more serious dysrhythmia.

WANDERING JUNCTIONAL PACEMAKER

A *wandering junctional pacemaker dysrhythmia* originates from at least three sites within the junctional area (Fig. 4-15). The size and shape of each complex is determined by the site of origin for each complex.

The individual complexes are characterized by P waves that are inverted, buried, or retrograde. Any PR intervals that are seen are usually less than 0.12 second, but the QRS complexes are usually normal; less than 0.12 second.

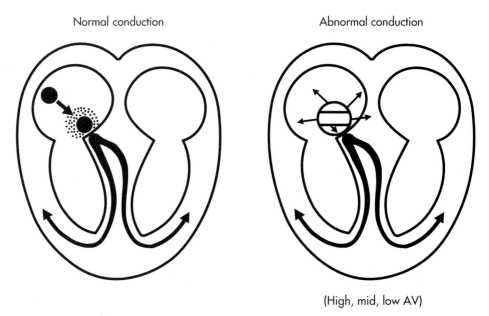

Normal conduction   Abnormal conduction

(High, mid, low AV)

Fig. 4-15 Left heart shows normal electrical conduction pathway. Right heart shows conduction pathway of a wandering junctional pacemaker.

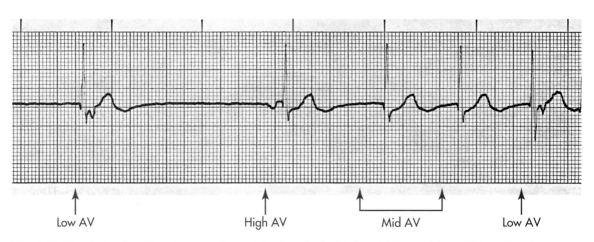

Low AV   High AV   Mid AV   Low AV

Fig. 4-16 Wandering junctional pacemaker originating in the high, middle, and low AV junctional areas; heart rate, 50.

The rhythm is irregular with varying P to P intervals and R to R intervals. The rate may also vary but is usually 40 to 60 impulses per minute (Fig. 4-16).

This dysrhythmia is not usually serious. However, it is frequently treated, because it indicates increased irritability within the junctional area that may progress to a more serious dysrhythmia.

A wandering junctional pacemaker dysrhythmia may be caused by heart disease, myocardial infarction, or drug toxicity.

A wandering junctional pacemaker dysrhythmia has three or more **junctional** sites. However, a rhythm that has both atrial and junctional sites is identified as a wandering atrial pacemaker.

Review Questions

1. True or false? The AV node is located in the lower, right atrium, near the septum.

2. True or false? A junctional bradycardia has a heart rate of less than 40 impulses per minute.

3. True or false? A wandering junctional pacemaker dysrhythmia originates from the atria and AV junction.

4. True or false? In a junctional rhythm, if the electrical impulse is initiated high in the AV junctional area, the P wave will be buried.

5. The inherent AV junctional heart rate is _____ to _____ electrical impulses per minute.

6. In an AV junctional rhythm the QRS complex usually measures

7. Junctional tachycardia has a heart rate between _____ and .

8. The rate of a wandering junctional pacemaker may vary but usually remains between _____ and _____ impulses per minute.

9. What are the two definitions of the term retrograde, as used to describe AV junctional rhythms?

   a. _____

   b. _____

10. Define the term premature junctional contraction._____

    _____

    _____

11. List the three types of P waves that can be seen with a junctional rhythm:

    a. _____

    b. _____

    c. _____

12. PJCs are usually followed by what type of pause? _____

Rhythm Strip Review

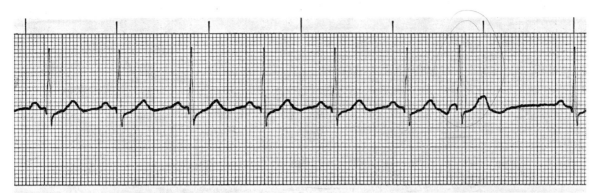

1. MEASURE: PR interval:_____   Rhythm: _____

    QRS complex: _____   Heart rate: _____

    INTERPRETATION: _____

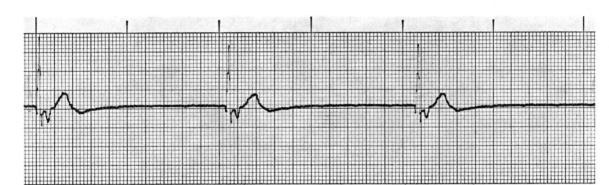

2. MEASURE: PR interval:_____   Rhythm: _____

    QRS complex: _____   Heart rate: _____

    INTERPRETATION: _____

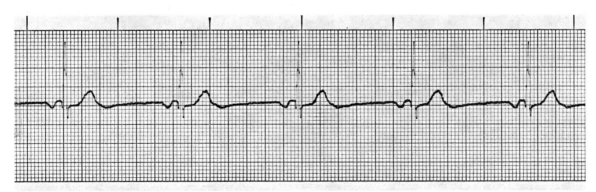

3. MEASURE: PR interval:_____   Rhythm: _____

    QRS complex: _____   Heart rate: _____

    INTERPRETATION: _____

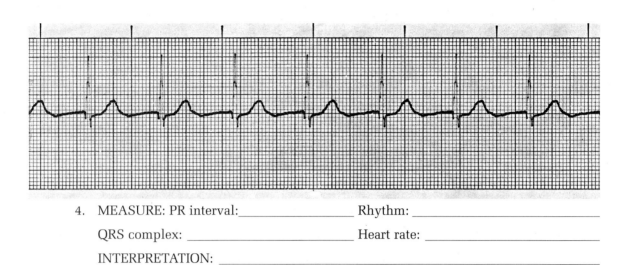

4. MEASURE: PR interval:_____ Rhythm: _____

QRS complex: _____ Heart rate: _____

INTERPRETATION: _____

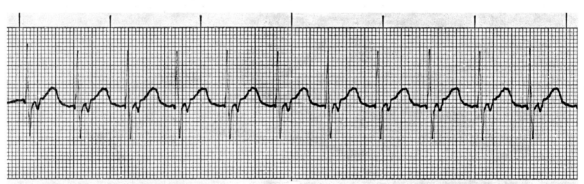

5. MEASURE: PR interval:_____ Rhythm: _____

QRS complex: _____ Heart rate: _____

INTERPRETATION: _____

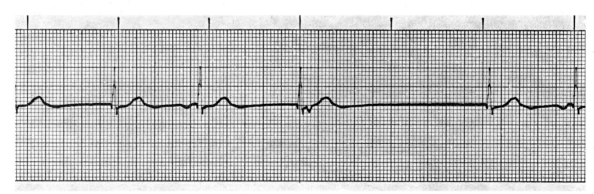

6. MEASURE: PR interval:_____ Rhythm: _____

QRS complex: _____ Heart rate: _____

INTERPRETATION: _____

Heart Blocks

Chapter Five

Objectives On completion of this chapter, the reader should be able to:

1. Describe first-degree heart block, including measurements of the components.
2. Explain the appearance of Mobitz I heart block, including measurements of the components.
3. Describe the appearance of Mobitz II heart block, including measurements of the components for 2:1, 3:1, and 4:1 blocks.
4. Describe third-degree heart block, including the appearance and measurements of the components.
5. Explain the appearance of a bundle branch block, including measurements of the components.
6. Define the terms prolonged PR interval, progressive block, Wenckebach, complete AV dissociation.

Outline **Heart Blocks**

A. Heart Blocks
1. First-Degree Heart Block
2. Mobitz I Heart Block
3. Mobitz II Heart Block
4. Third-Degree Heart Block
5. Bundle Branch Block

B. Chapter Review Questions

C. Rhythm Strip Review

HEART BLOCKS

Heart blocks occur when there is a *partial* or *complete interruption* in the cardiac electrical conduction system. This interruption can occur anywhere in the atria, between the sinoatrial (SA) node and the atrioventricular (AV) junction, or in the ventricles between the AV junction and the Purkinje's fibers.

The appearance of the P wave and the QRS complex varies, depending on the type of heart block. The rate and the rhythm also may vary.

The location of the block and the resulting patient symptoms determine if the dysrhythmia is lethal.

First-Degree Heart Block

A *first-degree heart block* is caused by a delay in the conduction of an electrical impulse between the atria and the bundle of His. This delay occurs when there is a partial interruption anywhere in the atrial or AV junctional conduction system (Fig. 5-1).

Although all electrical impulses are eventually conducted to the ventricles, the interruption causes the impulse to be delayed. Therefore, a first-degree heart block is **not** a true block, but simply a **delay** in the electrical conduction system. The delay is seen on the monitor screen or rhythm strip as a prolonged PR interval, greater than 0.20 second (Fig. 5-2).

A P wave occurs before every QRS complex; however, the PR interval is always greater than 0.20 second. The size and shape of both the P wave and QRS complex may vary, depending on the underlying rhythm. The P to P and the R to R intervals are usually regular, also depending on the underlying rhythm.

Because a first-degree heart block may be found in any rhythm that has a P wave before the QRS complex, the rate may be normal, bradycardic, or tachycardic. When describing a rhythm containing a first-degree heart block, identify the underlying rhythm first; for example, sinus bradycardia with a first-degree heart block (Fig. 5-3).

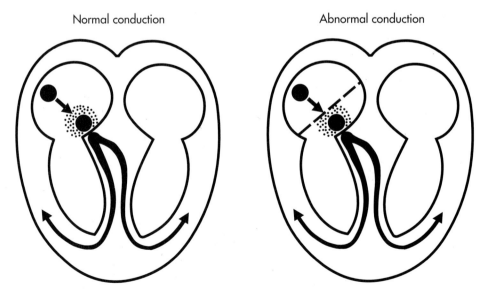

Normal conduction   Abnormal conduction

Fig. 5-1 Left heart shows normal electrical conduction pathway. Right heart shows pathway of a first-degree heart block with a delay between the atria and AV junction.

Although a first-degree heart block is not usually a serious dysrhythmia, it **is** important to assess the patient carefully when the block indicates a recent change in the patient's electrical conduction system. This change may indicate damage to the myocardium, which can lead to a more serious dysrhythmia.

First-degree heart block may be caused by myocardial infarction or drugs.

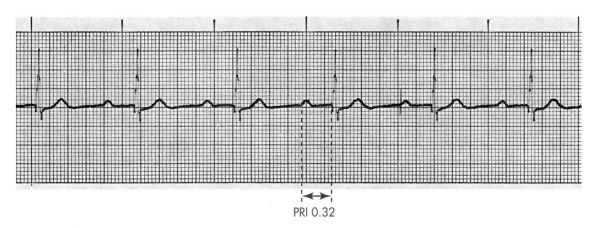

PRI 0.32

Fig. 5-2 PR interval greater than 0.20 second. The delay is seen on the monitor screen or rhythm strip as a prolonged PR interval.

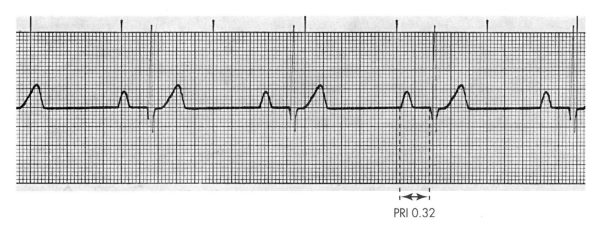

PRI 0.32

Fig. 5-3 Sinus bradycardia with first-degree heart block. PR interval, 0.32 second; heart rate, 40.

Mobitz I Heart Block

Mobitz I (Wenckebach or second-degree heart block, type I) is a **progressive** block. This block occurs when the electrical impulse traveling from the atria is interrupted at the AV junction, slowing the conduction of the impulse to the ventricles.

The interruption becomes longer with each impulse, delaying the depolarization of the ventricles, until the interruption completely blocks the conduction to the ventricles. The cycle of **progressively delayed conduction** is then repeated (Fig. 5-4).

The delay is seen on the rhythm strip as PR intervals becoming longer with each QRS complex, until a *dropped*, or *absent*, QRS complex occurs (P wave is seen without a QRS complex). This pattern is repeated throughout the dysrhythmia.

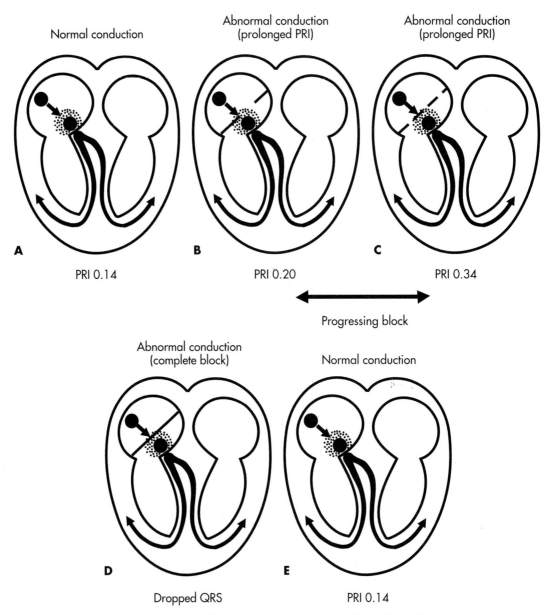

Normal conduction

Abnormal conduction
(prolonged PRI)

Abnormal conduction
(prolonged PRI)

A

B

C

PRI 0.14

PRI 0.20

PRI 0.34

Progressing block

Abnormal conduction
(complete block)

Normal conduction

D

E

Dropped QRS

PRI 0.14

Fig. 5-4A-E Hearts show the cycle of progressive delay of a Mobitz I heart block.

A P wave occurs before every QRS complex, and the P waves are the same size and shape. A QRS complex follows each P wave until a QRS is dropped. The QRS complex is usually less than 0.12 second.

Although the PR interval becomes progressively longer, the R to R intervals usually become progressively shorter, until the QRS complex is dropped. The pattern then repeats itself. The P to P interval remains regular; however, the overall rhythm is irregular. The rate may vary (Fig. 5-5).

Although Mobitz I is not a lethal dysrhythmia, the patient may become medically unstable due to a bradycardic rate, recent injury to the cardiac muscle, or prior illness. Mobitz I heart block may be serious when it indicates a recent change in the conduction system following an injury to the cardiac muscle. Mobitz I heart block may be caused by infection, myocardial infarction, or drug toxicity.

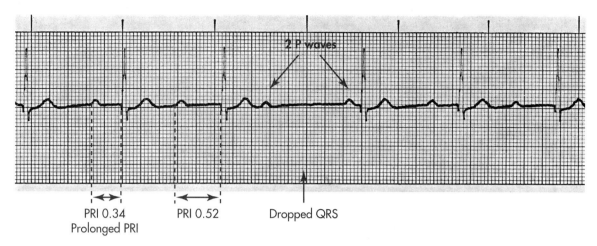

PRI 0.34   PRI 0.52   Dropped QRS
Prolonged PRI

Fig. 5-5 Mobitz I heart block. Atrial heart rate, 60; ventricular heart rate, 50.

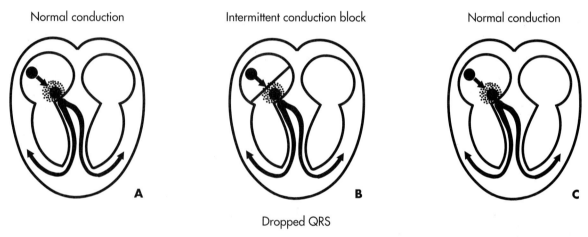

Dropped QRS

Fig. 5-6 (A) Heart shows normal electrical conduction pathway. Hearts in **(B) (C)** show conduction pathway of a Mobitz II heart block with an intermittent interruption at the AV junction.

As with any rhythm, **patient assessment** is necessary to determine the patient's tolerance of the dysrhythmia.

Mobitz II Heart Block

Mobitz II (second-degree heart block, type II) occurs when there is an **intermittent interruption** in the electrical conduction system near or below the AV junction. This interruption is **not** progressive, but occurs **suddenly and without warning**, blocking the conduction of the impulse to the ventricles (Fig. 5-6).

The rhythm strip shows a P wave before every QRS complex, and all P waves are the same size and shape. A QRS complex follows every P wave until an interruption occurs and a QRS is dropped (absent). The PR intervals of the underlying rhythm usually remain the same length and measure within the normal limits of 0.12 to 0.20 second. Although the QRS complex usually measures less than 0.12 second, the complex may be wider if the block occurs near the bundle of His.

A Mobitz II heart block can occur in any rhythm that has a P wave followed by a QRS complex. The P to P intervals are usually regular, and the R to R intervals are usually regular until a QRS complex is dropped. The overall rhythm is usually irregular, and the heart rate varies, also depending on the underlying rhythm (Fig. 5-7).

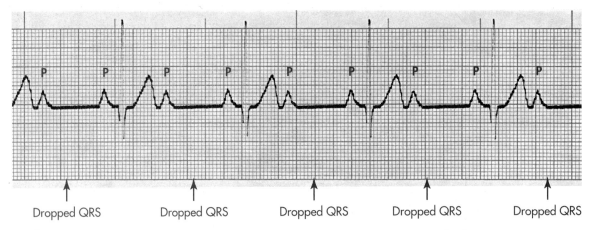

Fig. 5-7 Sinus rhythm with a Mobitz II heart block. Atrial heart rate, 90; ventricular heart rate, 40.

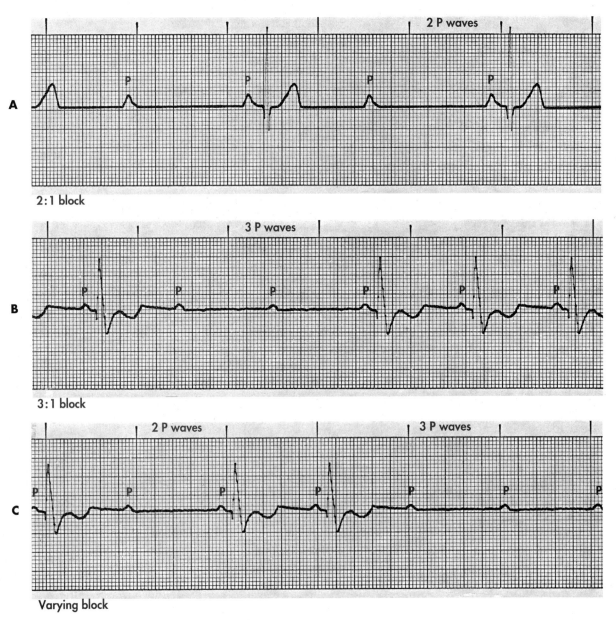

Fig. 5-8 **(A)** Mobitz II with a 2:1 block. **(B)** Mobitz II with a 3:1 block. **(C)** Mobitz II with a varying block.

When interpreting a dysrhythmia containing a Mobitz II block, it is important to:

1. Identify the underlying rhythm.
2. Determine the ratio of P waves to each QRS complex. The number of P waves before each QRS complex helps to determine the severity of the block.

    Example: Two P waves before one QRS complex = 2:1 block
    Three P waves before one QRS complex = 3:1 block
    Four P waves before one QRS complex = 4:1 block

    This ratio may be constant or may vary. Mobitz II heart block becomes more serious as the ratio of P waves to QRS complexes increases or if the ratio varies.
3. Determine the frequency of occurrence. Mobitz II heart block may occur in a pattern or at random. A Mobitz II block with no pattern (varying block) is more dangerous, since this lack of a pattern indicates the block is irregular and may progress to a more serious dysrhythmia (Fig. 5-8).

Mobitz II heart block is a dangerous dysrhythmia because of the increased irritability of the myocardium, which may lead to a more serious dysrhythmia such as third-degree heart block. If the block is severe enough, the ventricular rate may become bradycardic. A ventricular rate of 40 impulses per minute or less is not sufficient to maintain adequate circulation to the vital organs of the body. Frequent assessment is very important to determine the patient's tolerance of the dysrhythmia.

Mobitz II heart block may be caused by myocardial infarction, heart disease, or drug toxicity.

Third-Degree Heart Block

Third-degree heart block (complete heart block or complete AV dissociation) occurs when the electrical impulse is completely blocked between the atria and the ventricles. The interruption usually takes place between the AV junction and the bundle of His (Fig. 5-9).

The electrical impulse causes depolarization of the atria; however, the impulse is blocked before it can reach the ventricles. Because the electrical conduction system is completely interrupted, the ventricles must initiate

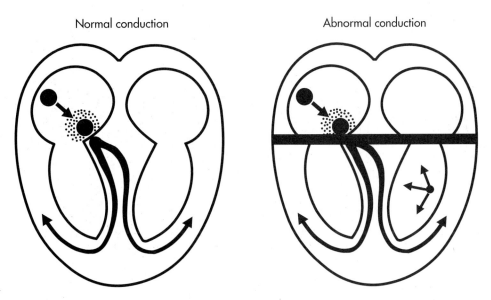

Normal conduction   Abnormal conduction

Fig. 5-9 Left heart shows normal electrical conduction pathway. Right heart shows conduction pathway of a third-degree heart block with a complete interruption between the atria and the ventricles.

their own impulses to cause cardiac muscle contraction. Both the atria and the ventricles function independently, as if they were two separate hearts (Fig. 5-10).

The rhythm strip shows both P waves and QRS complexes, as well as what appear to be PR intervals that are constantly changing in length. However, the PR intervals do **not** become progressively longer as they do in Mobitz I block.

On closer inspection of the rhythm strip, one can see that no relationship exists between the P waves and the QRS complexes. Because the atria and the ventricles are each functioning independently, no true PR interval occurs (Fig. 5-11).

The P waves are the same size and shape. The QRS complexes are wide, longer than 0.12 second, and bizarre in appearance, but are usually the same size and shape. Occasionally, the QRS complexes will measure less than 0.12 second, if the block occurs at the AV junction.

Because both the atria and the ventricles are generating their own impulses, each will depolarize at its own inherent rate causing the P to P intervals to be equal and the R to R intervals to be equal. However, the P to P intervals are not equal to the R to R intervals (Fig. 5-12).

The atrial rate is usually 60 to 100 impulses per minute, and the ventricular rate is usually 20 to 40, however the ventricular rate may be faster.

Third-degree heart block is a **lethal** dysrhythmia because it may progress to asystole (no heart beat). It is also lethal because the ventricular rate is usually so slow and inefficient, the heart cannot maintain a cardiac output adequate to sustain life.

Third-degree block is often caused by a myocardial infarction or severe heart disease.

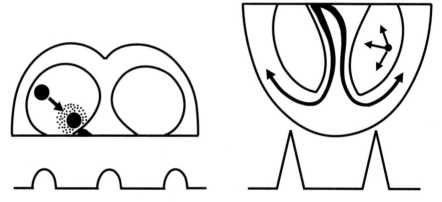

Fig. 5-10 Third-degree heart block with separate atrial and ventricular responses.

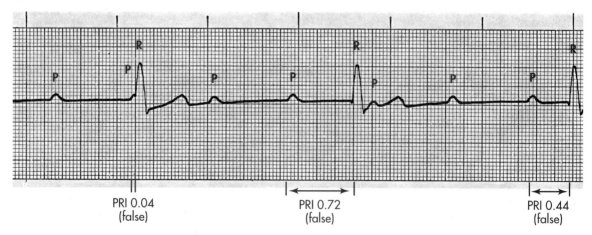

PRI 0.04
(false)

PRI 0.72
(false)

PRI 0.44
(false)

Fig. 5-11 Separate P waves and QRS complexes of third-degree heart block. Atrial heart rate, 70; ventricular heart rate, 30.

Bundle Branch Block

A *bundle branch block* (BBB) occurs when there is an interruption in the cardiac electrical conduction system of either the right, the left, or both bundle branches. This interruption causes a delay in the conduction of the electrical impulse to the ventricle of the blocked bundle branch (Fig. 5-13A-D).

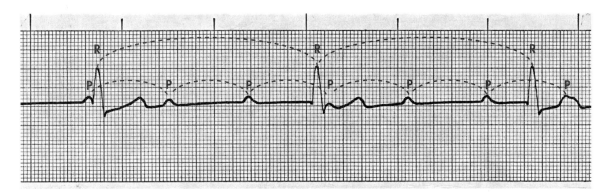

Fig. 5-12 Third-degree heart block. Atrial heart rate, 70; ventricular heart rate, 30.

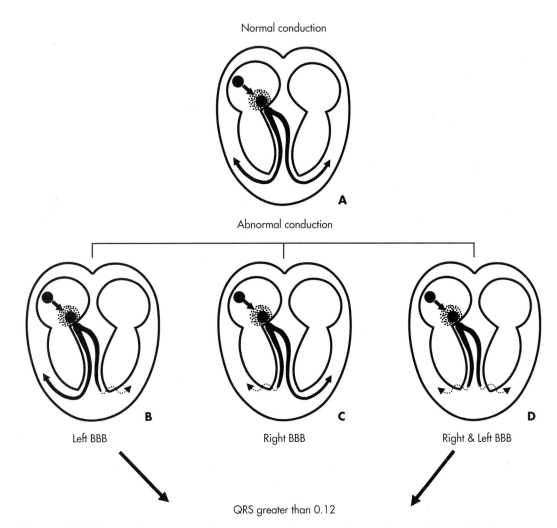

Fig. 5-13A-D Heart A shows normal electrical conduction pathway. Hearts B, C, and D show, respectively, the delayed conduction pathway of a left bundle, right bundle, and both a left and right bundle branch block (BBB).

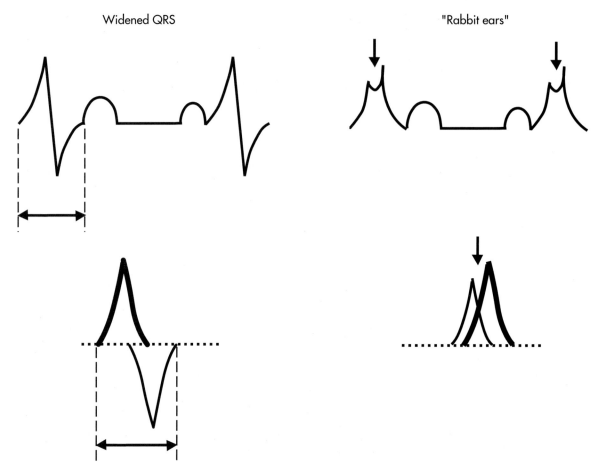

Fig. 5-14 The two types of ventricular depolarizations seen with a BBB; either a widened QRS or a "rabbit ears."

The atria are usually depolarized in a normal manner. The electrical impulse then follows the normal conduction pathway until it reaches the interruption in the bundle branch. The interruption in the conduction system forces the impulse to "detour" and take an alternate route.

As with any detour, the alternate route takes more time to travel. This extra time causes the electrical impulse to reach the ventricle of the blocked bundle branch later than the ventricle of the normal bundle branch.

As a result, the blocked ventricle depolarizes slightly later than the normal ventricle, causing two separate depolarizations (Fig. 5-14). The two depolarizations are shown on the rhythm strip as a single notched or widened QRS complex. The notched QRS is frequently referred to as "rabbit ears." The QRS complex is wider than normal, measuring more than 0.12 second (Fig. 5-15).

If both bundle branches are blocked, the electrical impulse must detour around both interruptions, causing the electrical impulse to reach both ventricles later than normal. The electrical impulse rarely reaches both ventricles at the same time.

Bundle branch blocks may occur in any rhythm. The presence of P waves and PR intervals is determined by the underlying rhythm. The rate and rhythm also may vary, depending on the underlying rhythm.

When interpreting a rhythm strip containing a bundle branch block, you must first identify the underlying rhythm; for example, sinus rhythm with a bundle branch block (Fig. 5-16).

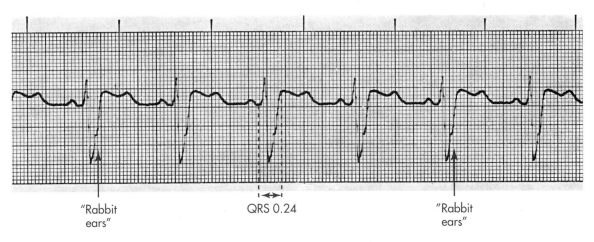

"Rabbit
ears"

QRS 0.24

"Rabbit
ears"

Fig. 5-15 Typical "rabbit ears" QRS complex seen with BBB.

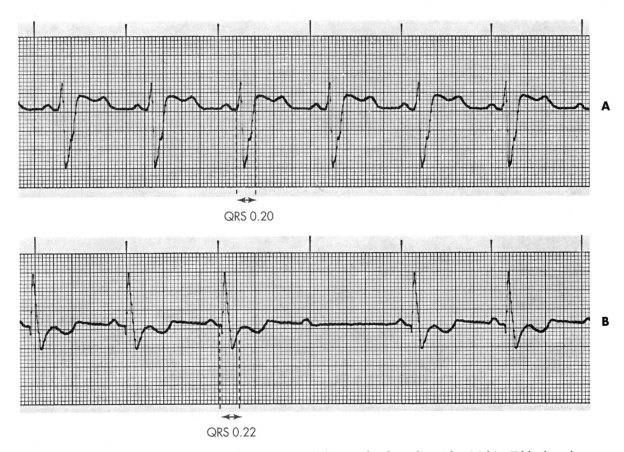

A

QRS 0.20

B

QRS 0.22

Fig. 5-16 (A) Sinus rhythm with a BBB; heart rate, 60. **(B)** Sinus bradycardia with a Mobitz II block and a BBB; overall heart rate, 50.

These blocks are not lethal dysrhythmias. They are important only as an indication of a problem in the cardiac conduction system. As with all dysrhythmias, patient assessment is required to determine the patient's tolerance of the block.

A 12-Lead electrocardiogram (EKG, ECG) is required to determine if the block is in the right or left bundle branch.

Bundle branch blocks may be caused by heart disease or myocardial infarction.

Review Questions

1. True or false? Heart blocks occur when there is a partial or complete interruption in the cardiac electrical conduction system.

2. True or false? A first-degree heart block occurs when there is a partial or complete interruption anywhere in the ventricles.

3. True or false? A third-degree heart block may progress to a Mobitz II block.

4. True or false? A third-degree heart block exists when the atria and ventricles function independently.

5. In a bundle branch block, the two depolarizations are seen on the rhythm strip as a notched or widened:

   a. T wave

   b. PR interval

   c. QRS complex

   d. ST segment

6. A third-degree heart block is a lethal dysrhythmia because:

   a. the additional force of the ventricular contraction can cause cardiac exhaustion

   b. it can progress to asystole

   c. the electrical impulse cannot be transmitted to the Purkinje's fibers

   d. the atria do not depolarize

7. Second-degree heart block, type I is also known as:

   a. Mobitz II

   b. AV dissociation

   c. Wenckebach

   d. bundle branch block

8. In a first-degree heart block the PR interval is greater than _____ second.

9. Complete heart block, or AV dissociation, is also known as _____ _____.

10. In a Mobitz I block, the PR intervals become progressively _____, until a P wave is followed by a dropped or absent _____.

11. Explain why a Mobitz II block is considered a dangerous dysrhythmia.

    _____

    _____

12. When identifying a Mobitz II heart block, which three aspects of a rhythm are important to evaluate?

    a. _____

    b. _____

    c. _____

Rhythm Strip Review

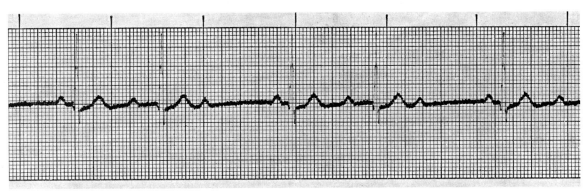

1. MEASURE: PR interval: _____ Rhythm: _____

    QRS complex: _____ Heart rate: _____

    INTERPRETATION: _____

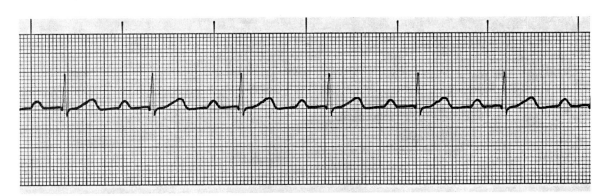

2. MEASURE: PR interval: _____ Rhythm: _____

    QRS complex: _____ Heart rate: _____

    INTERPRETATION: _____

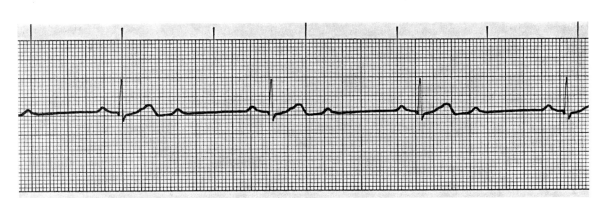

3. MEASURE: PR interval: _____ Rhythm: _____

    QRS complex: _____ Heart rate: _____

    INTERPRETATION: _____

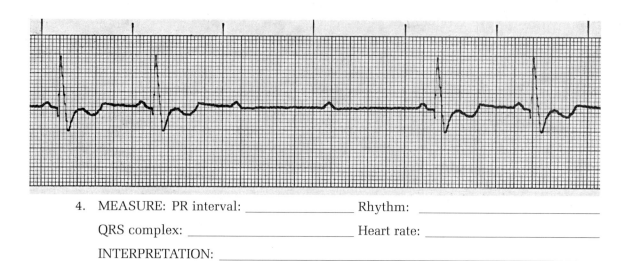

4. MEASURE: PR interval: _____ Rhythm: _____

    QRS complex: _____ Heart rate: _____

    INTERPRETATION: _____

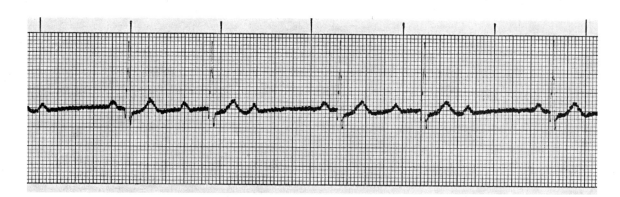

5. MEASURE: PR interval: _____ Rhythm: _____

    QRS complex: _____ Heart rate: _____

    INTERPRETATION: _____

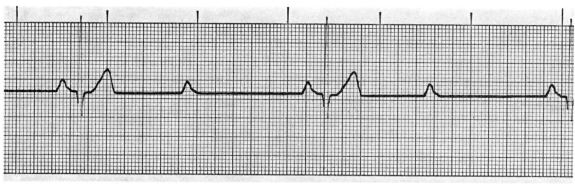

6. MEASURE: PR interval: _____ Rhythm: _____

    QRS complex: _____ Heart rate: _____

    INTERPRETATION: _____

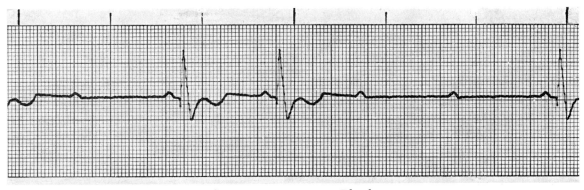

7. MEASURE: PR interval: _____   Rhythm: _____

QRS complex: _____   Heart rate: _____

INTERPRETATION: _____

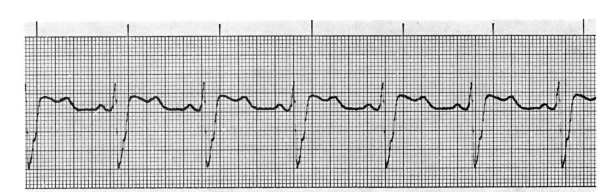

8. MEASURE: PR interval: _____   Rhythm: _____

QRS complex: _____   Heart rate: _____

INTERPRETATION: _____

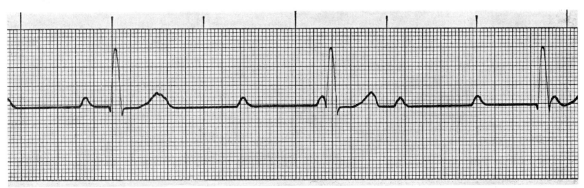

9. MEASURE: PR interval: _____   Rhythm: _____

QRS complex: _____   Heart rate: _____

INTERPRETATION: _____

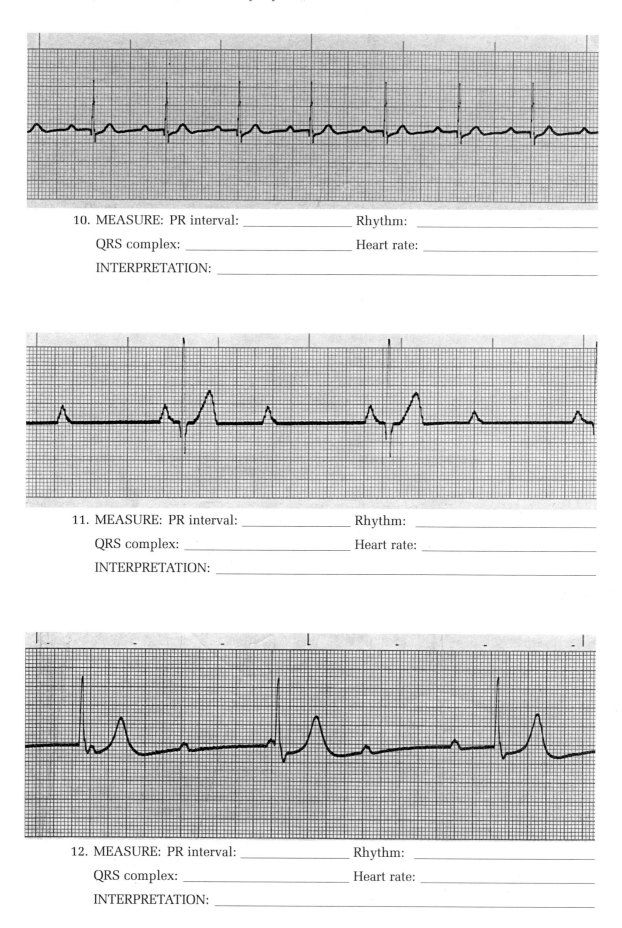

10. MEASURE: PR interval: _____ Rhythm: _____

    QRS complex: _____ Heart rate: _____

    INTERPRETATION: _____

11. MEASURE: PR interval: _____ Rhythm: _____

    QRS complex: _____ Heart rate: _____

    INTERPRETATION: _____

12. MEASURE: PR interval: _____ Rhythm: _____

    QRS complex: _____ Heart rate: _____

    INTERPRETATION: _____

Ventricular Dysrhythmias

Chapter Six

Objectives On completion of the chapter, the reader should be able to:

1. Describe a premature ventricular contraction, including measurements of the components.
2. Define compensatory pause, unifocal and multifocal premature ventricular contractions, bigeminy, trigeminy, quadrigeminy, couplet, run of VT, and R on T phenomenon.
3. Explain the difference between ventricular tachycardia and torsades de pointes.
4. Describe ventricular fibrillation, including coarse and fine fibrillation waves.
5. Describe an idioventricular rhythm.
6. Explain the difference between ventricular standstill and asystole, including measurements of the components.

Outline **Ventricular Dysrhythmias**

A. Ventricular Dysrhythmias
1. Premature Ventricular Contraction
   a. Site of origin
   b. Frequency of occurrence
   c. R on T phenomenon
   d. Other aspects
2. Ventricular Tachycardia
3. Torsades de Pointes
4. Ventricular Fibrillation
5. Idioventricular and Agonal Dysrhythmia
6. Ventricular Standstill
7. Asystole

B. Chapter Review Questions

C. Rhythm Strip Review

VENTRICULAR DYSRHYTHMIAS

When the sinoatrial (SA) node, the atria, and the atrioventricular (AV) junction fail to initiate an electrical impulse, the ventricles may become the pacemaker of the heart. The electrical stimulus can be initiated from any pacemaker cell in the ventricles, including the bundle branches, the Purkinje's fibers, or the ventricular muscle.

Because the electrical impulse begins in the lower portion of the heart, the impulse must take an alternate conduction pathway. The electrical impulse must travel in a retrograde (backward) direction to depolarize the atria **and** also in a forward direction to depolarize the ventricles (Fig. 6-1).

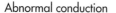

Abnormal conduction

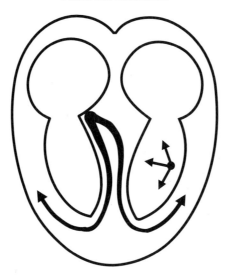

Fig. 6-1 Ventricular conduction pathway.

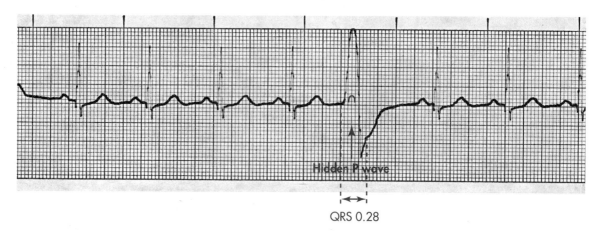

QRS 0.28

Fig. 6-2 Ventricular response with hidden P wave within QRS complex.

Since the atria depolarize at about the same time as the ventricles, the P wave is usually hidden in the QRS complex and will not be seen (Fig. 6-2). The QRS complex is wide, bizarre in appearance, and greater than 0.12 second.

Because the ventricles are the least efficient pacemaker of the heart, they usually generate 20 to 40 electrical impulses per minute (inherent ventricular heart rate). Ventricular dysrhythmias are usually considered life threatening. However, as with any rhythm, **patient assessment** is essential to determine the patient's tolerance of the dysrhythmia.

Premature Ventricular Contraction

A *premature ventricular contraction* (PVC) is an individual complex that originates from an area below the bundle of His and occurs earlier than the next expected complex of the underlying rhythm (Fig. 6-3). PVCs are very common and can occur in any cardiac rhythm.

Although PVCs are *individual* complexes and not rhythms, they are included in this chapter because they originate from the ventricles.

When the ventricles initiate a PVC, the atria may or may not depolarize. If the atria do not depolarize, a P wave will not be formed. When atrial depolarization does occur, the P wave is usually hidden in the QRS complex because the ventricles depolarize at about the same time.

The QRS complex has a wide and bizarre appearance, is greater than 0.12 second, and may deflect in the opposite direction of the QRS complex in the underlying rhythm.

The T wave immediately following the PVC is usually deflected in the opposite direction of the QRS complex of the PVC. The ST segment of the PVC appears abnormal because of this opposite direction.

A PVC is usually followed by a complete compensatory pause. This pause allows the underlying rhythm to continue again at its normal rate, as if the PVC had never occurred (Fig. 6-4).

You can check the complete compensatory pause by measuring the R to R intervals before and after the PVC. Measure from the R wave of the complex be-

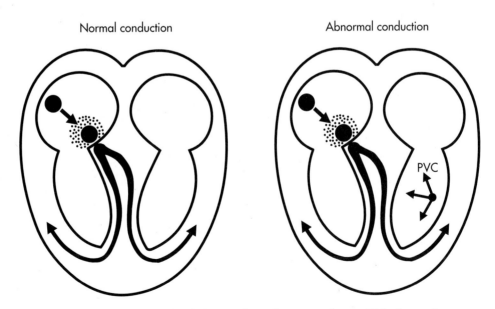

Normal conduction   Abnormal conduction

PVC

Fig. 6-3 Left heart shows normal electrical conduction pathway. Right heart shows conduction pathway of a premature ventricular contraction (PVC).

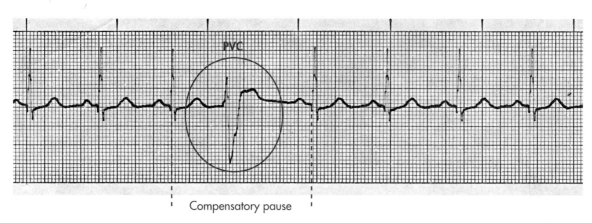

Fig. 6-4 PVC with a complete compensatory pause.

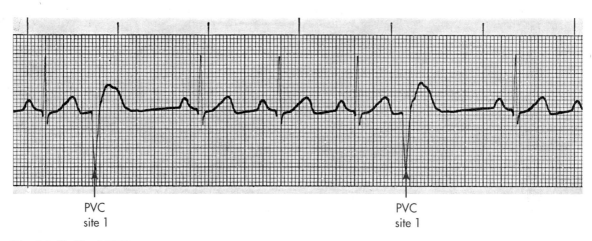

Fig. 6-5 Unifocal PVCs.

fore the PVC to the R wave of the complex after the PVC. The distance will be equal to two times the R to R interval of the underlying rhythm.

The P to P and R to R intervals of the underlying rhythm vary, depending on that rhythm. A PVC, in even the most regular rhythm, may cause the P to P and R to R intervals to be irregular.

The rate of the rhythm also varies, depending on the underlying rhythm and the number of PVCs within that rhythm. When determining the rate of a rhythm that contains PVCs, the number of PVCs are included in the total count of R waves.

Site of Origin
PVCs are further classified by the site of origin and the frequency of their occurrence.

1. *Unifocal* PVCs originate from a single site within the ventricles and therefore look alike (Fig. 6-5).
2. *Multifocal* PVCs originate from different ventricular sites and have varying sizes and shapes. These PVCs are more dangerous because they are the result of increased irritability within the ventricles (Fig. 6-6).

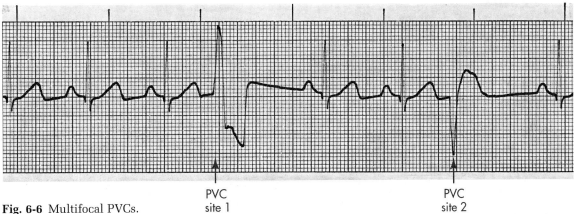

Fig. 6-6 Multifocal PVCs.

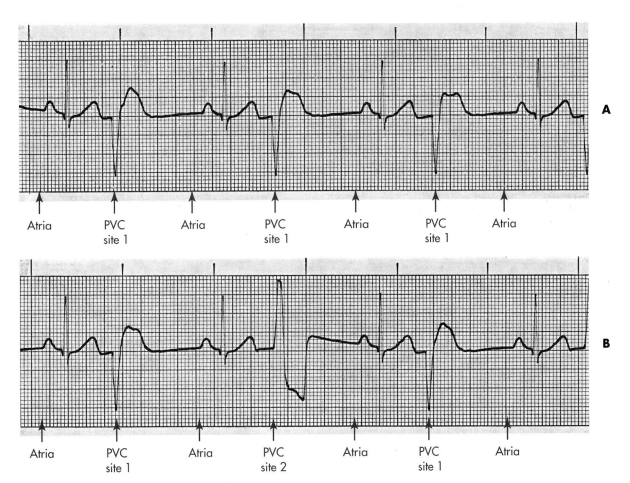

Fig. 6-7 Bigeminy. **(A)** Sinus rhythm with unifocal bigeminy PVCs; heart rate, 70. **(B)** Sinus rhythm with multifocal bigeminy PVCs; heart rate, 70.

Frequency of Occurrence

1. *Bigeminy* occurs when every other complex is a PVC. This rate of occurrence is the most serious, since it usually means a high degree of irritability exists within the ventricles (Fig. 6-7).
2. *Trigeminy* occurs when every third complex is a PVC (Fig. 6-8).
3. *Quadrigeminy* occurs when every fourth complex is a PVC (Fig. 6-9).

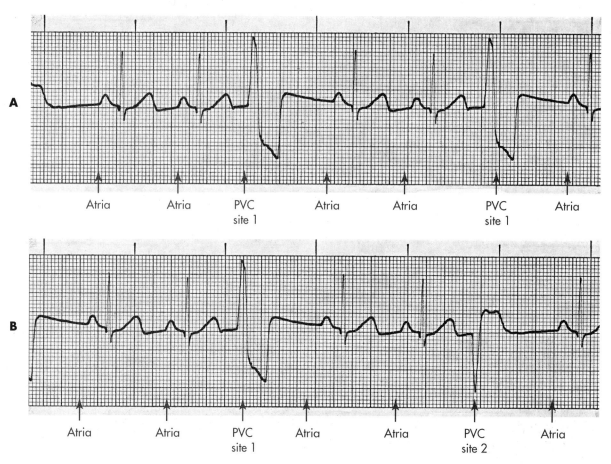

Fig. 6-8 Trigeminy. **(A)** Sinus rhythm with an episode of unifocal trigeminy PVCs; heart rate, 70. **(B)** Sinus rhythm with an episode of multifocal trigeminy PVCs; heart rate, 70.

> NOTE: In the clinical setting, to identify bigeminy, trigeminy, and quadri-geminy, there must be at least three episodes in a row on the monitor or rhythm strip.

4. *Couplet* describes two PVCs in a row that are not separated by a complex of the underlying rhythm (Fig. 6-10).
5. *Run of ventricular tachycardia* (run of VT) occurs when three or more PVCs exist in a row, not separated by a QRS complex of the underlying rhythm. A run of VT is of short duration (less than 30 seconds), and the PVCs are usually all unifocal. Both couplets and runs of VT indicate a high degree of irritability in the ventricles and may lead to a lethal dys-rhythmia (Fig. 6-11). A run of VT may be called a *salvo* in some parts of the country.

R on T Phenomenon

R on T phenomenon (R on T) is an additional term used to describe PVCs. It oc-curs when the R wave of the PVC falls on the T wave of the previous complex. R on T phenomenon may lead to a lethal dysrhythmia, since the PVC occurs during the vulnerable period of ventricular repolarization (Fig. 6-12). (To review vulnerable period, *see* page 28, relative refractory period.)

Other aspects

When the rate of the underlying rhythm is bradycardic, the PVCs may also be the heart's attempt to increase the cardiac rate and maintain adequate circula-tion and cardiac output.

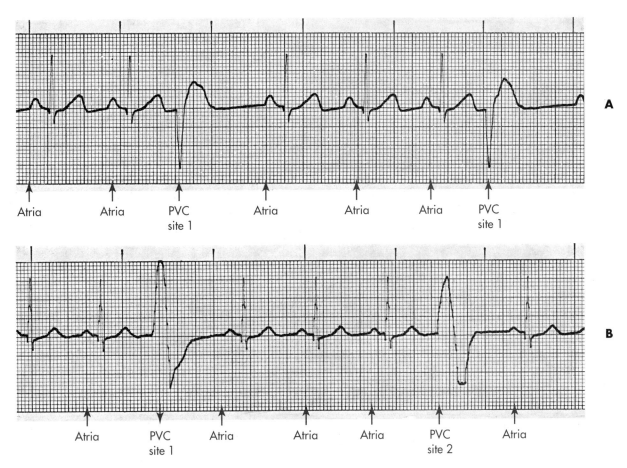

Atria   Atria   PVC   Atria   Atria   Atria   PVC
                  site 1   site 1

Atria   PVC   Atria   Atria   Atria   PVC   Atria
         site 1   site 2

Fig. 6-9 Quadrigeminy. **(A)** Sinus rhythm with an episode of unifocal quadrigeminy PVCs; heart rate, 70. **(B)** Sinus rhythm with an episode of multifocal quadrigeminy PVCs; heart rate, 80.

Patients with PVCs do not always require treatment. However, PVCs are usually considered dangerous, and patients may require treatment, if one or more of the following occur:

1. More than six PVCs on a 1-minute rhythm strip
2. Multifocal PVCs
3. Couplets
4. Run of VT
5. R on T phenomenon
6. A medically unstable patient

Assessment of the patient is essential to evaluate the patient's tolerance of the dysrhythmia and to determine the possible need for treatment.

PVCs can be caused by heart disease, myocardial infarction, or stimulants such as caffeine or nicotine. Stress and anxiety also can cause PVCs.

Ventricular Tachycardia

Ventricular tachycardia (VT, V tach) is a dysrhythmia that usually originates from a single site in the ventricles at a rate of 100 to 250 electrical impulses per minute (Fig. 6-13). A ventricular tachycardia with a rate of 40 to 100 is considered a slow ventricular tachycardia or an accelerated idioventricular rhythm. Because the inherent rate of the ventricles is 20 to 40 impulses per minute, any ventricular rate greater than 40 can be considered ventricular tachycardia.

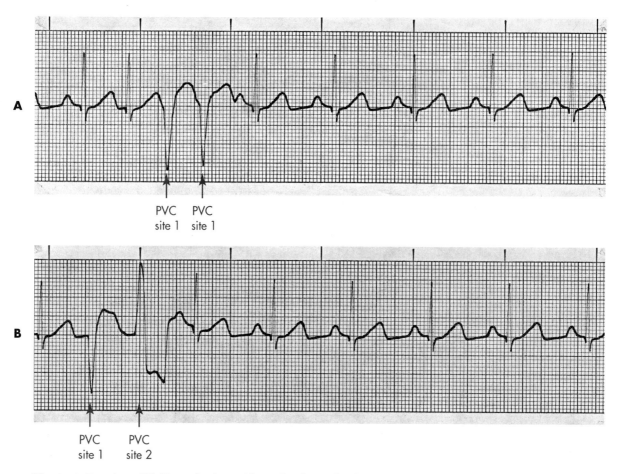

Fig. 6-10 Couplets. **(A)** Sinus rhythm with unifocal couplet; heart rate, 90. **(B)** Sinus rhythm with multifocal couplet; heart rate, 80.

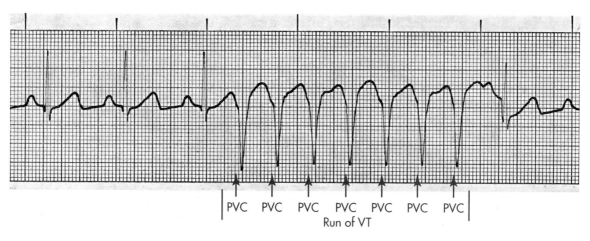

Fig. 6-11 Sinus rhythm with a run of ventricular tachycardia; heart rate, 110.

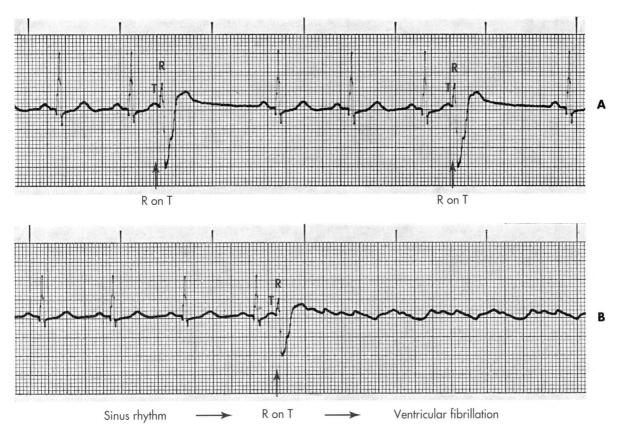

Fig. 6-12 R on T phenomenon. **(A)** Sinus rhythm with unifocal PVCs with R on T; heart rate, 80. **(B)** Sinus rhythm; heart rate, 100, with an R on T PVC, progressing to ventricular fibrillation.

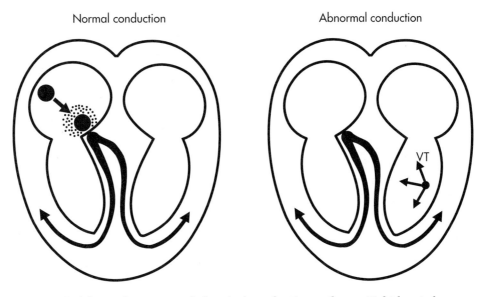

Fig. 6-13 Left heart shows normal electrical conduction pathway. Right heart shows conduction pathway of ventricular tachycardia (VT).

P waves, if present, are from the underlying rhythm, not from the ventricular tachycardia. PR intervals and P to P intervals are not measurable.

The QRS complex is wide, bizarre, and longer than 0.12 second. The R to R interval is usually regular, although it may be slightly irregular (Fig. 6-14).

This dysrhythmia starts suddenly and is frequently triggered by a PVC. Although the definition of ventricular tachycardia is more than three PVCs in a row, a ventricular tachycardia that lasts 30 seconds or less is usually called a *run of VT*, while *sustained* (prolonged) ventricular tachycardia is longer than 30 seconds.

Ventricular tachycardia is a **life-threatening** dysrhythmia. As the heart rate increases, the ventricles do not have time to completely empty and refill. Therefore, cardiac output is decreased and adequate amounts of blood are not circulated to vital organs, such as the heart and brain.

Patient symptoms vary, depending on the duration of the ventricular tachycardia. For example, with a run of VT, the patient may only feel slightly weak

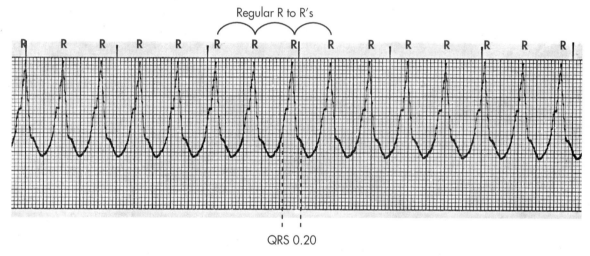

Fig. 6-14 Ventricular tachycardia with regular R to R intervals and QRS greater than 0.12 second; heart rate, 150.

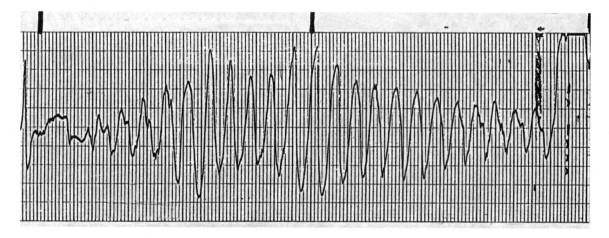

Fig. 6-15 Torsade de pointes; heart rate, 240-250.

or complain of occasional "palpitations" or a "racing heart." However, in *sustained VT* the patient's condition may become unstable, leading to unresponsiveness and **loss of pulse**, requiring immediate treatment. Again, the patient **must** be assessed frequently to determine the patient's tolerance of the dysrhythmia and the appropriate treatment.

Torsades de Pointes

Torsades de pointes is a dysrhythmia that looks similar to ventricular tachycardia. The dysrhythmia originates from the ventricles, but it is unclear whether it is from a single site or multiple sites.

Unlike ventricular tachycardia, the wave amplitude (height) of torsades de pointes begins close to the baseline, gradually increasing and decreasing in a repeating pattern. The rhythm resembles a twisting and turning motion along the baseline (Fig. 6-15). It is important to determine if the dysrhythmia is ventricular tachycardia or torsades de pointes because these dysrhythmias are each treated differently (*see* Chapter 9, "Medication Review and Adult Treatment Guidelines").

This dysrhythmia usually starts suddenly and is frequently preceded by a prolonged QT interval (more than one half the R to R interval of that complex). P waves, if seen, are from the underlying rhythm, not the torsades de pointes. PR intervals and P to P intervals are not measurable. The QRS complex is wide, bizarre, and greater than 0.12 second. The R to R interval is usually regular, although it may be slightly irregular. The ventricular rate is often greater than 150 impulses per minute.

The duration of the torsades de pointes will affect the patient's tolerance of the dysrhythmia. The patient may complain of symptoms such as a slight weakness, occasional palpitations, or a feeling of a "racing" heart if the torsades de pointes lasts only a few seconds. However a torsades de pointes with a longer duration may lead to unstable conditions, such as low blood pressure, unresponsiveness, and **loss of pulse**.

Torsades de pointes is a **life-threatening** dysrhythmia. As the heart rate increases, the ventricles do not have enough time to completely empty and refill. Therefore, good cardiac output is not maintained, and adequate amounts of blood and oxygen are **not** circulated to the vital organs, such as the heart and brain.

Patient assessment **must** be performed frequently to determine the patient's tolerance of the dysrhythmia and the proper treatment protocol.

Ventricular Fibrillation

Ventricular fibrillation (VF, V Fib) is a **lethal** dysrhythmia that originates from many different sites within the ventricles (Fig. 6-16). Because so many ventricular sites initiate electrical impulses, the cardiac cells do not have time to completely depolarize and repolarize. Therefore, electrical impulses are not transmitted through **any** normal conduction pathway of the heart.

Neither the atria nor the ventricles depolarize; therefore, P waves, QRS complexes, PR intervals, P to P intervals, and R to R intervals are **not** present. Only a chaotic, wavy line is seen on the monitor or rhythm strip. Because QRS complexes are not seen, it is impossible to measure a heart rate (Fig. 6-17).

The ventricles make ineffective quivering movements, not actual contractions. Consequently, blood is not being pumped throughout the body, and the patient **does not** have a pulse. Death will occur if treatment is not begun immediately.

Ventricular fibrillation is further described as either coarse or fine. The *coarse ventricular fibrillation* waves have a higher amplitude (height) and are

Normal conduction   Abnormal conduction

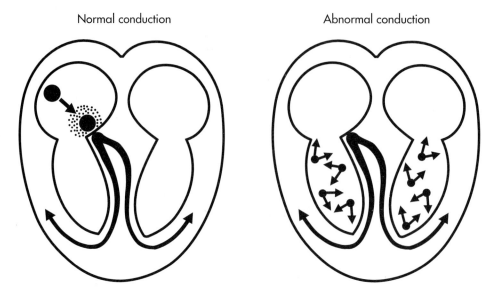

Fig. 6-16 Left heart shows normal electrical conduction pathway. Right heart shows conduction pathway of ventricular fibrillation (VF).

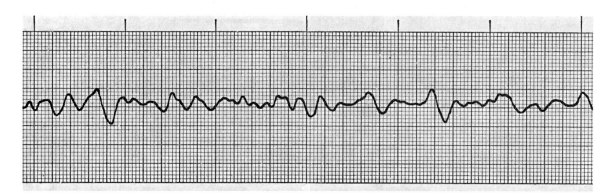

Fig. 6-17 Coarse ventricular fibrillation; heart rate, not measurable.

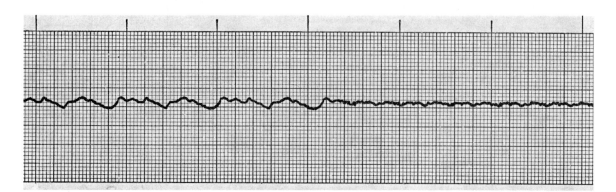

Fig. 6-18 Coarse VF progressing to fine VF; heart rate, not measurable.

more irregular than the fine VF waves. This difference indicates that a greater number of cardiac cells are able to respond to the electrical stimulation. Coarse ventricular fibrillation may progress to fine VF, which responds less easily to treatment (Fig. 6-18).

Fine ventricular fibrillation waves have less amplitude, indicating fewer cardiac cells are able to respond to an electrical impulse (Fig. 6-19).

Ventricular fibrillation is usually the result of severe heart disease, electrical shock, or drug toxicity. Patients with this dysrhythmia do not have a pulse and require immediate treatment.

> NOTE OF CAUTION: Assessment of the patient before beginning treatment is very important, since loose leads or artifact can mimic this dysrhythmia on the monitor screen or rhythm strip.

Idioventricular and Agonal Dysrhythmia

Idioventricular dysrhythmia (agonal or dying heart) is a **lethal** dysrhythmia that usually originates from a single site in the ventricles.

The atria, AV junction, bundle of His, and bundle branches can no longer function as pacemakers. This is the **final attempt** of the conduction system to initiate an electrical impulse from the ventricular muscle. However, the cardiac muscle is so damaged that it **cannot** respond effectively (Fig. 6-20).

The atria do not depolarize. Therefore, P waves, PR intervals, and P to P intervals are not present. Ventricular depolarization is slow and ineffective, causing QRS complexes that are very wide and bizarre and measure more than 0.12 second (Fig. 6-21A). R to R intervals may be irregular.

The ventricular rate is usually less than 40 impulses per minute. When the ventricular rate becomes less than 20 impulses per minute, the rhythm is known as *agonal* (dying heart) rhythm (Fig. 6-21B). As the ventricles weaken and the ventricular impulses become slower, the QRS complexes progressively show less amplitude and become wider, until all cardiac electrical activity stops.

The heart muscle is so damaged that the cardiac contractions are ineffective, and cardiac output is so poor that oxygen is not reaching the body cells in sufficient amounts to maintain life. Idioventricular rhythm is a **lethal** rhythm, and treatment **must** be started immediately.

Idioventricular rhythm is usually seen in the end stage of advanced heart disease.

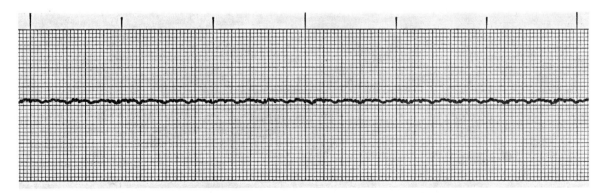

Fig. 6-19 Fine ventricular fibrillation; heart rate, not measurable.

Ventricular Standstill

Ventricular standstill occurs when only atrial depolarization exists and there is no ventricular depolarization (Fig. 6-22).

P waves are present, and the P to P intervals are regular. The ventricles do not depolarize; therefore, QRS complexes, PR intervals, and R to R intervals are not present (Fig. 6-23).

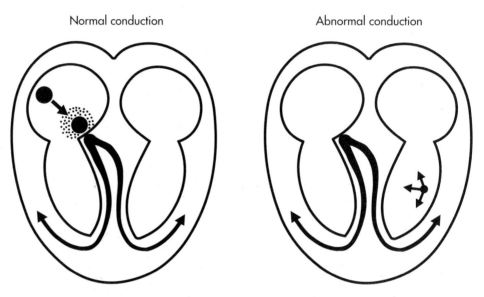

Normal conduction   Abnormal conduction

Fig. 6-20 Left heart shows normal electrical conduction pathway. Right heart shows conduction pathway of idioventricular/agonal rhythm.

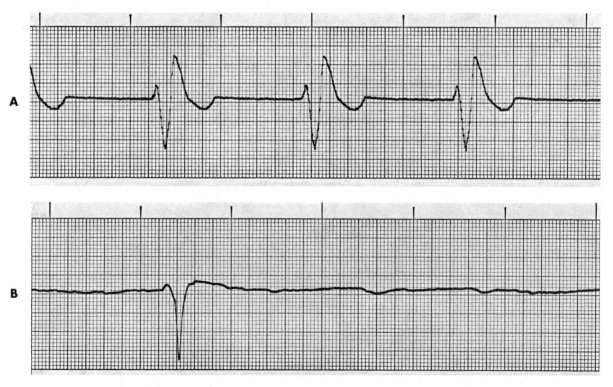

Fig. 6-21 (A) Idioventricular rhythm; ventricular heart rate, 30. **(B)** Agonal rhythm; heart rate, 10.

Normal conduction   Abnormal conduction

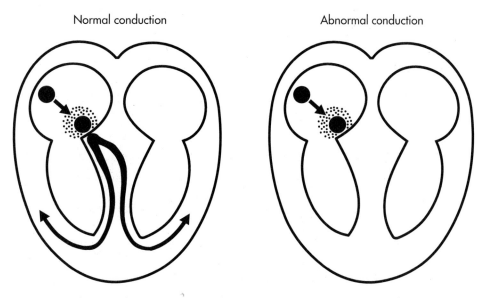

Fig. 6-22 Left heart shows normal electrical conduction pathway. Right heart shows conduction pathway of ventricular standstill.

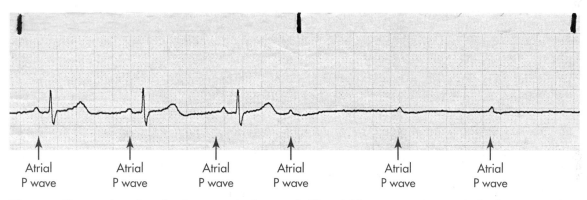

| Atrial | Atrial | Atrial | Atrial | Atrial | Atrial |
| P wave | P wave | P wave | P wave | P wave | P wave |

Fig. 6-23 Sinus rythm changing into ventricular standstill; atrial heart rate, 60; ventricular heart rate, 30.

The atrial heart rate usually varies from 60 to 100 electrical impulses per minute, while the ventricular rate is 0. Because the ventricles do **not** depolarize, there is **no** ventricular contraction. Blood does not circulate to any part of the body. The patient does not have a pulse. This dysrhythmia is **lethal** and requires immediate treatment.

Ventricular standstill may be the result of third-degree heart block, massive myocardial infarction, or a ventricular rupture.

Asystole

Asystole occurs when there is a complete lack of electrical activity in both the atria and the ventricles. Therefore, the atria and ventricles do not depolarize (Fig. 6-24).

No P waves, PR intervals, QRS complexes, P to P intervals, or R to R intervals exist. Asystole appears as a slightly wavy or straight line on the monitor screen or rhythm strip (Fig. 6-25). Because it may be difficult to distinguish asystole from very fine VF, two different leads should be used to identify asystole (e.g.: Lead II and MCL I).

Normal conduction   Abnormal conduction

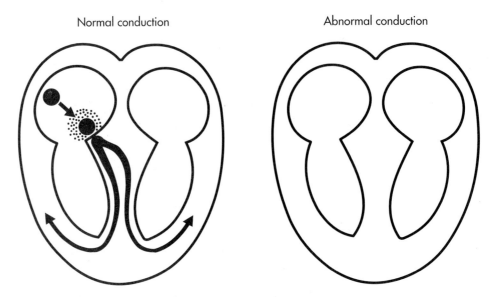

Fig. 6-24 Left heart shows normal electrical conduction pathway. Right heart shows conduction pathway of asystole.

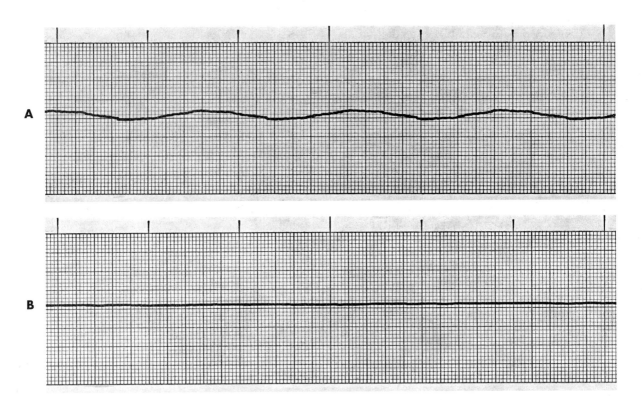

Fig. 6-25 Asystole. **(A)** Lead II, slightly wavy line, possibly fine VF. **(B)** MCL I, straight line. Rhythm, is asystole.

This dysrhythmia is **lethal**. The patient will **not** have a pulse, and immediate assessment and treatment are required.

Asystole usually follows untreated ventricular tachycardia or ventricular fibrillation. It also may be caused by massive myocardial infarction, advanced cardiac disease, or electrocution.

Review Questions

1. True or false? Ventricular tachycardia is a dysrhythmia that originates from many ventricular sites.

2. True or false? Asystole occurs when there is no electrical activity in the atria or ventricles.

3. True or false? PVCs are a common ventricular dysrhythmia and can occur in any cardiac rhythm.

4. True or false? If two PVCs occur in a row, the dysrhythmia is called a run of VT.

5. True or false? In ventricular fibrillation, the QRS complex usually measures more than 0.12 second.

6. The heart rate of agonal rhythm is usually less than _____ impulses per minute.

7. Explain the difference between the appearance of ventricular tachycardia and torsades de pointes on the monitor or rhythm strip.

   _____

   _____

   _____

8. Define the following terms:

   a. Multifocal PVCs _____

   b. Couplet _____

   c. Bigeminy_____

9. List three causes of ventricular fibrillation:

   a. _____

   b. _____

   c. _____

10. In an idioventricular dysrhythmia, the heart rate usually varies from:
    a. The heart rate can not be measured
    b. 20 to 40 impulses per minute
    c. 60 to 100 impulses per minute
    d. 80 to 100 impulses per minute

11. The QRS complex of a PVC usually measures:
    a. 0.04 to 0.08 second
    b. 0.04 to 0.12 second
    c. Less than 0.12 second
    d. Greater than 0.12 second

12. The rate of a rhythm containing a PVC varies depending on the underlying rhythm and:
    a. Cause of the PVC in the underlying rhythm
    b. Site of origin of the PVC
    c. Width of the QRS complex
    d. Number of PVCs in the underlying rhythm

RHYTHM STRIP REVIEW

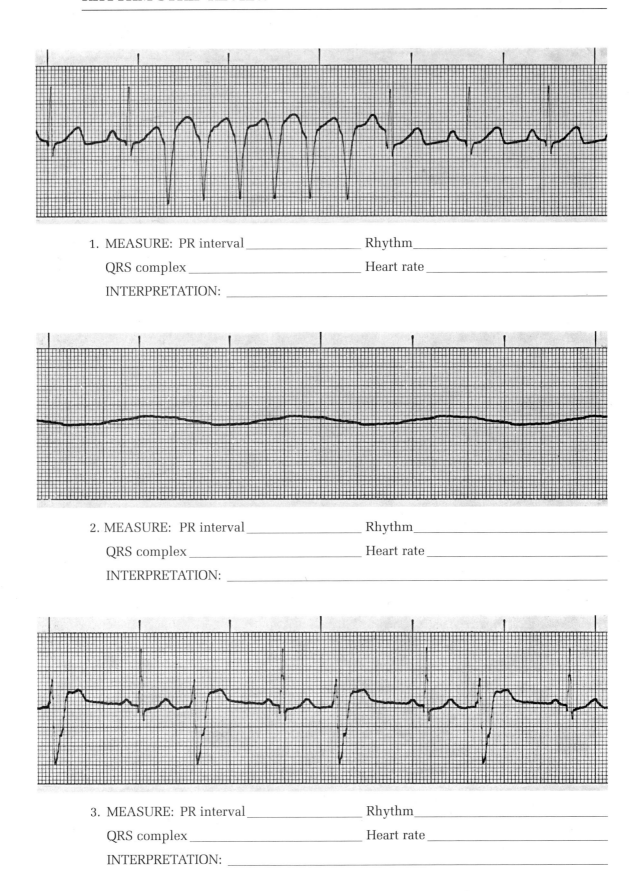

1. MEASURE: PR interval_____ Rhythm_____

   QRS complex_____ Heart rate_____

   INTERPRETATION: _____

2. MEASURE: PR interval_____ Rhythm_____

   QRS complex_____ Heart rate_____

   INTERPRETATION: _____

3. MEASURE: PR interval_____ Rhythm_____

   QRS complex_____ Heart rate_____

   INTERPRETATION: _____

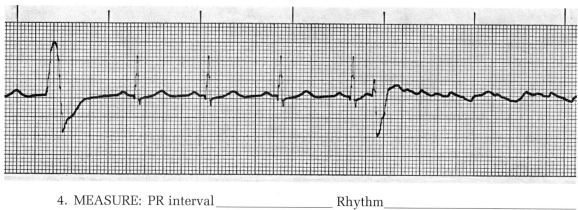

4. MEASURE: PR interval_____ Rhythm_____

QRS complex_____ Heart rate_____

INTERPRETATION: _____

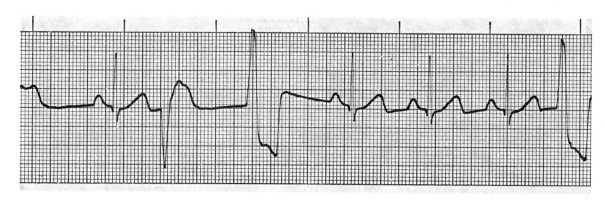

5. MEASURE: PR interval_____ Rhythm_____

QRS complex_____ Heart rate_____

INTERPRETATION: _____

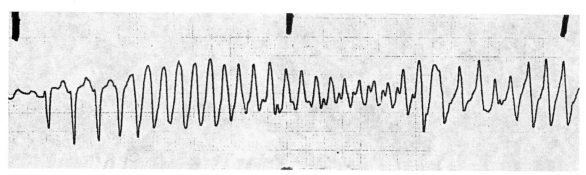

6. MEASURE: PR interval_____ Rhythm_____

QRS complex_____ Heart rate_____

INTERPRETATION: _____

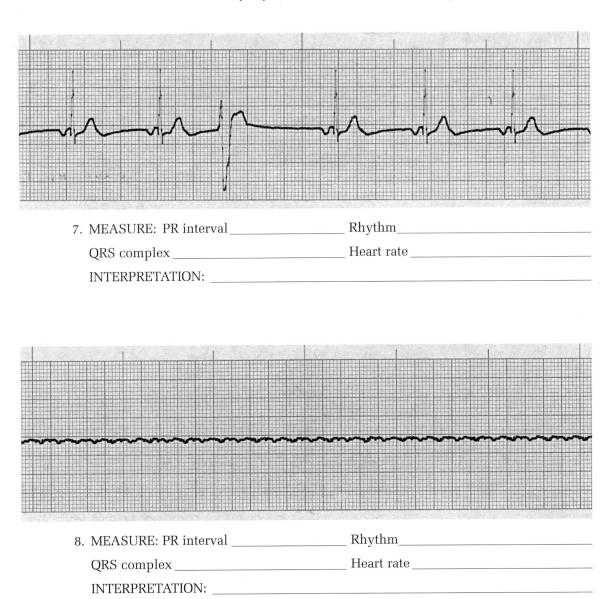

7. MEASURE: PR interval_____ Rhythm_____

QRS complex_____ Heart rate_____

INTERPRETATION: _____

8. MEASURE: PR interval _____ Rhythm_____

QRS complex_____ Heart rate_____

INTERPRETATION: _____

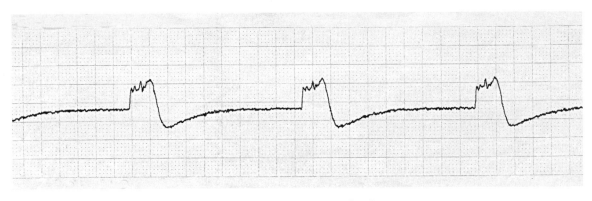

9. MEASURE: PR interval_____ Rhythm_____

QRS complex_____ Heart rate_____

INTERPRETATION: _____

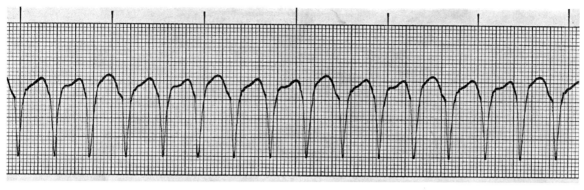

10. MEASURE: PR interval_____ Rhythm_____

QRS complex _____ Heart rate _____

INTERPRETATION: _____

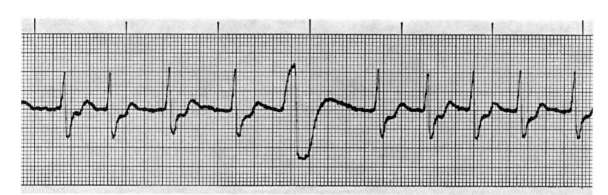

11. MEASURE: PR interval_____ Rhythm_____

QRS complex _____ Heart rate _____

INTERPRETATION: _____

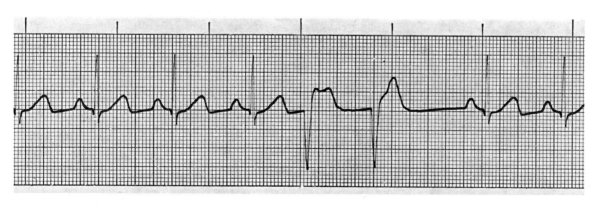

12. MEASURE: PR interval_____ Rhythm_____

QRS complex _____ Heart rate _____

INTERPRETATION: _____

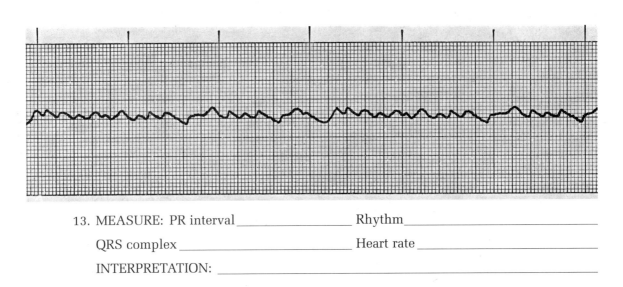

13. MEASURE: PR interval_____ Rhythm_____

        QRS complex_____ Heart rate_____

        INTERPRETATION: _____

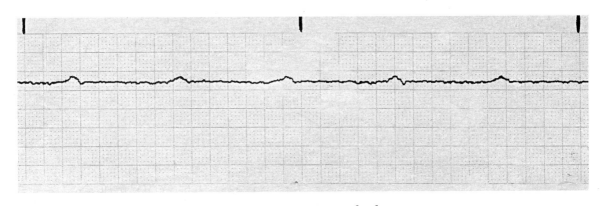

14. MEASURE: PR interval_____ Rhythm_____

        QRS complex_____ Heart rate_____

        INTERPRETATION: _____

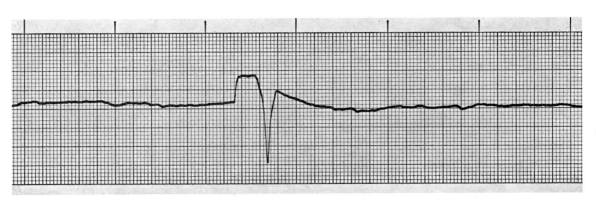

15. MEASURE: PR interval_____ Rhythm_____

        QRS complex_____ Heart rate_____

        INTERPRETATION: _____

"Funny Looking" Beats (FLBs)

Chapter Seven

Objectives On completion of this chapter, the reader should be able to:

1. Describe an escape beat and an escape rhythm, including measurements of all components.
2. Describe an aberrantly conducted complex.
3. Explain pulseless electrical activity.
4. Explain the difference between permanent and temporary pacemakers and the indications for the use of each type.
5. Explain the differences between atrial, ventricular, and sequential pacemakers.
6. Define capture and pacing and give examples of 50% pacing and 75% capture.
7. Describe an automatic implantable cardioverter defibrillator and its use.

Outline "Funny Looking" Beats

A. "Funny Looking" Beats
1. Escape Beats
2. Aberrantly Conducted Complexes
3. Pulseless Electrical Activity

B. Pacemaker Rhythms
1. Temporary Pacemakers
2. Permanent Pacemakers
   a. Atrial pacemakers
   b. Ventricular pacemakers
   c. Sequential pacemakers
3. Capture and Pacing

C. Automatic Implantable Cardioverter Defibrillator

D. Chapter Review Questions

E. Rhythm Strip Review

"FUNNY LOOKING" BEATS

Some complexes and wave formations do not fall into any of the specific patterns discussed in the previous chapters. In many parts of the United States, the slang expression for these complexes is *"funny looking beats"* or *FLB*.

Escape Beats

When the cardiac electrical conduction system is interrupted for a brief period of time (sinus arrest) or when the heart rate is bradycardic, an impulse may "escape" from a site other than the sinoatrial (SA) node and cause depolarization of the myocardium (Fig. 7-1).

Escape beats are one way the heart tries to maintain a normal rate or rhythm. For example, if the inherent heart rate of the SA node falls below 60, an electrical impulse may be initiated from outside the SA node. This escape beat is the heart's attempt to maintain normal cardiac output by increasing the heart rate. Usually the escape beat will occur later than the next expected complex of the underlying rhythm. The complex that ends a sinus arrest or sinus exit block is an example of an escape beat.

An escape beat may originate from the atria, the atrioventricular (AV) junction, or the ventricles and is named by the approximate point of origin. The rate of a rhythm containing an escape beat will vary, depending on the underlying rhythm.

Atrial escape beats can originate from anywhere in the atria and usually meet the same criteria as other atrial complexes: an upright P wave before the QRS complex, a PR interval of 0.12 to 0.20 second, and a QRS complex of less than 0.12 second. An atrial complex that ends a sinus arrest or sinus exit block is usually the only atrial complex referred to as an "escape beat" (Fig. 7-2A).

If the SA node and atria fail to generate an electrical impulse or if the impulse is not conducted, the AV junctional area can initiate an impulse that "escapes" to increase the heart rate. This impulse is a *junctional escape beat* and will have the same characteristics as all junctional complexes. The P wave is

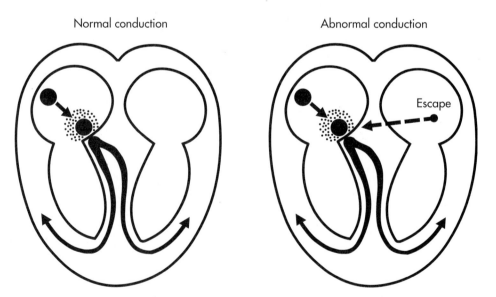

Normal conduction   Abnormal conduction

Escape

Fig. 7-1 Left heart shows normal electrical conduction pathway. Right heart shows conduction pathway of atrial escape beats.

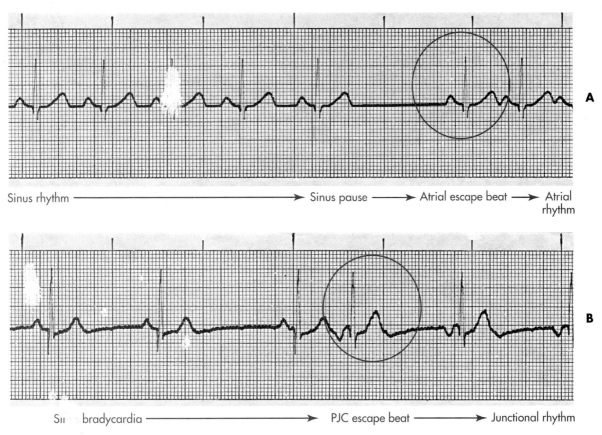

Sinus rhythm ⟶ Sinus pause ⟶ Atrial escape beat ⟶ Atrial rhythm

Si___ bradycardia ⟶ PJC escape beat ⟶ Junctional rhythm

Fig. 7-2 Escape beats and escape rhythms. **(A)** Sinus rhythm with sinus exit block ended by an atrial escape beat. **(B)** Sinus bradycardia with PJC escape beat beginning a junctional rhythm.

either inverted, hidden, or retrograde, and the QRS complex is usually less than 0.12 second (Fig. 7-2B).

If the SA node, the atria, and the AV junction fail to generate an electrical impulse and the heart rate falls below the junctional inherent rate of 40, a *ventricular escape beat* may be initiated from anywhere in the ventricles. As with all other ventricular complexes, the QRS complex of a ventricular escape beat is greater than 0.12 second and a P wave is usually not seen.

An escape beat can either remain a single complex or progress to an escape rhythm, if the myocardial pacemaker cells do not initiate enough electrical impulses to maintain an adequate cardiac output. Junctional tachycardia and idioventricular dysrhythmias are examples of escape rhythms.

Aberrantly Conducted Complexes

An *aberrantly conducted complex* is formed when one ventricle repolarizes at a slower rate than the other. One ventricle is then able to accept an electrical impulse causing depolarization earlier than the other ventricle.

Aberrantly conducted complexes are individual complexes that appear different than the complexes of the underlying rhythm because they do not follow the same electrical conduction pathway as the underlying rhythm (Fig. 7-3). Examples of aberrantly conducted complexes include:

1. an aberrantly conducted complex that has a negative QRS when the underlying rhythm has a positive QRS complex

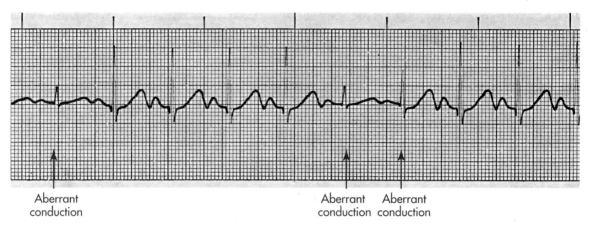

Aberrant
conduction

Aberrant   Aberrant
conduction conduction

Fig. 7-3 Aberrantly conducted complexes. Sinus rhythm with three aberrantly conducted complexes; heart rate, 90.

2. the QRS of the aberrantly conducted complex is wider or shorter than the complexes of the underlying rhythm

Aberrantly conducted complexes can originate from anywhere in the atria, the AV junction, or the ventricles. The origin of the aberrantly conducted complex will determine its size and shape. Because most aberrant complexes have a wide QRS, they may be hard to distinguish from a bundle branch block. However, aberrantly conducted complexes usually occur as individual complexes, not entire rhythms.

The presence of P waves, PR intervals, and QRS complexes in the underlying rhythm varies. The rate and regularity of the rhythm containing the aberrantly conducted complex also vary, depending on the underlying rhythm.

Pulseless Electrical Activity

Pulseless electrical activity (PEA) is the current term used to describe any dysrhythmia that shows the conduction of electrical impulses, without contraction of the myocardium. Electrical depolarization of cardiac cells appears to occur throughout the heart, but the patient **does not** have a pulse or blood pressure.

Almost any cardiac rhythm may be seen on the monitor screen or rhythm strip. The rhythm usually appears bradycardic and may have either wide or narrow QRS complexes (Fig. 7-4).

Since the patient does not have a pulse and cardiac output has ceased, this dysrhythmia is **lethal,** and treatment **must** be started immediately. Patient assessment is the **only** means of determining the presence or absence of a pulse. The patient, **not** the monitor, must be treated.

Electromechanical dissociation (EMD) is one type of PEA dysrhythmia. Other types of pulseless electrical activity include idioventricular rhythms, ventricular escape rhythms, and bradyasystolic (bradycardic rhythm without a pulse) rhythms. These dysrhythmias all show complexes on the monitor indicating electrical activity. However, because there is no mechanical cardiac activity, blood is not being circulated and the patient does not have a pulse.

PEA may be caused by hypovolemia (loss of blood volume), hypoxia (decrease in oxygen), cardiac tamponade (excess fluid or blood in pericardial sac), or tension pneumothorax (air in the pleural cavity that prevents one lung from expanding). PEA may also occur when the cardiac muscle is too damaged to contract, although electrical impulses are being conducted by the electrical conduction pathways.

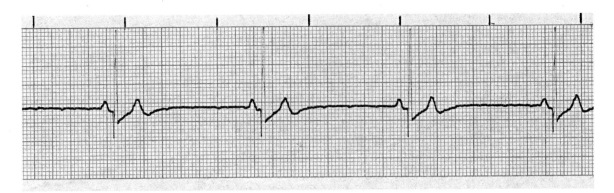

Fig. 7-4 Pulseless electrical activity. Rhythm strip shows sinus bradycardia (heart rate, 40) but the patient does not have a pulse.

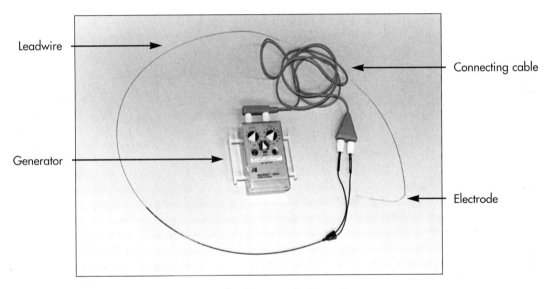

Fig. 7-5 External pacemaker generator, leadwire, and electrode.

PACEMAKER RHYTHMS

Many dysrhythmias have bradycardic rates that are too slow to maintain a normal cardiac output. Other dysrhythmias may be too rapid to allow complete filling of the ventricles before each contraction, resulting in poor cardiac output and decreased circulation to the vital organs of the body. These are **lethal** dysrhythmias. Although many patients with these dysrhythmias respond to drug therapy, others will require assistance from an artificial pacemaker.

These pacemakers are small, battery-operated devices that initiate electrical impulses in the myocardium. The two main parts of a pacemaker are the generator and the leadwires (Fig. 7-5). The *generator* is a small box that initiates and controls the rate and strength of each electrical impulse. The *leadwire* has an electrode at its tip that transmits the electrical impulse from the generator to the myocardium.

Temporary Pacemakers

Pacemakers may be either temporary or permanent. *Temporary pacemakers* are used to maintain a patient's heart rate in an emergency situation or until a permanent pacemaker can be surgically implanted.

There are two types of temporary pacemakers. Although the generator remains outside the patient's body with both types of pacemakers, the electrical

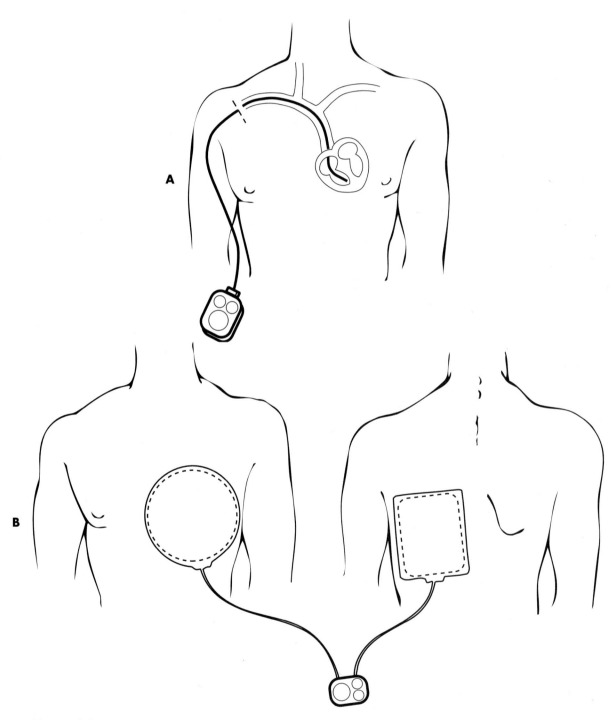

Fig. 7-6 (A) Temporary transvenous pacemaker placement. **(B)** Temporary transcutaneous (transdermal) pacemaker placement.

impulse used to stimulate the cardiac muscle is delivered by two different means.

A method for delivery of the electrical impulse that has been used for many years is *transvenous* (through a vein). The leadwire is inserted through the skin and threaded through a large vein into the right side of the heart. The electrical impulses stimulate the atrium and then are conducted through the cardiac electrical conduction system, causing depolarization (Fig. 7-6A).

A more recent method is *transdermal* or *transcutaneous* (through the skin). This method uses two large pads as electrodes to conduct the electrical impulses. There are two leadwires, each connected to a pad. One pad is placed on the front of the patient's chest and the other pad on the patient's back (Fig. 7-6B). The electrical impulses are then conducted through the body and heart, stimulating the entire cardiac muscle and causing depolarization of the cardiac cells to occur in a normal manner. Transdermal (transcutaneous) pacing has a great advantage. It is quickly and easily positioned and does not require piercing the patient's skin to position the electrodes.

All pacemakers can be preset to initiate electrical impulses in one of two ways:

1. Fixed—set to generate impulses at a constant rate, usually 72 to 80 impulses per minute.
2. Demand—set to generate electrical impulses only when the patient's heart rate falls below a predetermined rate, usually less than 70 beats per minute.

NOTE: The terms *fire* and *pace* are often used in a clinical setting to mean the initiation of an electrical impulse from an artificial pacemaker.

Permanent Pacemakers

A *permanent pacemaker* is necessary when the patient is unable to maintain a normal heart rate or a normal cardiac output, even with the aid of medications.

The generator of a permanent pacemaker is surgically implanted under the patient's skin, usually in the upper left chest or upper abdominal area. The leadwire is then inserted into the heart through a large vein (Fig. 7-7).

There are three main types of permanent pacemakers: atrial, ventricular, and sequential.

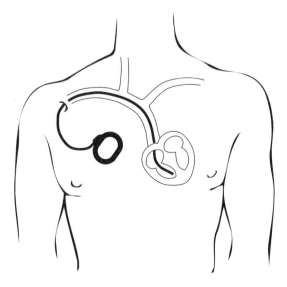

Fig. 7-7 Permanent pacemaker placement.

Normal conduction   Abnormal conduction

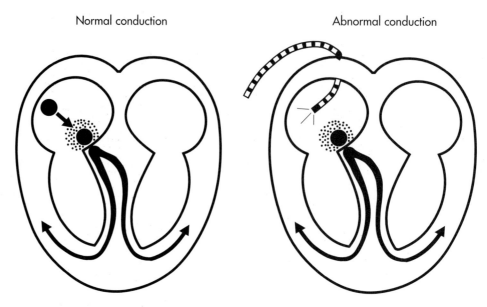

Fig. 7-8 Left heart shows normal electrical conduction pathway. Right heart shows conduction pathway of atrial pacemaker.

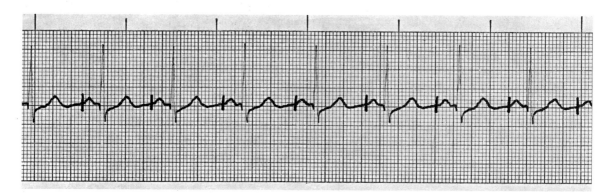

Fig. 7-9 Atrial pacemaker rhythm showing pacer spikes.

Atrial Pacemakers

The leadwire and electrode of an *atrial pacemaker* are inserted into the right atrium. The electrical impulse that is generated by the pacemaker stimulates the atria, then follows the normal electrical conduction pathway through the heart to the ventricles (Fig. 7-8).

The discharge of electrical energy from the pacemaker is represented on the rhythm strip by a vertical line, called a *pacer spike*, or *spike*. The pacer spike is usually followed by a P wave and a QRS complex, although the P wave may not be seen unless the electrode is positioned high in the right atrium (Fig. 7-9). The P wave that follows a pacer spike is usually not measured.

An atrial pacemaker can only be used if the AV junction and ventricular conduction pathways are functioning. Atrial pacemakers are rarely used today because they are less efficient than ventricular or sequential pacemakers.

Normal conduction

Abnormal conduction

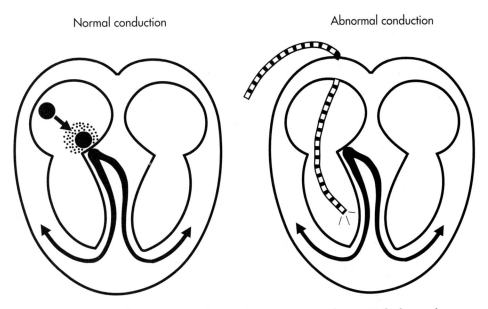

Fig. 7-10 Left heart shows normal electrical conduction pathway. Right heart shows conduction pathway of ventricular pacemaker.

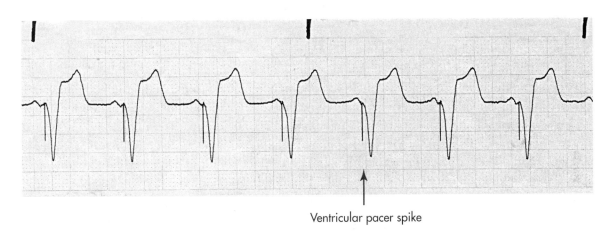

Ventricular pacer spike

Fig. 7-11 Ventricular pacemaker rhythm with pacer spikes.

Ventricular Pacemakers

With *ventricular pacemakers*, the leadwire and electrode are placed in the right ventricle (Fig. 7-10). The pacemaker impulse causes the depolarization of the ventricular muscle. The atria may not depolarize if the atrial myocardium is extensively damaged.

A pacer spike, immediately followed by a QRS complex, will appear on the monitor or rhythm strip. Because the electrode is usually positioned low in the right ventricle, depolarization may not occur in a normal manner and the QRS is usually greater than 0.12 second (Fig. 7-11).

Sequential Pacemakers

One of the most commonly used type of pacemaker is the *sequential pacemaker.* While the other two types of pacemakers initiate depolarization of **either** the atria **or** the ventricles, the sequential pacemaker stimulates the depolarization of **both** the atria **and** the ventricles.

Normal conduction   Abnormal conduction

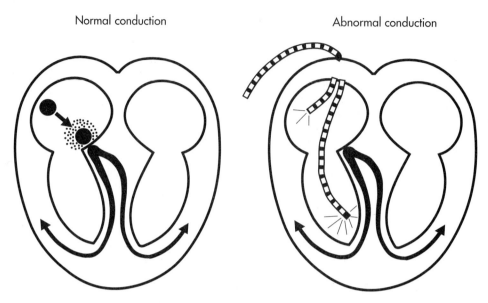

Fig. 7-12 Left heart shows normal electrical conduction pathway. Right heart shows conduction pathway of sequential pacemaker.

Ventricular pacer spike

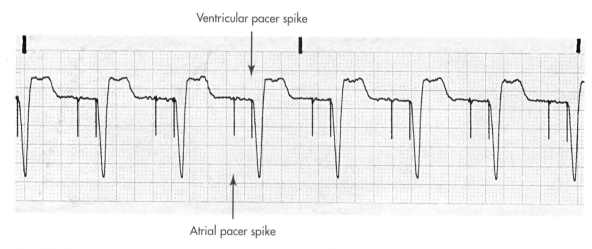

Atrial pacer spike

Fig. 7-13 Sequential pacemaker rhythm with two pacer spikes.

The leadwire has two electrodes, one positioned in the right atrium and one positioned in the right ventricle. The use of two electrodes allows the atria and the ventricles to depolarize in a normal sequential manner (Fig. 7-12).

The rhythm strip of a sequential pacemaker usually shows two pacer spikes before each QRS complex (Fig 7-13). The spikes may occur so closely together that they appear as one long spike. The first spike represents the firing of the atrial electrode, and the second spike represents the firing of the ventricular electrode. A P wave may be seen, and the QRS is typically greater than 0.12 second.

Capture and Pacing

When interpreting a pacemaker rhythm, the percentage of capture and the percentage of pacing must be determined.

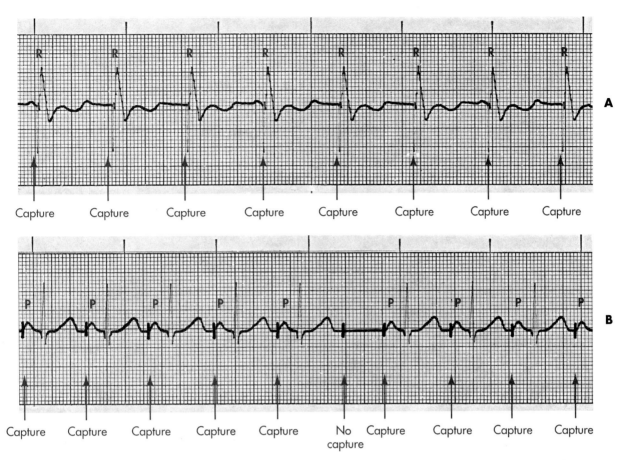

Fig. 7-14 Pacemaker capture. **(A)** Ventricular pacemaker with 100% capture **(B)** Loss of capture; atrial pacemaker with 90% capture.

Capture refers to the cardiac muscle's ability to conduct the electrical impulse generated by a mechanical pacemaker. This conduction is indicated by a P wave or QRS complex following **every** pacer spike. The presence of a complex following a pacer spike **does not** always indicate the **contraction** of the myocardium, only the **conduction** of an electrical impulse through the cardiac muscle. The patient **must** be assessed to determine the presence of a pulse.

The *percentage of capture* is determined by the number of pacer spikes that are followed by a complex in relationship to the total number of pacer spikes on the entire rhythm strip. For example, the rhythm strip will show 100% capture if every pacer spike is followed by a P wave or QRS complex (Fig. 7-14A). If only nine out of 10 pacer spikes are followed by a complex, the rhythm strip will show 90% capture.

Loss of capture occurs when a QRS complex does not follow a pacer spike (Fig. 7-14B). Loss of capture indicates that the electrical impulse generated by the artificial pacemaker has not been conducted and the cardiac cells have not depolarized. This situation may simply indicate that the voltage of the pacemaker electrical impulse needs to be increased. However, loss of capture may indicate that the myocardium is so damaged, it is unable to respond to every electrical impulse.

Pacing refers to the percentage of complexes generated by the mechanical pacemaker. For example, if every QRS complex is preceded by a pacer spike,

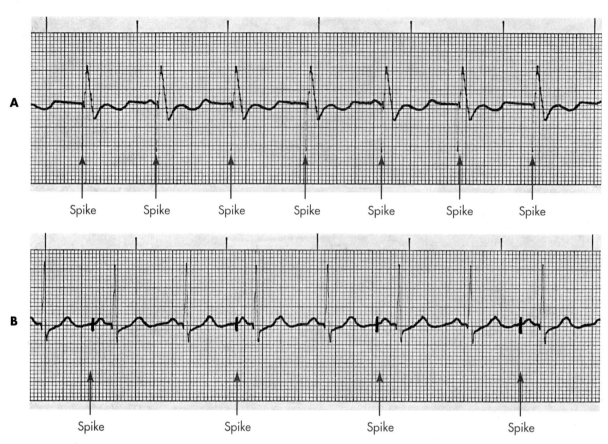

Fig. 7-15 Pacemaker pacing. **(A)** Ventricular pacemaker with 100% pacing **(B)** Atrial pacemaker with 50% pacing.

the rhythm is 100% paced (Fig. 7-15A). If a pacer spike occurs before only half of the QRS complexes, the strip is 50% paced (Fig. 7-15B). Complexes that do not have a pacer spike are generated by the patient's heart, not the mechanical pacemaker. These complexes may appear normal or bizarre depending on whether they follow the normal cardiac electrical conduction pathway.

The *percentage of pacing* depends on the pacemaking ability of the patient's own heart as well as the type of pacemaker in use (demand or fixed-rate pacemaker).

The percentage of capture should **always** be 100%, regardless of the percent of pacing. For example, every pacer spike should be **followed** by a QRS complex. However, every QRS complex does **not** have to be **preceded** by a pacer spike. Complexes that appear without a pacer spike indicate that the patient's heart, not the pacemaker, has initiated the electrical impulse.

AUTOMATIC IMPLANTABLE CARDIOVERTER DEFIBRILLATOR

Automatic implantable cardioverter defibrillators (AICDs) are one of the newest types of pacemaker/defibrillators on the market. They can identify and treat some rapid lethal dysrhythmias, such as ventricular tachycardia.

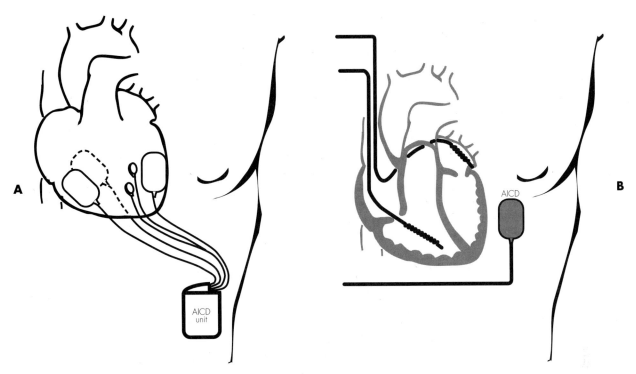

Fig. 7-16 AICD units **(A)** Electrode pads sewn on to heart muscle **(B)** Electrodes inserted into ventricles.

The AICD unit is surgically implanted under the skin (similar to a pacemaker), and pads containing electrodes are sewn to the front and back of the heart muscle (Fig. 7-16A), with electrodes or sensing units inserted into the ventricles (Fig. 7-16B). The newest AICD offers the option of electrodes that can be inserted into the heart chambers through transvenous placement, instead of pads requiring major surgery.

The AICD can be programmed to initiate low-voltage electrical impulses when the heart rate becomes very fast (more than 160). The impulse from the AICD attempts to force the heart into a normal rate. If the first electrical impulse from the AICD is not strong enough, the AICD may be programmed to increase the voltage and initiate an additional one to two impulses, raising the voltage slightly each time. The patient usually does not feel these impulses.

If the patient's heart rate continues to increase, or if the rhythm becomes ventricular fibrillation or ventricular tachycardia, the AICD will deliver an electrical impulse that is strong enough to defibrillate (*see* glossary) the heart. This defibrillation is an attempt to allow the SA node to again initiate electrical impulses at a normal rate.

The AICD will defibrillate the patient until the heart has recovered its normal rate or until the AICD is turned off by medical personnel.

The patient may complain of a feeling of getting "kicked" in the chest while defibrillation is occurring. Anyone touching the patient while the AICD is defibrillating may also feel a mild, tingling sensation. The patient may "jump" or "jerk" slightly as an effect of the defibrillation.

On the monitor or rhythm strip, the firing of the AICD appears similar to a pacing spike, but it may have a greater amplitude.

Some of the newer models of AICDs can temporarily pace bradycardic dysrhythmias that may occur after defibrillation.

Review Questions

1. True or false? Sequential pacemakers are used to stimulate either the atria or the the ventricles.

2. True or false? Escape beats are usually named for the approximate point of origin.

3. True or false? PEA can be identified on a 12-Lead electrocardiogram.

4. List the two ways that pacemakers can be preset to initiate impulses.

   a. _____

   b. _____

5. Explain the following terms:

   a. Pacer spike _____ _____

   b. Capture _____

6. The three types of permanent pacemakers are atrial, ventricular, and _____

   _____.

7. If every pacer spike is followed by a QRS complex, the percent of capture is _____ %.

8. The QRS complex of an escape beat usually measures _____ second.

9. List two types of temporary pacemakers:

   a. _____

   b. _____

10. Describe PEA. _____

    _____

Rhythm Strip Review

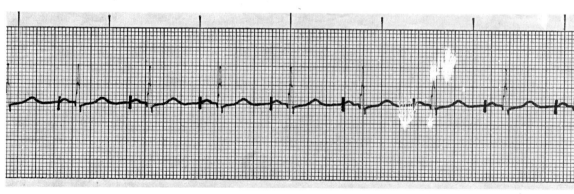

1. MEASURE: PR interval_____ Rhythm_____ _____

   QRS complex_____ _____ Heart rate_____ _____

   INTERPRETATION: _____

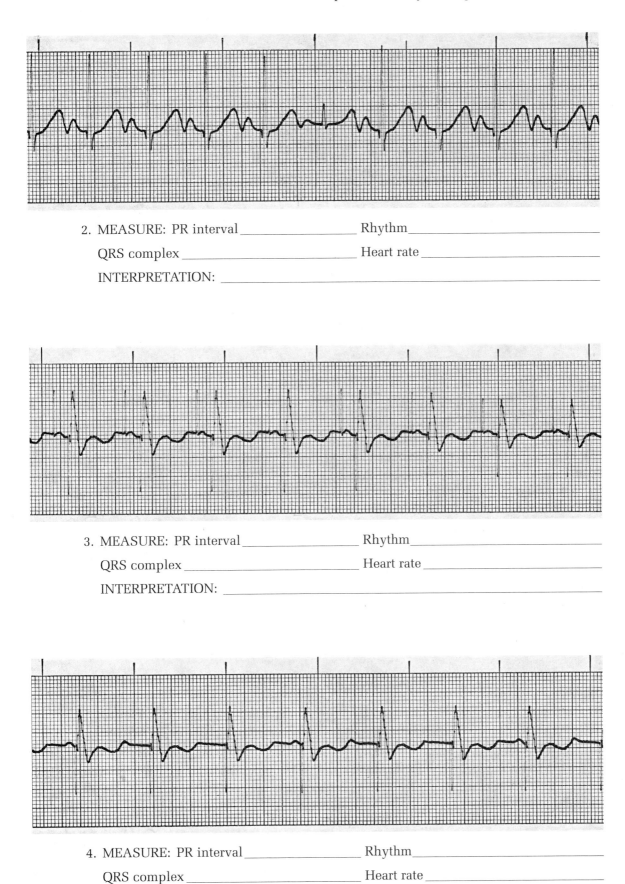

2. MEASURE: PR interval _____ Rhythm _____

   QRS complex _____ Heart rate _____

   INTERPRETATION: _____

3. MEASURE: PR interval _____ Rhythm _____

   QRS complex _____ Heart rate _____

   INTERPRETATION: _____

4. MEASURE: PR interval _____ Rhythm _____

   QRS complex _____ Heart rate _____

   INTERPRETATION: _____

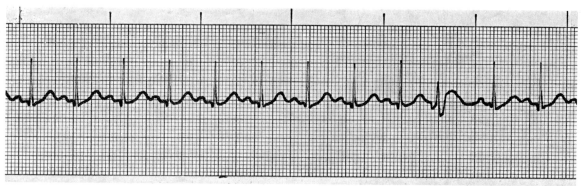

5. MEASURE: PR interval_____ Rhythm_____

QRS complex _____ Heart rate _____

INTERPRETATION: _____

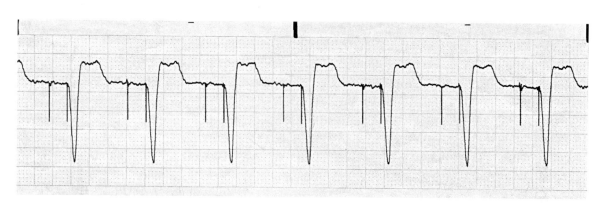

6. MEASURE: PR interval_____ Rhythm_____

QRS complex _____ Heart rate _____

INTERPRETATION: _____

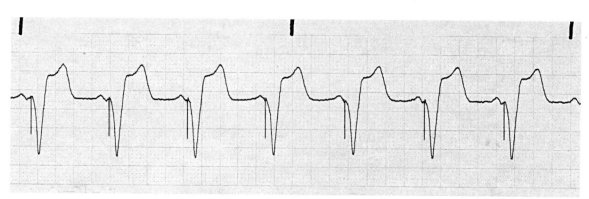

7. MEASURE: PR interval_____ Rhythm_____

QRS complex _____ Heart rate _____

INTERPRETATION: _____

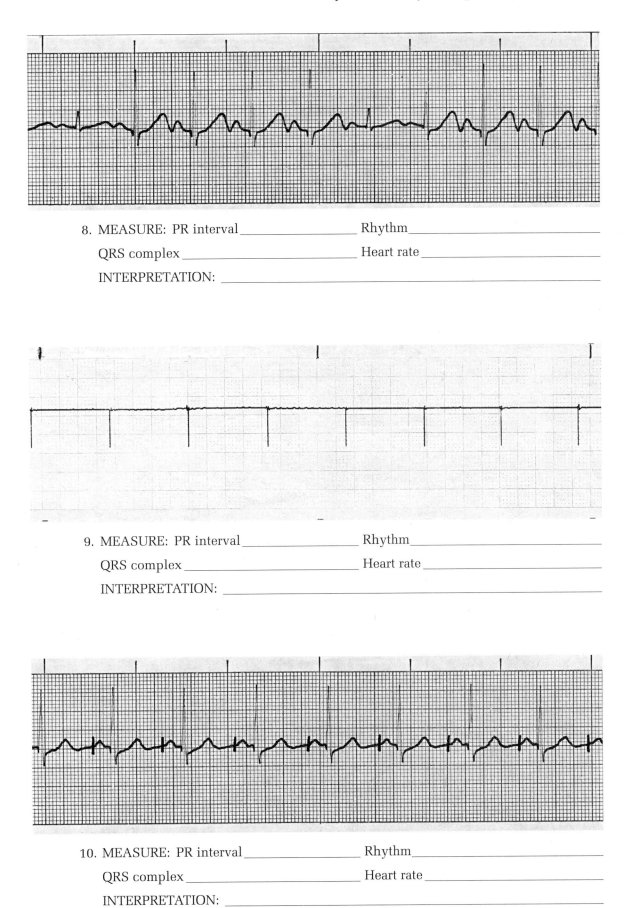

8. MEASURE: PR interval_____ Rhythm_____

    QRS complex _____ Heart rate _____

    INTERPRETATION: _____

9. MEASURE: PR interval_____ Rhythm_____

    QRS complex _____ Heart rate _____

    INTERPRETATION: _____

10. MEASURE: PR interval_____ Rhythm_____

    QRS complex _____ Heart rate _____

    INTERPRETATION: _____

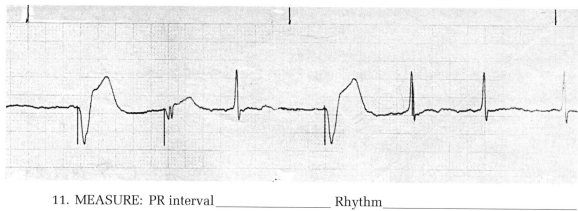
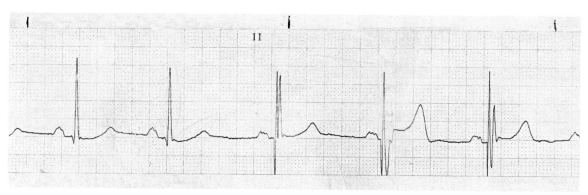

11. MEASURE: PR interval_____ Rhythm_____

    QRS complex_____ Heart rate _____

    INTERPRETATION: _____

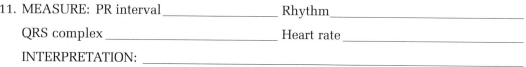
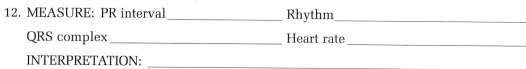

12. MEASURE: PR interval_____ Rhythm_____

    QRS complex_____ Heart rate _____

    INTERPRETATION: _____

Dysrhythmia Review

Chapter Eight

This chapter is designed as a review of all the dysrhythmias discussed in Chapters 3 to 7. Each dysrhythmia is presented with a rhythm strip followed by the criteria for that dysrhythmia.

SINUS DYSRHYTHMIAS

Normal Sinus Rhythm

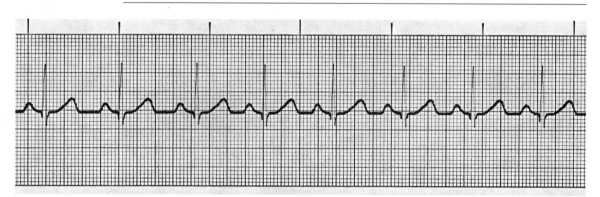

1. Site of origin: SA node
2. P wave: before every QRS; same size and shape
3. PR interval: 0.12 to 0.20 second
4. QRS: same size and shape; less than 0.12 second
5. Rhythm: a) P to P interval regular; b) R to R interval regular
6. Rate: 60 to 100

Sinus Bradycardia

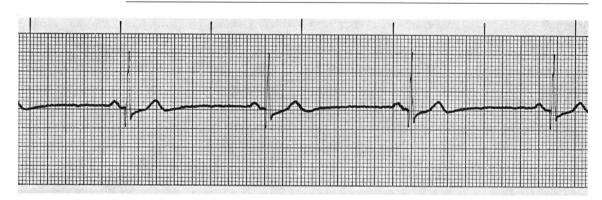

1. Site of origin: SA node
2. P wave: before every QRS; same size and shape
3. PR interval: 0.12 to 0.20 second
4. QRS: same size and shape; less than 0.12 second
5. Rhythm: a) P to P interval regular; b) R to R interval regular
6. Rate: less than 60

Sinus Tachycardia

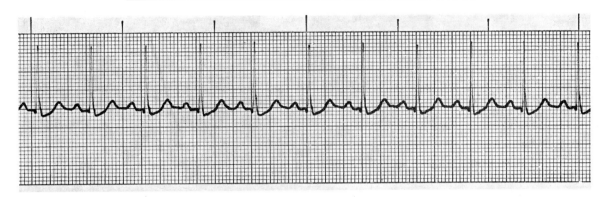

1. Site of origin: SA node
2. P wave: before every QRS; same size and shape
3. PR interval: 0.12 to 0.20 second
4. QRS: same size and shape; less than 0.12 second
5. Rhythm: a) P to P interval regular; b) R to R interval regular
6. Rate: 101 to 150

Sinus Arrhythmia

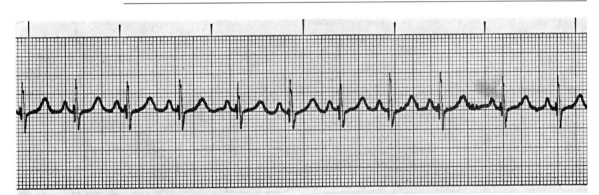

1. Site of origin: SA node
2. P wave: before every QRS; same size and shape
3. PR interval: varies slightly within normal limits of 0.12 to 0.20 second
4. QRS: same size and shape; less than 0.12 second
5. Rhythm: a) P to P interval irregular; b) R to R interval irregular
6. Rate: overall rate varies with respirations; a) increases as patient inhales; b) Decreases as patient exhales

Sinus Exit Block and Sinus Arrest

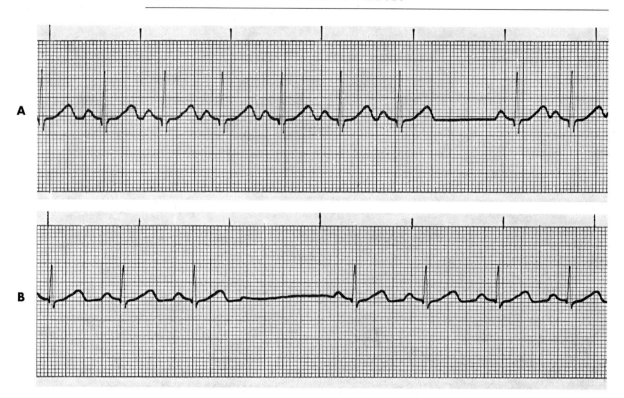

1. Site of origin: SA node fails to fire for at least two cardiac cycles
2. P wave: before every QRS; same size and shape
3. PR interval: varies slightly within normal limits of 0.12 to 0.20 second
4. QRS: same size and shape; less than 0.12 second
5. Rhythm: a) P to P interval regular, except during pause; b) R to R interval regular, except during pause
6. Rate: varies according to underlying rhythm
7. Pause: a) sinus exit block: the distance from the last normal beat to the next beat is equal to exactly two or more cardiac cycles, able to divide pause equally; b) sinus arrest: equal to less than or more than two cardiac cycles; not able to divide pause equally

ATRIAL DYSRHYTHMIAS

Premature Atrial Contraction

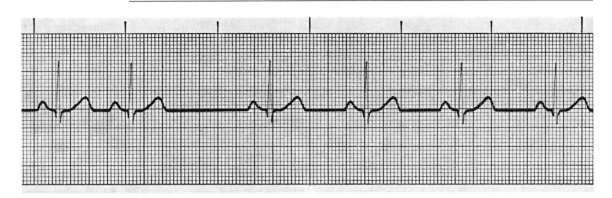

1. Site of origin: atria
2. P wave: before every QRS; may be buried in preceding T wave; may vary in size and shape
3. PR interval: varies within normal limits of 0.12 to 0.20 second
4. QRS: same size and shape; less than 0.12 second
5. Rhythm: a) P to P interval varies according to the underlying rhythm and the number of PACs; b) R to R interval varies according to the underlying rhythm and the number of PACs
6. Rate: varies according to the underlying rhythm, including the number of PACs
7. Occurs: premature; usually followed by a noncompensatory pause

Paroxysmal Atrial Tachycardia

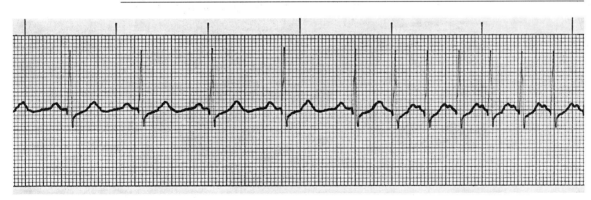

1. Site of origin: atria
2. P wave: before every QRS; may be buried in preceding T wave; same size and shape
3. PR interval: 0.12 to 0.20 second
4. QRS: same size and shape; less than 0.12 second
5. Rhythm: a) P to P interval regular; b) R to R interval regular
6. Rate: 151 to 250
7. Onset: starts suddenly; onset must be observed

Supraventricular Tachycardia

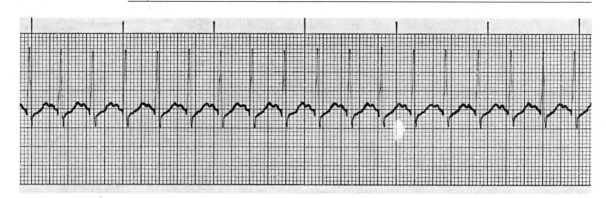

1. Site of origin: above the bundle of His
2. P wave:
   a) Atrial: before every QRS or buried in preceding T wave; same size and shape
   b) Junction: inverted, hidden, or retrograde; same size and shape
3. PR interval: normal to not measurable
4. QRS: same size and shape; less than 0.12 second
5. Rhythm: a) P to P interval regular, if present; b) R to R interval regular
6. Rate: 151 to 250
7. Onset: starts suddenly; onset is not observed

Wandering Atrial Pacemaker

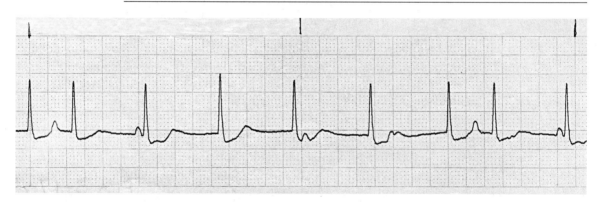

1. Site of origin: must be combination of three or more sites from above bundle of His
2. P wave: varies according to site of origin
3. PR interval: varies, if present
4. QRS: varies according to site of origin; may be greater than 0.12 second
5. Rhythm: a) P to P interval irregular; b) R to R interval irregular
6. Rate: varies

Atrial Flutter

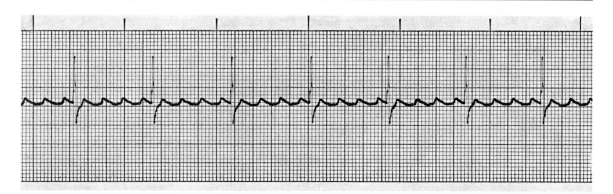

1. Site of origin: one atrial site
2. P wave: not present
3. Flutter waves: "saw-toothed" in shape; size may vary
4. PR interval: cannot be measured
5. QRS: same size and shape; less than 0.12 second
6. Rhythm: a) P to P interval not present; b) F to F interval regular; c) R to R interval regular, except in varying block
7. Rate: a) atrial: 250 to 350; b) ventricular: usually 60 to 100 but may vary
8. Ratio of block: a) 2 F waves to 1 QRS = 2:1 block; b) 3 F waves to 1 QRS = 3:1 block; c) 4 F waves with 1 QRS = 4:1 block; d) varying number of F waves to 1 QRS = varying block

Atrial Fibrillation

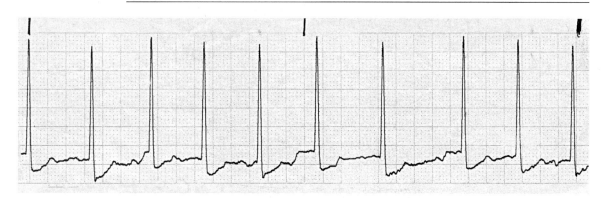

1. Site of origin: atria
2. P wave: no distinctive P wave
3. PR interval: cannot be measured
4. QRS: same size and shape; less than 0.12 second
5. Rhythm: a) P to P interval cannot be measured; b) R to R interval irregular
6. Rate:
   a) Atrial: 350 to 500 or more
   b) Ventricular:
      (1) Less than 60; slow ventricular response
      (2) 60 to 100; controlled A Fib
      (3) 101 to 150; rapid ventricular response
      (4) Greater than 150; uncontrolled A Fib

JUNCTIONAL DYSRHYTHMIAS

Junctional Rhythm

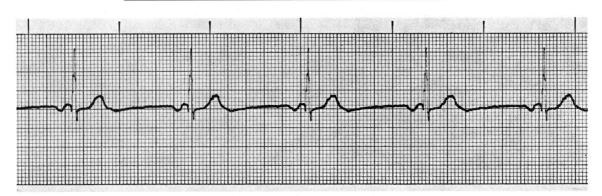

1. Site of origin: AV junction
2. P wave: inverted, buried, or retrograde; same size and shape, if present
3. PR interval: usually less than 0.12 second, if upright P wave is present
4. QRS: same size and shape; less than 0.12 second
5. Rhythm: a) P to P interval regular if present; b) R to R interval regular
6. Rate: 40 to 60

Junctional Bradycardia

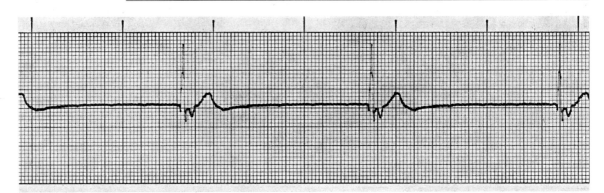

1. Site of origin: AV junction
2. P wave: inverted, buried, or retrograde; same size and shape, if present
3. PR interval: usually less than 0.12 second if upright P wave is present
4. QRS: same size and shape, less than 0.12 second
5. Rhythm: a) P to P interval regular, if present; b) R to R interval regular
6. Rate: less than 40

Accelerated Junctional Rhythm and Junctional Tachycardia

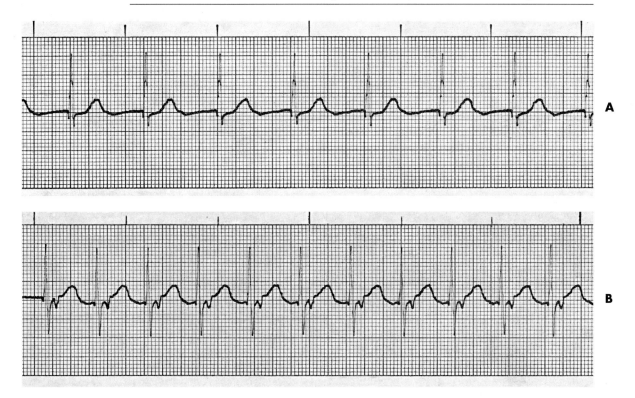

1. Site of origin: AV junction
2. P wave: inverted, buried, or retrograde; same size and shape, if present
3. PR interval: usually less than 0.12 second, if upright P wave is present
4. QRS: same size and shape, less than 0.12 second
5. Rhythm: a) P to P interval regular, if present; b) R to R interval regular
6. Rate: a) accelerated junctional rhythm 61 to 100; b) junctional tachycardia 101 to 150

Premature Junctional Contraction

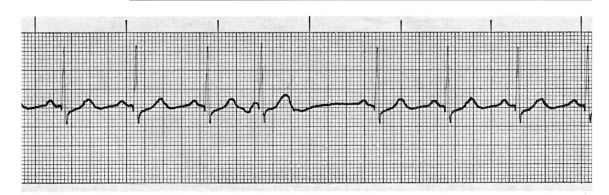

1. Site of origin: AV junction
2. P wave: inverted, buried, or retrograde
3. PR interval: usually less than 0.12 second, if upright P wave is present
4. QRS: less than 0.12 second
5. Rhythm: a) P to P interval varies according to the underlying rhythm; b) R to R interval varies according to the underlying rhythm and number of PJCs
6. Rate: varies according to underlying rhythm
7. Occurs: prematurely; usually followed by a compensatory pause

Wandering Junctional Pacemaker

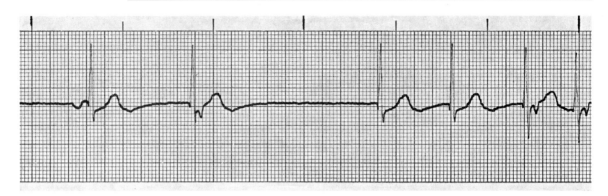

1. Site of origin: at least three junctional sites
2. P wave: inverted, buried, or retrograde; varies in size and shape, if present
3. PR interval: usually less than 0.12 second, if present
4. QRS: less than 0.12 second; size and shape may vary
5. Rhythm: a) P to P interval irregular, if present; b) R to R interval irregular
6. Rate: varies, usually 40 to 60

HEART BLOCKS

First-Degree Heart Block

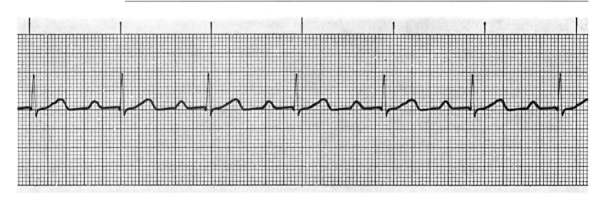

1. Site of origin: atria
2. Site of delay: between atria and bundle of His
3. P wave: before every QRS; same size and shape
4. PR interval: greater than 0.20 second
5. QRS: same size and shape; usually less than 0.12 second
6. Rhythm: a) P to P interval varies according to underlying rhythm; b) R to R interval varies according to underlying rhythm
7. Rate: varies according to underlying rhythm

Mobitz I (Wenkebach, Second-Degree Heart Block, Type I)

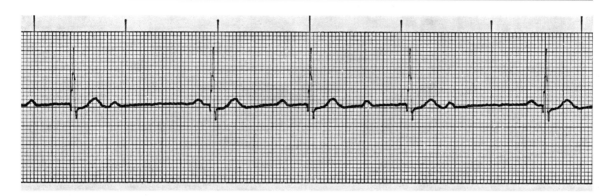

1. Site of origin: atria
2. Site of block: AV junction; progressive
3. P wave: at least one for every QRS; same size and shape
4. PR interval: becomes progressively longer, until QRS is dropped
5. QRS: same size and shape; less than 0.12 second
6. Rhythm: a) P to P interval regular; b) R to R interval irregular
7. Rate: varies

Mobitz II (Second-Degree Heart Block, Type II)

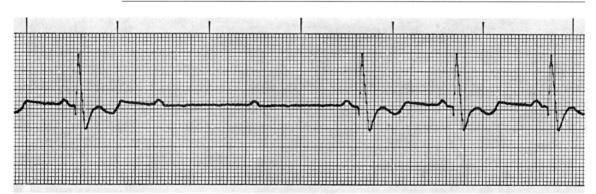

1. Site of origin: atria
2. Site of block: AV junction; intermittent block
3. P wave: at least one for every QRS; same size and shape
4. PR interval: usually 0.12 to 0.20 second and equal throughout
5. QRS: same size and shape; less than 0.12 second
6. Rhythm: a) P to P interval varies according to underlying rhythm; b) R to R interval irregular
7. Rate: varies according to underlying rhythm
8. Ratio of block:
    a) 2 P waves to 1 QRS = 2:1 block
    b) 3 P waves to 1 QRS = 3:1 block
    c) 4 P waves to 1 QRS = 4:1 block
    d) Varying number of P waves to 1 QRS = varying block

Third-Degree Heart Block

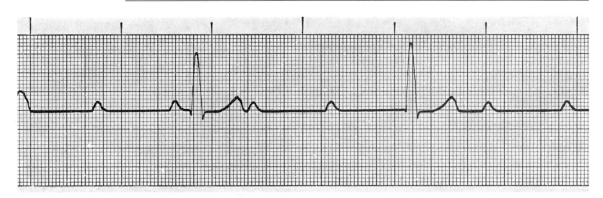

1. Site of origin: atria and ventricles
2. Site of block: between atria and ventricles
3. P wave: no relationship to QRS; same size and shape
4. PR interval: appears to vary; no true PR interval
5. QRS: same size and shape; usually wide, bizarre, and greater than 0.12 second
6. Rhythm: a) P to P interval: regular; b) R to R interval: regular
7. Rate: a) atrial: usually 60 to 100; b) ventricular: usually 20 to 40

Bundle Branch Block

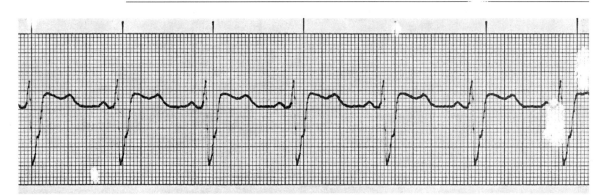

1. Site of origin: usually atria
2. Site of block: bundle branch (right, left, or both)
3. P wave: varies according to underlying rhythm
4. PR interval: varies according to underlying rhythm
5. QRS: usually same size and shape; notched appearance; usually greater than 0.12 second
6. Rhythm: a) P to P interval: varies according to the underlying rhythm
   b) R to R interval: varies according to the underlying rhythm
7. Rate: varies according to the underlying rhythm

VENTRICULAR DYSRHYTHMIAS

Premature Ventricular Contraction

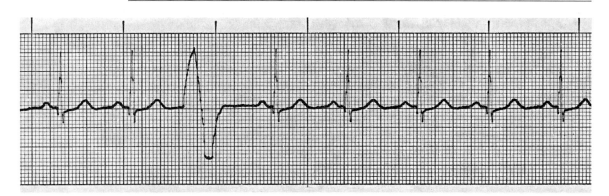

1. Site of origin: ventricles
2. P waves: not present, or hidden in PVC
3. PR interval: not measurable
4. QRS: may vary in size and shape; wide, bizarre, greater than 0.12 sec
5. Rhythm: a) P to P interval not measurable in PVC; b) R to R interval: varies according to the underlying rhythm and number of PVCs
6. Rate: varies according to the underlying rhythm; includes PVCs
7. Occurs: premature; followed by a compensatory pause
8. T wave: deflected in the opposite direction of the QRS
9. Classification
   a) **Unifocal PVC**

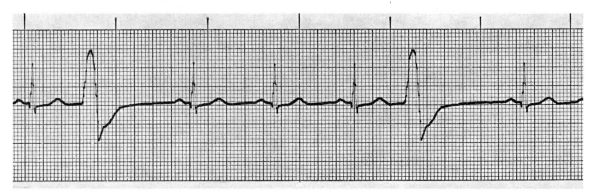

   (1) Site of origin: one ventricular site
   (2) QRS: same size and shape
   (3) Other characteristics: same as PVC

Premature Ventricular Contraction—cont'd

9. Classification—cont'd
   b) **Multifocal PVC**

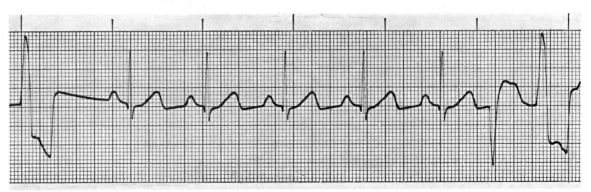

(1) Site of origin: two or more ventricular sites
(2) QRS: varies in size and shape
(3) Other characteristics: same as PVC

c) **Bigeminy**

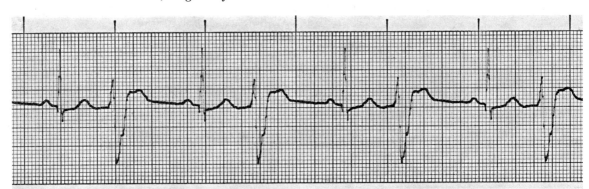

(1) Site of origin: one or more ventricular sites
(2) QRS: unifocal or multifocal
(3) Occurs: every other complex is a PVC
(4) Other characteristics: same as PVC

d) **Trigeminy**

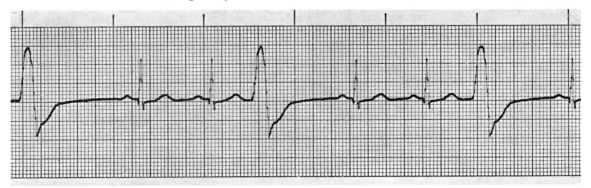

(1) Site of origin: one or more ventricular sites
(2) QRS: unifocal or multifocal
(3) Occurs: every third complex is a PVC
(4) Other characteristics: same as PVC

e) **Quadrigeminy**

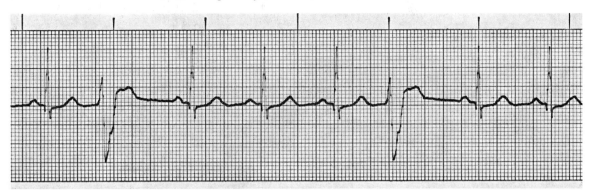

    (1) Site of origin: one or more ventricular sites
    (2) QRS: unifocal or multifocal
    (3) Occurs: every fourth complex is a PVC
    (4) Other characteristics: same as PVC

f) **Couplet**

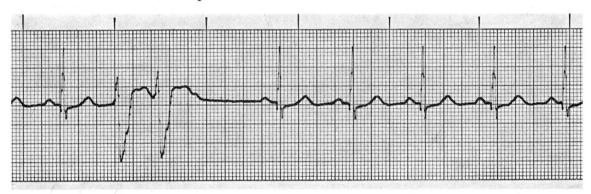

    (1) Site of origin: one or more ventricular sites
    (2) QRS: unifocal or multifocal
    (3) Occurs: two PVCs in a row
    (4) Other characteristics: same as PVC

g) **R on T phenomenon**

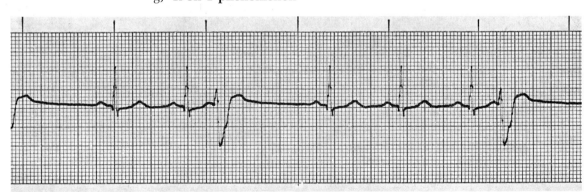

    (1) Site of origin: one or more ventricular sites
    (2) QRS: unifocal or multifocal
    (3) Occurs: R wave of PVC falls on the T wave of the preceding QRS
    (4) Other characteristics: same as PVC

Premature Ventricular Contraction—cont'd

9. Classification—cont'd
h) **Run of ventricular tachycardia**

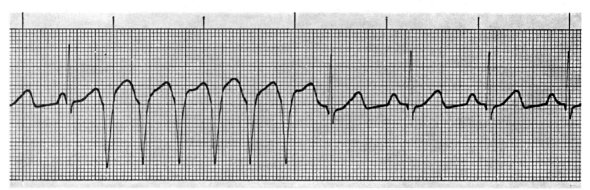

(1) Site of origin: one or more ventricular sites
(2) QRS: usually unifocal
(3) Occurs: three or more PVCs in a row
(4) Duration: less than 30 seconds
(5) Other characteristics: same as PVC

Ventricular Tachycardia

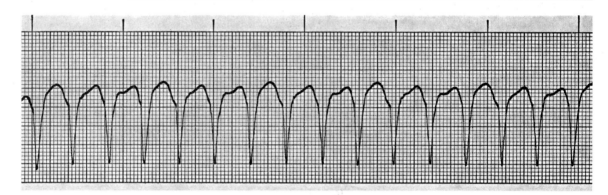

1. Site of origin: one or more ventricular sites
2. P wave: usually not present
3. PR interval: not measurable
4. QRS: usually same size and shape; wide, bizarre, greater than 0.12 second
5. Rhythm: a) P to P interval not measurable; b) R to R interval usually regular
6. Rate: 41 to 250, usually greater than 150
7. Occurs: three or more PVCs in a row; sudden onset
8. Duration: greater than 30 seconds

Torsades de Pointes

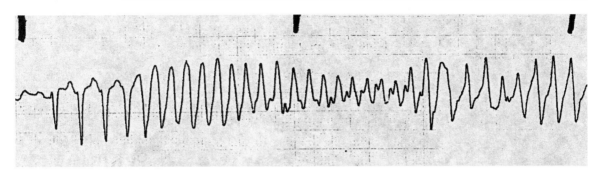

1. Site of origin: one or more ventricular sites
2. P wave: usually not present
3. PR interval: not measurable
4. QRS: usually same shape; varies in size, going from low to high and back to low amplitude
5. Rhythm: a) P to P interval: not measurable; b) R to R interval: usually regular
6. Rate: usually greater than 150
7. Occurs: sudden onset; frequently seen in a rhythm with prolonged QT intervals
8. Duration: varies

Ventricular Fibrillation

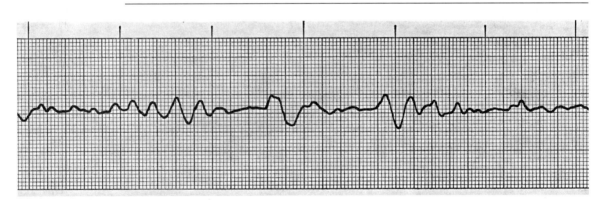

1. Site of origin: many ventricular sites
2. P wave: not present
3. PR interval: not measurable
4. QRS: not present; only chaotic, wavy line
5. Rhythm: a) P to P interval: not present; b) R to R interval: not present
6. Rate: not measurable
7. Wave amplitude: coarse or fine

Idioventricular and Agonal Dysrhythmias (dying heart)

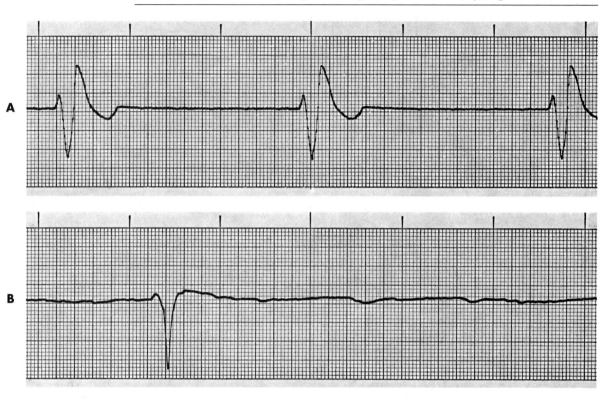

1. Site of origin: usually one ventricular site
2. P wave: not present
3. PR interval: not measurable
4. QRS: gradually *decreases* in amplitude and *increases* in width; wide, bizarre, greater than 0.12 second
5. Rhythm: a) P to P interval not present; b) R to R interval usually irregular
6. Rate: a) idioventricular: 20-40; b) agonal: less than 20; becoming slower until completely stopped

Ventricular Standstill

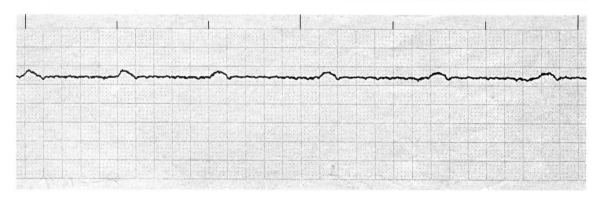

1. Site of origin: atria
2. P wave: seen without QRS; usually same size and shape
3. PR interval: not measurable
4. QRS: not present
5. Rhythm: a) P to P interval: usually regular; b) R to R interval not present
6. Rate: a) atrial: usually 60 to 100; b) ventricular: 0

Asystole

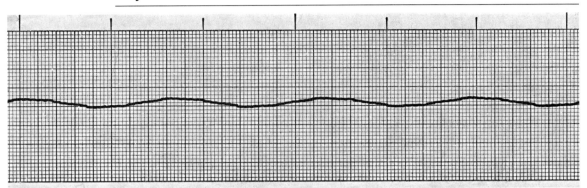

1. Site of origin: no electrical activity in heart muscle
2. P wave: not present
3. PR interval: not present
4. QRS: not present; only straight or slightly wavy line
5. Rhythm: a) P to P interval: not present; b) R to R interval: not present
6. Rate: 0

"FUNNY LOOKING" BEATS

Escape beats

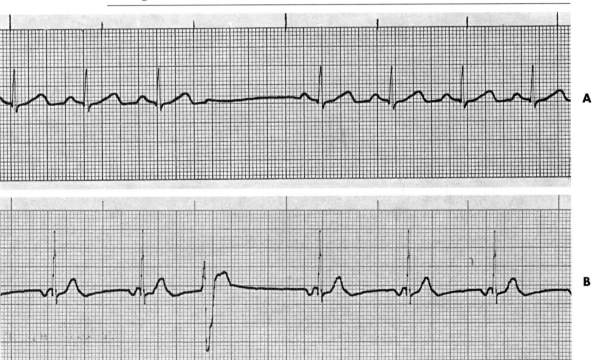

1. Site of origin: single atrial, junctional, or ventricular site; other than the SA node
2. P wave: varies according to site of origin
3. PR interval: varies according to site of origin
4. QRS: varies according to site of origin
5. Rhythm: a) P to P interval irregular, if present; b) R to R interval irregular
6. Rate: varies according to site of origin and underlying rhythm
7. Occurs: a) complex that ends the pause of a sinus exit block or sinus arrest; b) premature complexes that increase the rate of a bradycardic rhythm

Aberrantly Conducted Complex

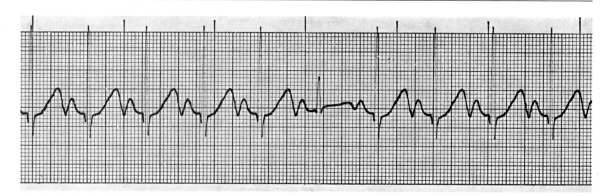

1. Site of origin: varies
2. P wave: varies according to site of origin
3. PR interval: varies according to site of origin
4. QRS: varies according to site of origin
5. Rhythm: a) P to P interval: varies according to underlying rhythm; b) R to R interval: varies according to underlying rhythm
6. Rate: varies according to underlying rhythm
7. Occurs: a) single complex that follows different electrical conduction pathway than the underlying rhythm; b) complex usually does not occur prematurely

Pulseless Electrical Activity

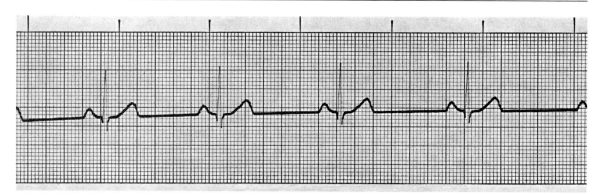

1. Site of origin: mimics **any rhythm**
2. P wave: mimics any rhythm
3. PR interval: mimics any rhythm
4. QRS: mimics any rhythm
5. Rhythm: a) P to P interval: mimics any rhythm; b) R to R interval mimics any rhythm
6. Rate: mimics any rhythm; patient **does not** have a pulse
7. Includes: electromechanical dissociation; idioventricular dysrhythmias, bradyasystole dysrhythmias

Pacemaker Rhythms

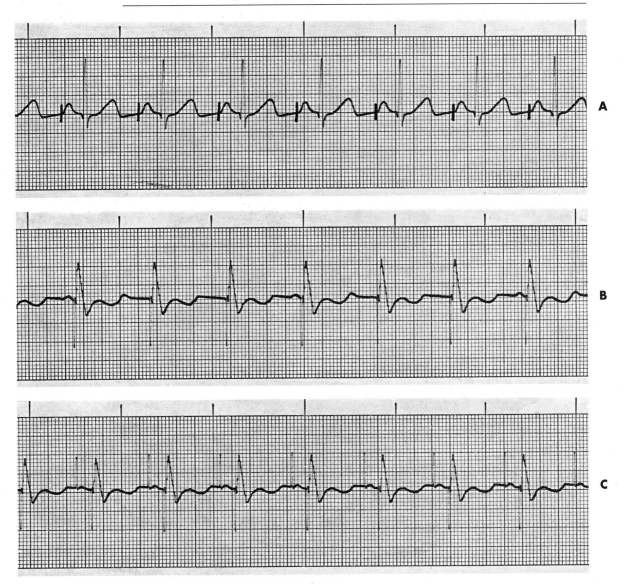

1. Site of origin:
   a) Atrial pacemaker: right atria
   b) Ventricular pacemaker: right ventricle
   c) Sequential pacemaker: right atria and right ventricle
2. P wave: may be replaced by pacer spike
3. PR interval: not measurable in paced rhythm
4. QRS: usually greater than 0.12 second; occurs after pacer spike
5. Rhythm:
   a) P to P interval: varies if present
   b) R to R interval:
      (1) Fixed rate pacemaker: regular
      (2) Demand pacemaker: varies
   c) Pacer spike to pacer spike
      (1) Fixed rate: regular
      (2) Demand rate: varies
6. Rate: varies according to pacemaker; fixed rate or demand rate
7. Pacing: varies

Pacemaker Rhythms—cont'd

8. Capture: 100 %
9. Types:
    a) Temporary
        (1) Transvenous
        (2) Transcutaneous
    b) Permanent

Chapter Nine

Medication Review and Adult Treatment Guidelines

This chapter is a brief and simplified summary of the most common drugs used to treat cardiac dysrhythmias in the adult patient. This chapter does **not** include all medications that might be used in the treatment of any dysrhythmia or cardiac disease. This review is not meant to take the place of a pharmacology course. Anyone administering medication should do so only after certification by his/her institution and as governed by the laws of his/her state.

The medication review and treatment guidelines are based on the American Heart Association's advanced cardiac life support (ACLS) protocols of 1994 and include the most recent updates including the *1996 Handbook of Emergency Cardiac Care for Healthcare Providers.*

The treatments outlined in this chapter are only general guidelines. They should be used in conjunction with, *not instead of,* your institution's policies and procedures. All treatments **MUST** be performed under the guidance of a physician.

For the purpose of treatment, it is assumed that all patients are being monitored in Lead II, all patients are adult, and no contraindications exist to any of the treatment protocols. Anyone wishing to learn pediatric treatment protocols is encouraged to attend a pediatric advanced life support (PALS) course offered by the American Heart Association.

As with any dysrhythmia, ongoing assessment of the patient's condition is essential. The patient's tolerance of the dysrhythmia and any subsequent symptoms will determine the appropriate treatment. Patients should be assessed **before** and **after** administering any medication and **before** and **after** each cardioversion attempt.

Patient assessment involves observing the patient's overall condition in addition to monitoring vital signs and interpreting the dysrhythmia on the monitor.

Patients who are symptomatic will show signs and symptoms of poor cardiac output. These signs and symptoms include cool, sweaty skin; hypotension (low blood pressure); pallor (pale, grayish skin); cyanosis (bluish tint to lips, nailbeds, skin); dyspnea (difficulty breathing); dizziness; nausea or vomiting; a decrease in urinary output; and a decrease in the level of consciousness (responsiveness).

Any one of these symptoms by itself may not indicate poor cardiac output. However, if these symptoms occur with either tachycardia or a bradycardia, it strongly suggests poor cardiac output and treatment should be started immediately.

The terms *poor cardiac output* and *medically unstable* are **both** used to describe a patient who is unable to tolerate a dysrhythmia.

MEDICATION REVIEW

Oxygen (O$_2$)

Action: Increases oxygen available to all tissue cells; helps to reduce shortness of breath; may help to decrease ischemia.

Indications: For all patients with respiratory distress, chest pains, dysrhythmias, decreased cardiac output, and in all cardiopulmonary arrests.

Dosage: 2 to 4 L/min (liters per minute) for alert patients with only mild distress, delivered by nasal cannula; 6 to 8 L/min by mask for patients with moderate respiratory distress; 10 to 15 L/min of 100% oxygen for patients with severe respiratory distress, delivered by a nonrebreather mask, by bag-valve mask, or endotracheal tube during CPR.

Oxygen (O_2), continued   Precautions: Flammable, do not use in presence of flames or sparks. Use with caution in alert patients with chronic lung disease. Should be used at 100% in all resuscitation attempts.

Intravenous Fluids   Actions: Replaces lost body fluids; provides intravenous (IV) access for administration of medications; used to dilute and deliver medications.

Indications: Hypovolemia; patients who require administration of IV medications to treat symptoms.

Dosage: 1000 cc of 0.9 normal saline (NS) or lactated ringers (LR) administered IV; Hypovolemia: Bolus (rapid infusion) of 300 cc/hr or greater; IV access only, usually 60 cc/hr or less. IV rate of infusion varies since the rate is titrated (adjusted) to the patient's needs.

Precautions: Must be used with caution in elderly patients or patients with chronic lung problems to prevent complications such as congestive heart failure. Must be used with caution in patients with brain injury. Monitor IV site to prevent infiltration (IV catheter slips out of vein and solution infuses into skin and muscle tissue).

Epinephrine Hydrochloride (Adrenalin®)   Action: Increases rate and force of cardiac contractions; increases coronary and cerebral blood flow; increases automaticity.

Indications: During CPR and cardiac resuscitation; during ventricular fibrillation; severe bradycardia.

Dosage: IV: 1:10,000 dilution; 1 mg (milligram); may be repeated at 3- to 5-minute intervals; Endotracheal tube: 2 to 2.5 mg diluted in 10cc NS; may be repeated at 3- to 5-minute intervals; continuous intravenous infusion: 1 mg epinephrine in 250 cc of 5% dextrose in water, starting at a rate of 2 mcg/min (microgram per minute) and titrated (adjusted) as needed. Intermediate dosage: 2-5 mg IV every 3 to 5 minutes; escalating dosage: 1 mg—3 mg—5mg IV, 3 minutes apart; high dosage: 0.1 mg/kg (milligram/kilogram) IV every 3 to 5 minutes.

Precautions: Do not mix with sodium bicarbonate; continuous infusion not used in cardiac arrests until the patient has a pulse; may increase ischemia due to increased rate and force of contractions (increasing work of myocardium will increase the need for oxygen); may cause or increase ventricular ectopy (abnormal rhythm).

Atropine Sulfate   Action: Increases heart rate; increases sinus node automaticity; improves AV conduction.

Indications: To correct symptomatic bradycardia; asystole; pulseless electrical activity; to increase heart rate to at least 60 beats/min in a bradycardic rhythm with PVCs.

Dosage: Symptomatic bradycardia: 0.5 to 1 mg IV, repeated at 5-minute intervals to a total of 0.04 mcg/kg (microgram per kilogram of body weight) for a total of 3 mg; asystole: 1 mg IV, repeated in 5 minutes for a total of 0.04 mcg/kg or 3 mg total; endotracheal administration: 2 to 3 mg diluted in 10 cc sterile water or sterile saline.

Atropine Sulfate, continued	Precautions:	May cause tachycardia; may increase ischemia due to increased need for oxygen by the myocardium.

Lidocaine Hydrochloride (Xylocaine®, Xylocard®, LidoPen®)	Action:	Decreases automaticity, helping to decrease ventricular dysrhythmias.
	Indications:	To control ventricular dysrhythmias such as PVCs, ventricular tachycardia, or ventricular fibrillation.
	Dosage:	1 to 1.5 mg/kg (milligram per kilogram of body weight) IV repeated at 5- to 10-minute intervals in doses of 0.5 to 0.75 mg/kg IV until a total of 3 mg/kg has been given; if the ventricular ectopy has been suppressed and the patient has a pulse, begin a continuous infusion at 2 to 4 mg/min (milligram per minute). In cardiac arrest, a single dose of 1.5 mg/kg may be used.
	Precautions:	Signs of toxicity include drowsiness, decreased hearing, numbness in hands or feet, confusion, muscle twitching or tremors, agitation; in severe cases of toxicity, seizures may occur; large doses of lidocaine may cause heart block or AV conduction dysrhythmias.

Procainamide Hydrochloride (Pronestyl®)	Action:	Suppresses ventricular ectopy when lidocaine has not been effective.
	Indications:	To control PVCs and ventricular tachycardia when lidocaine has not been effective.
	Dosage:	20 to 30 mg/min IV until any of the following occur: 1) the dysrhythmia is suppressed; 2) the patient becomes hypotensive; 3) the QRS complex widens by 50% of its original width; 4) a total of 17 mg/kg has been given. A continuous IV infusion of procainamide at a rate of 1 to 4 mg/min should be started if the ventricular dysrhythmia has been suppressed and the patient has a pulse.
	Precautions:	Avoid using in patients with pre-existing prolonged QT intervals and in torsades de pointes; monitor blood pressure closely; may cause hypotension if administered too quickly; decrease maintenance dose if patient has renal failure.

Bretylium Tosylate (Bretylium®, Bretylate®, Bretylol®)	Action:	Decreases incidence of ventricular fibrillation and ventricular tachycardia when lidocaine, procainamide, and defibrillation have not been effective.
	Indications:	To treat ventricular fibrillation and ventricular tachycardia when lidocaine and procainamide have not been effective.
	Dosage:	Ventricular fibrillation: 5 mg/kg IV administered rapidly, then repeated every 15 to 30 minutes at a dose of 10 mg/kg up to a total dose of 30 mg/kg. Ventricular tachycardia: dilute 500 mg of bretylium and administer 5 to 10 mg/kg IV over 8 to 10 minutes slowly; repeat in 5 min. A continuous IV infusion can be administered at a rate of 2 mg/min if the dysrhythmia is suppressed and the patient has a pulse.
	Precautions:	May cause hypotension, nausea, and vomiting; use with caution for dysrhythmias caused by digitalis toxicity.

Dopamine Hydrochloride
(Intropin®, Dopastat®, Revimine®)

Actions: Increases cardiac output by improving myocardial contractility; increases blood pressure by constricting peripheral arterial and venous vessels.

Indications: To treat hypotension accompanied by other symptoms, when there is no hypovolemia.

Dosage: To improve urine output: 1 to 2 mcg/kg/min continuous IV infusion; to improve cardiac output: 2 to 10 mcg/kg/min continuous IV infusion; to improve blood pressure: greater than 10 mcg/kg/min continuous IV infusion.

Precautions: Increased heart rate may produce supraventricular and ventricular dysrhythmias. Increased heart rate and increased blood pressure may increase need for oxygen by the myocardium, which may lead to ischemia; may cause nausea and vomiting; use with an infusion pump; monitor vital signs and cardiac rhythm frequently; do not mix with sodium bicarbonate.

Nitroglycerin
(Nitro-bid®, Nitrol®, Nitrostat®, Tridil®)

Action: Relieves cardiac chest pain by relaxing smooth muscle in blood vessels and increasing circulation of oxygenated blood to myocardium.

Indications: To treat acute angina pectoris, unstable angina, and congestive heart failure associated with myocardial infarctions (MIs). May also be used to reduce pain in MIs; used to reduce hypertension associated with MIs.

Dosage: Sublingual (under the tongue): one tablet (0.3 or 0.4 mg); repeat at 3- to 5-minute intervals; if no relief with three tablets, seek emergency medical help immediately.
Spray: 0.4 mg under or on the tongue by metered dose canister (patient should wait 10 seconds before swallowing); maximum dose, three sprays in 15 minutes.
IV: an initial bolus of 50 mcg IV may be given or a continuous IV infusion of 5 to 20 mcg/min; increase by 5 to 10 mcg/min every 3 to 5 minutes, until desired effect is obtained.

Precautions: May cause severe hypotension soon after administration of medication; monitor vital signs frequently; headache, nausea, and vomiting may occur; administer with an infusion pump; incompatible with Dobutamine; be aware of other drug incompatibilities when administering IV nitroglycerin; absorbed by plastic; must be administered in glass bottles with polyethylene tubing.

Morphine Sulfate
(Astramorph®, Astromorph PF®, Duramorph PF®)

Action: Provides relief for severe chest pain; reduces need for oxygen in the myocardium.

Indications: Pain relief of choice for MIs.

Dosage: 1 to 3 mg titrated intravenously over 1 to 5 minutes; may repeat in 5 to 30 minutes until pain is relieved; may dilute morphine to a 1 mg per 1 ml solution with sterile normal saline for ease in administration.

Precautions: Monitor respirations frequently because morphine may depress respiratory function; use with caution in patients with impaired respiratory function; follow your institution's guidelines for use of a schedule II controlled narcotic.

Thrombolytic Therapy ("Clot Busters")   Streptokinase (Kabikinase®, Streptase®); Alteplase, tissue plasminogen activator, recombinant; t-PA (Activase®); Anistreplase, anisoylated plasminogen-streptokinase activator complex: APSAC (Eminase®); Urokinase (Abbokinase®, Ukidan®, Win-Kinase®).

Action: Dissolves clots in the coronary arteries that cause ischemia and infarction; may reduce number of deaths from MI.

Indications: All patients with symptoms and EKG findings of acute MI, within less than 12 hours of onset of symptoms; patients must meet specific criteria determined by the manufacturer and your institution.

Dosage: Varies with specific thrombolytic agent; follow manufacturer's instructions or the policy of your institution, and specific instructions of the physician.

Precautions: Should be used only if patient meets specific criteria; all patients receiving thrombolytic therapy should receive 150 to 325 mg of aspirin as soon as possible; patients may require heparinization to help keep blood vessels open after thrombolytic therapy; may lead to increased bleeding, decreased clot formation, and intercranial bleeding; should not be used in patients with bleeding disorders, recent surgery, recent CVAs (strokes); streptokinase should not be used in patients with recent streptococcal infections.

Adenosine (Adenocard®)   Action: Decreases heart rate by depressing the SA node and AV node activity.

Indications: To treat paroxysmal atrial tachycardia and supraventricular tachycardia.

Dosage: 6 mg IV push rapidly over 1 to 3 seconds, followed immediately by a 20-ml saline flush; if no response in 1 to 2 minutes, repeat adenosine at 12 mg IV rapidly, followed by 20-ml saline flush; may repeat once more at 12 mg IV, if there is no response in 1 to 2 minutes.

Precautions: Side effects usually last only 1 to 2 minutes and include flushing, difficulty breathing, and mild chest pain; may also have short-lasting episodes of sinus bradycardia and ventricular ectopy (abnormal beats); PAT and SVT may recur because the effects of this medication last only a short time; may interact with theophylline (aminophylline), dipyridamole (Persantine®), or carbamazepine (Tegretol®).

Verapamil Hydrochloride (Calan®, Isoptin®)

Diltiazem Hydrochloride (Cardizem®, Cardizem SR®)   Action: Both decrease the heart rate by slowing conduction of the AV node and by lengthening the refractory periods.

Indications: To treat SVTs, PATs, and rapid ventricular responses in atrial flutter and atrial fibrillation.

Dosage: **Verapamil** initial dose: 0.075 to 0.15 mg/kg (2.5 to 5 mg) IV over 1 to 2 minutes; maximum dose 10 mg. Repeat dose: 0.15 mg/kg (5 to 10 mg) 15 to 30 minutes after first dose, if necessary; total maximum dosage of 30 mg. **Diltiazem** initial bolus: 0.25 mg/kg (average 20 mg) IV over 2 minutes; repeat dose: 0.35 mg/kg (average 25 mg) over 2 to 5 minutes, 15 minutes after the first dose; maintenance dose: continuous infusion of 5 to 15 mg per hour, titrated to heart rate, not to exceed 15 mg per hour and not to infuse more than 24 hours.

Verapamil Hydrochloride, continued	Precautions:	Older patients should have Verapamil administered over 3 minutes; do not use in patients with Wolff-Parkinson-White syndrome; do not use in wide QRS tachycardias; may cause a short period of hypotension; may cause bradycardia; do not use with ßeta blockers; do not use in patients with an AV block, unless a temporary pacemaker is available.
Isoproterenol Hydrochloride (Isuprel®)	Action:	Increases force and rate of myocardial contractions, improving cardiac output and systolic blood pressure.
	Indications:	Bradycardia, third-degree heart block.
	Dosage:	Continuous infusion at 2 to 10 mcg/min, titrated to patient's blood pressure and pulse.
	Precautions:	Use with extreme caution. Do not use with tachycardic dysrhythmias; must be used with infusion pump; incompatible with aminophylline and sodium bicarbonate; use lower doses in the elderly; use with caution in patients with sulfite allergy, may contain sulfite preservative; do not use with epinephrine—can cause VF/VT.
Magnesium Sulfate (Slow-Mag®)	Actions:	Reduces ventricular dysrhythmias that may follow an MI (decreased magnesium levels may cause ventricular fibrillation and may also prevent ventricular tachycardia from responding to treatment).
	Indications:	Treatment of choice in torsades de pointes; should be used whenever magnesium levels are decreased; may be used following MIs.
	Dosage:	Torsade de pointes: higher doses, up to 5 to 10 gm, may be administered IV; ventricular tachycardia: 1 to 2 gm magnesium sulfate, diluted in 10 ml of 5% dextrose in water (D$_5$W), administered IV over one to two minutes; ventricular fibrillation: 1 to 2 gm magnesium sulfate, diluted in 10 ml of 5% dextrose in water, given IV push; magnesium deficiency: continuous infusion of 0.5 to 1 gm magnesium sulfate for 24 hours may be used.
	Precautions:	May cause flushing, sweating, slight bradycardia, and hypotension. Use with caution in patients with renal failure.
Calcium Chloride (Kalcinate®)	Actions:	Increases myocardial contractility.
	Indications:	Replace and maintain calcium levels; hyperkalemia (increased potassium level); calcium channel blocker toxicity.
	Dosage:	8 to 16 mg/kg of a 10% solution IV; may repeat if necessary.
	Precautions:	Rapid administration may cause slowing of the heart rate; may cause spasms of the coronary and cerebral arteries; use with caution in patients receiving digitalis; incompatible with sodium bicarbonate.
Dobutamine Hydrochloride (Dobutrex®)	Actions:	Increases force of contraction of heart muscle, increasing cardiac output and increasing coronary artery blood flow.
	Indications:	Short-term treatment of heart disease.
	Dosage:	2 to 20 mcg/kg/min IV. Titrate so heart rate does not increase by more than 10% of HR prior to treatment.
	Precautions:	Monitor vital signs and patient's rhythm continuously; administer with infusion pump; use with caution in patients who have: 1) atrial fibrillation: increases AV conduction and rapid ventricular

Dobutamine Hydrochloride, continued		response; 2) myocardial infarction: high doses may increase my-ocardium's need for oxygen and increase ischemia; 3) PVCs: may increase incidence of PVCs. Incompatible with aminophylline, verapamil, bretylium, and heparin.
Sodium Nitroprusside (Nipride®, Nitropress®)	Action:	Decreases blood pressure by relaxing smooth muscle of blood vessels; increases cardiac output; reduces myocardium's need for oxygen (may reduce ischemia); relieves chest pain.
	Indications:	Hypertensive emergencies (when high blood pressure will not respond to other drugs).
	Dosage:	50 mg diluted in 500 ml 5% dextrose in water (D_5W) for a concentration of 100 mcg/ml; initial IV dose: 0.5 mcg/kg/min (micrograms per kilograms of body weight per min); titrate (adjust rate) to desired blood pressure or maximum dose of 10 mcg/kg/min.
	Precautions:	Monitor vital signs frequently because medication may decrease blood pressure rapidly; solution must be protected from light, cover IV bottle with foil or dark plastic; follow your institution's policy regarding covering IV tubing; incompatible with bacteriostatic water and saline solution; use D_5W to reconstitute medication; do not add any other drugs or preservatives to nitroprusside solution.
Norepinephrine Bitartrate (Levophed®)	Action:	Constricts blood vessels, increasing coronary artery flow, blood pressure, and cardiac output; increases force of cardiac contraction and increases heart rate, which may increase the myocardium's need for oxygen.
	Indications:	To treat acute hypotension, and severe hypotension following cardiac arrest.
	Dosage:	0.5 to 1.0 mcg/min IV, titrate infusion to patient's blood pressure up to 30 mcg/min.
	Precautions:	May cause an increased need for oxygen in myocardium; monitor rhythm strip continuously for development of dysrhythmias; monitor vital signs frequently, at least every 5 minutes; assess infusion site frequently, because infiltration (leaking IV solution into tissue) may cause death of tissues around the IV site; incompatible with aminophylline, lidocaine, sodium bicarbonate, and normal saline; use only with 5% dextrose in water.
Digitalis Glycoside (Digoxin®, Lanoxin®)	Action:	Increases myocardial contractility; helps control ventricular response to atrial dysrhythmias.
	Indications:	Atrial flutter, atrial fibrillation, atrial tachycardias including PAT and SVT; used in treatment of chronic congestive heart failure.
	Dosage:	10 to 15 mcg/kg of lean body weight administered IV.
	Precautions:	Contraindicated for patients with digitalis toxicity, ventricular tachycardia, or ventricular fibrillation; use with caution in patients with acute MI because the drug may cause AV block, sinus bradycardia, or ventricular tachycardia; incompatible with dobutamine;

Digitalis Glycoside, continued		do not administer if heart rate is less than 60 beats per minute (a heart rate of below 60 may indicate digitalis toxicity); usually not used outside hospital setting because of slow onset of action.

Furosemide (Lasix®, Lasix Special®)	Action:	Dilates blood vessels; removes excess fluid from tissues; increases formation of urine.
	Indications:	Acute pulmonary edema; congestive heart failure; cerebral edema following MI.
	Dosage:	0.5 to 1 mg/kg IV, over 1 to 2 minutes; if there is no response, double the dose to 2.0 mg/kg IV slowly over 1 to 2 minutes.
	Precautions:	May cause severe dehydration, loss of potassium, or hyperglycemia (high blood sugar).

Beta Blockers Atenolol (Tenormin®, Noten®), Metoprolol tartrate (Lopressor®), Propranolol hydrochloride (Inderal®), and Esmolol hydrochloride (Brevibloc®)

Action:	May reduce cardiac ischemia in patients receiving thrombolytics; may reduce occurrence of V fib after MI.
Indications:	Recurrent V tach and V fib; after emergency treatment of MI.
Dosage:	**Atenolol:** 5 mg IV over 5 minutes; give second dose of 5 mg IV slowly over 10 minutes; **metoprolol:** 5 mg slow IV over 2 to 5 minutes, repeated at 5 minute intervals to a total of 15 mg; **propranolol:** initial dose of 1 to 3 mg IV over 2 to 5 minutes (not more than 1 mg/min), may be repeated in 2 minutes, until a total dose of 0.1 mg/kg has been given; **Esmolol:** initial dose: mix 2.5 gm in 250 ml of IV solution; administer 250 to 500 mcg/kg for 1 minute, then 25 to 50 mcg/kg for 4 minutes; the maintenance dose may be titrated at 5- to 10-minute intervals to a maximum dose of 300 mcg/kg/min.
Precautions:	May cause bradycardia, AV conduction delays, and hypotension; should not be used in patients with bradycardias, second- or third-degree heart block, conduction delays, hypotension, congestive heart failure, or bronchospasm; use with caution in patients with renal failure; incompatible with furosemide and sodium bicarbonate.

Sodium Bicarbonate	Actions:	Reverses acidosis by working as an alkalinizing agent throughout the body.
	Indications:	Metabolic acidosis; prolonged cardiac arrest.
	Dosage:	1 mEq/kg (milliequivalent per kilogram) IV; repeat every 10 minutes at 0.5 mEq/kg, depending on arterial blood gas results.
	Precautions:	Flush IV before and after administering medication; do not use for patients with respiratory acidosis; monitor electrolytes, arterial blood gases, and renal function.

Amrinone Lactate (Inocor®)	Actions:	Improves cardiac output by increasing strength of cardiac contractions; decreases blood pressure by relaxing and dilating blood vessel walls.
	Indications:	Consider using in congestive heart failure that has not responded to other drug therapy.

Amrinone
Lactate,
continued

Dosage: Initial bolus: 0.75 to 1.0 mg/kg IV over 10 to 15 minutes; maintenance dose: 2 to 5 mcg/kg/min, titrated to a dose of 10 to 15 mcg/
kg/min.

Precautions: Increases myocardial demand for oxygen; may increase cardiac
ischemia; use an infusion pump to administer medication; may
reduce platelets; may cause stomach upset, fever, liver problems, or kidney failure; may increase ventricular irritability;
should not be used in patients who are allergic to sulfites; incompatible with furosemide, sodium bicarbonate, and dextrose.

ADULT TREATMENT GUIDELINES

Artifact

1. Artifact is not treated. Simply correct the cause of the artifact in order to
   identify the rhythm, and then initiate treatment if necessary.

Myocardial Infarction

1. Assess the patient.
2. Provide oxygen.
3. Begin IV fluids.
4. Give nitroglycerin for pain.
5. Obtain a 12-Lead electrocardiograph. Reassess the patient.
6. If no relief from repeated sublingual nitroglycerin, administer morphine
   IV, titrated to pain relief. Consider IV nitroglycerin.
7. Continue to assess and monitor the patient. Treat any dysrhythmias that occur.
8. Once diagnosis of MI has been confirmed, begin thrombolytic protocol if no
   contraindications exist and if within 12 hours of onset of symptoms; consider oral aspirin and IV heparin, if included in thrombolytic protocol.
9. Continued assessment and monitoring of the patient is essential. Transfer
   patient to care of cardiologist in coronary care unit.

Sinus Dysrhythmias

Normal sinus rhythm
1. Normal sinus rhythm does not require treatment.
2. **Remember**, the monitor is **not** the patient. The patient must be assessed,
   and, if symptomatic, treatment must be initiated.
3. Continue to assess and monitor the patient.

Sinus bradycardia
1. Assess the patient. If medically unstable, begin treatment.
2. Provide oxygen.
3. Begin IV fluids.
4. Administer atropine. Reassess the patient.
5. An artificial pacemaker (temporary or permanent) may be necessary.

Sinus bradycardia, continued

6. Dopamine may be administered for a systolic blood pressure less than 80 mm.
7. Epinephrine may be administered to patients who do not respond to atropine.
8. Isoproterenol may be helpful when used at low doses; use with caution.
9. Continue to assess and monitor the patient.

Sinus tachycardia

1. Assess the patient. If medically unstable, begin treatment.
2. Determine the cause of the tachycardia:
   a. Fever
      (1) administer antipyretics, such as aspirin or acetaminophen, to lower fever
      (2) provide cool to tepid bath
   b. Anxiety
      (1) acknowledge the patient's anxiety
      (2) offer reassurance in a calm manner
   c. Pain
      (1) administer pain medication as ordered
      (2) use relaxation techniques
   d. Hypovolemia
      (1) replace fluids or blood
3. Provide oxygen.
4. Begin IV fluids.
5. Consider using digoxin, beta blockers, or diltiazem if the patient's heart rate is greater than 100 but less than 150.
6. Continue to assess and monitor the patient.

Sinus arrhythmia

1. Assess the patient. If signs of poor cardiac output are present, begin treatment.
2. Provide oxygen.
3. Begin IV fluids.
4. If overall heart rate is bradycardic, administer atropine. Reassess the patient.
5. An artificial pacemaker (temporary or permanent) may be indicated.
6. Dopamine may be administered for a systolic blood pressure less than 80 mm.
7. Epinephrine may be administered to patients who do not respond to atropine.
8. Isoproterenol may be helpful when used at low doses; use with caution.
9. Continue to reassess and monitor the patient.

Sinus exit block and Sinus arrest

1. If the sinus exit block or sinus arrest is a new dysrhythmia, observe the patient closely for a change in the cardiac rhythm.
2. Sinus exit block and sinus arrest are both indications of damage or injury to the SA node. If the pauses are frequent, or long, the patient may become medically unstable and require an artificial pacemaker.
3. Continued assessment and monitoring of the patient is essential.

Atrial Dysrhythmias

Premature atrial contraction

1. Assess the patient. A PAC by itself does not require treatment. If the patient is medically unstable or showing signs of poor cardiac output, treat the underlying rhythm.

Premature atrial contraction, continued

2. If the cause of the PAC is caffeine or nicotine, decrease or eliminate the stimulant in the patient's daily intake.
3. If the PAC is a new occurrence, observe the patient closely for a change in the cardiac rhythm.
4. Continue to reassess and monitor the patient.

Paroxysmal atrial tachycardia

1. Assess the patient. If medically stable, continue to observe the patient. If medically unstable, begin treatment.
2. Provide oxygen.
3. Begin IV fluids.
4. The physician may perform vagal maneuvers, such as Valsalva's maneuver (have the patient bear down) or carotid massage. Reassess the patient.
5. Administer adenosine.
6. If PAT continues, repeat adenosine at higher dose; may repeat this dose once after 1 to 2 minutes.
7. If PAT continues, monitor blood pressure. If systolic pressure is normal or high, administer verapamil. Reassess the patient.
8. Wait 15 to 30 minutes; if PAT continues, repeat verapamil.
9. If systolic blood pressure is low or unstable, synchronized cardioversion may be necessary to convert the PAT to a normal or more stable rhythm. Reassess the patient.
10. If PAT continues, consider using digoxin, diltiazem, or beta blockers.
11. Reassess the patient. If the dysrhythmia has converted to another rhythm, reassess the patient; if necessary, treat the new dysrhythmia.

Supraventricular tachycardia

1. Assess the patient. If stable, continue to observe the patient. If the patient is medically unstable, begin treatment following the guidelines for the treatment of PAT.
2. Provide oxygen.
3. Begin IV fluids.
4. The physician may perform vagal maneuvers, such as Valsalva's maneuver (have the patient bear down) or carotid massage. Reassess the patient.
5. Administer adenosine. Must be pushed rapidly to be effective.
6. If SVT continues, administer adenosine again at higher dose. May repeat the higher dose once after 1 to 2 minutes.
7. If SVT continues, reassess the patient and monitor blood pressure. If systolic pressure is normal or high, administer verapamil.
8. Wait 15 to 30 minutes; if SVT continues, repeat verapamil.
9. If systolic blood pressure is low or unstable, synchronized cardioversion may be necessary to convert the SVT to a normal or more stable rhythm. Reassess the patient.
10. If SVT continues, consider using digoxin, diltiazem, or beta blockers.
11. Reassess the patient. If the dysrhythmia has converted to another rhythm, reassess the patient; if necessary, treat the new dysrhythmia.

Wandering atrial pacemaker

1. Assess the patient. If medically stable, continue to observe the patient; if showing signs of poor cardiac output, begin treatment.
2. Provide oxygen.
3. Begin IV fluids.

Wandering atrial pacemaker, continued
4. If overall heart rate is bradycardic, administer atropine.
5. An artificial pacemaker (temporary or permanent) may be indicated.
6. Dopamine may be administered for a systolic blood pressure less than 80 mm. Reassess the patient.
7. Epinephrine may be administered to patients who do not respond to atropine.
8. Isoproterenol may be helpful when used at low doses and when used with caution.
9. If heart rate is greater than 100 but less than 150, consider using diltiazem, digoxin, or beta blockers.
10. Reassess the patient. If the dysrhythmia has converted to another rhythm, reassess the patient; if necessary, treat the new dysrhythmia.

Atrial flutter
1. Assess the patient. If stable, continue to observe the patient. If medically unstable, begin treatment.
2. Provide oxygen.
3. Begin IV fluids.
4. If overall heart rate is bradycardic, administer atropine. Reassess the patient.
5. An artificial pacemaker (temporary or permanent) may be indicated.
6. Dopamine may be administered for a systolic blood pressure less than 80 mm.
7. Epinephrine may be administered to patients who do not respond to atropine.
8. Isoproterenol may be helpful when used at low doses and when used with caution.
9. If heart rate is greater than 100 but less than 150, consider using diltiazem, digoxin, or beta blockers.
10. Synchronized cardioversion may be indicated.
11. Reassess the patient. If the dysrhythmia has converted to another rhythm, reassess the patient; if necessary, treat the new dysrhythmia.

Atrial fibrillation
1. Assess the patient. If medically unstable, begin treatment.
2. Provide oxygen.
3. Begin IV fluids.
4. If overall heart rate is bradycardic, administer atropine. Reassess the patient.
5. An artificial pacemaker (temporary or permanent) may be indicated.
6. Dopamine may be administered for a systolic blood pressure less than 80 mm.
7. Epinephrine may be administered to patients who do not respond to atropine.
8. Isoproterenol may be helpful when used at low doses and when used with caution.
9. If heart rate is greater than 100 but less than 150, consider using diltiazem, digoxin, or beta blockers.
10. Synchronized cardioversion may be indicated.
11. Reassess the patient. If the dysrhythmia has converted to another rhythm, reassess the patient; if necessary, treat the new dysrhythmia.

Junctional Dysrhythmias

Junctional rhythm
1. Assess the patient. If the patient is medically stable, continue observing him or her.
2. If the patient is medically unstable, begin treatment, following the junctional bradycardia guidelines.

Junctional bradycardia
1. Assess the patient. If medically stable, continue to observe the patient. If medically unstable, begin treatment.
2. Provide oxygen.
3. Begin IV infusion.
4. Administer atropine. Reassess the patient.
5. An artificial pacemaker (temporary or permanent) may be necessary.
6. Dopamine may be administered for a systolic blood pressure less than 80 mm.
7. Epinephrine may be administered to patients who do not respond to atropine.
8. Isoproterenol may be helpful when used at low doses; use with caution.
9. Continue to monitor and reassess the patient.

Accelerated junctional rhythm and Junctional tachycardia
1. Assess the patient. If medically unstable, begin treatment.
2. Determine the cause of the tachycardia:
   a. Fever
      (1) administer antipyretics, such as aspirin or acetaminophen to lower fever
      (2) provide cool to tepid bath
   b. Anxiety
      (1) acknowledge the patient's anxiety
      (2) offer reassurance in a calm manner
   c. Pain
      (1) administer pain medication as ordered
      (2) use relaxation techniques
   d. Hypovolemia
      (1) replace fluids or blood
3. Provide oxygen.
4. Begin IV fluids.
5. Consider using digoxin, beta blockers, or diltiazem if the heart rate is greater than 100 but less than 150.
6. Continue to reassess and monitor patient.

Premature junctional contraction
1. Assess the patient. PJCs are not treated unless the patient becomes medically unstable.
2. If the cause of the PJC is caffeine or nicotine, decrease or eliminate the stimulant in the patient's daily intake.
3. If the PJCs are a new occurrence, observe the patient closely for a change in the cardiac rhythm.
4. If necessary, treat the underlying rhythm according to the patient's symptoms.
5. Continue to reassess and monitor the patient.

Wandering junctional pacemaker
1. Assess the patient. If medically stable, continue to observe the patient; if showing signs of poor cardiac output, begin treatment.
2. Provide oxygen.
3. Begin IV fluids. Reassess the patient.
4. If overall heart rate is bradycardic, administer atropine.
5. An artificial pacemaker (temporary or permanent) may be indicated.
6. Dopamine may be administered for a systolic blood pressure less than 80 mm.
7. Epinephrine may be administered to patients who do not respond to atropine.
8. Isoproterenol may be helpful when used at low doses and when used with caution.
9. If heart rate is greater than 100 but less than 150, consider using diltiazem, digoxin, or beta blockers.
10. Reassess the patient. If the dysrhythmia has converted to another rhythm, reassess the patient; if necessary, treat the new dysrhythmia.

Heart Blocks

First-degree heart block
1. Assess the patient. A first-degree block by itself does not require treatment.
2. If the first-degree block is a new occurrence, observe the patient closely for a change in the cardiac rhythm.
3. If the patient is medically unstable or showing signs of poor cardiac output, treat the underlying rhythm.
4. Continue to reassess and monitor the patient.

Mobitz I (Wenckebach, second-degree heart block, type I)
1. Assess the patient. A Mobitz I block by itself does not require treatment.
2. If the Mobitz I block is a new occurrence, observe the patient closely for a change in the cardiac rhythm.
3. If the patient is medically unstable or showing signs of poor cardiac output, treat the underlying rhythm.
4. If overall heart rate is bradycardic, administer atropine.
5. Continued assessment and monitoring of the patient is essential.

Mobitz II (Second-degree heart block, type II)
1. Assess the patient. If the patient is medically unstable or showing signs of poor cardiac output, treatment should be started immediately.
2. Provide oxygen.
3. Begin IV fluids. Reassess the patient.
4. If overall heart rate is bradycardic, administer atropine. (Atropine should be used with caution in a Mobitz II block because it may increase only the atrial rate, which may increase the block.)
5. An artificial pacemaker (temporary or permanent) may be indicated.
6. Dopamine may be administered for a systolic blood pressure less than 80 mm.
7. Epinephrine may be administered to patients who do not respond to atropine. Reassess the patient.
8. Isoproterenol may be helpful when used at low doses; use with caution.

Mobitz II, continued

9. If heart rate is greater than 100 but less than 150, consider using diltiazem, digoxin, or beta blockers.
10. Reassess the patient. If the dysrhythmia has converted to another rhythm, reassess the patient and, if necessary, treat the new dysrhythmia.

Third-degree heart block

1. Assess the patient. If medically stable, continue to observe the patient while setting up a pacemaker. If the patient shows signs of poor cardiac output, begin treatment immediately.
2. Provide oxygen.
3. Begin IV fluids.
4. If overall heart rate is bradycardic, administer atropine. (Atropine may be contraindicated if the QRS is wider than 0.12 seconds; atropine may worsen the block by increasing only the atrial rate.) Reassess the patient.
5. Dopamine may be administered for a systolic blood pressure less than 80 mm.
6. Epinephrine IV may be administered to patients who do not respond to atropine. Reassess the patient.
7. Isoproterenol may be helpful when used at low doses; use with caution.
8. An artificial pacemaker (temporary or permanent) should be initiated as soon as possible, if the patient is unstable or if the QRS is greater than 0.12 second.
9. Reassess the patient. If the dysrhythmia has converted to another rhythm, reassess the patient and, if necessary, treat the new dysrhythmia.

Bundle branch block

1. Assess the patient. A bundle branch block by itself does not require treatment.
2. If the bundle branch block is a new occurrence, observe the patient closely for a change in the cardiac rhythm.
3. If the patient is medically unstable or showing signs of poor cardiac output, treat the underlying rhythm.
4. Continue to monitor and reassess the patient.

Ventricular Dysrhythmias

Premature ventricular contraction

1. Assess the patient. Begin treatment if the patient is showing signs of poor cardiac output or if any of the following "danger signals" are present:
   a. More than six PVCs in 1 minute
   b. Bigeminy
   c. Multifocal PVCs
   d. R on T phenomenon
   e. Run of V tach
2. Provide oxygen.
3. Begin IV fluids.
4. If the rate is bradycardic, administer atropine. Reassess the patient.
5. If the heart rate is not bradycardic, administer lidocaine. Remember: the patient's heart rate must be at least 60 beats per minute without counting PVCs before starting lidocaine.
6. If the PVCs have been controlled and the patient has a pulse, start an IV infusion of lidocaine.

Premature ventricular contraction, continued

7. Reassess the patient. If lidocaine is not successful, administer procainamide until any one of the following occurs:
   a. Total of 17 mg/kg has been given
   b. The PVCs stop
   c. The patient becomes hypotensive
   d. The QRS becomes 50% wider than before administration of procainamide
8. Start a procainamide IV infusion if the PVCs have been controlled and the patient has a pulse.
9. If neither lidocaine nor procainamide control the PVCs, administer bretylium.
10. If bretylium has controlled the PVCs and the patient has a pulse, start a continuous bretylium infusion.
11. Reassess the patient. If the dysrhythmia has converted to another rhythm, reassess the patient; if necessary, treat the new dysrhythmia.

Ventricular tachycardia

1. Assess the patient. If the patient has a pulse and is medically stable, begin treatment. (If the patient is medically unstable, *see* # 10; if there is no pulse, *see* # 11.)
2. Provide oxygen.
3. Start IV fluids. Reassess the patient.
4. Administer lidocaine. Reassess the patient.
5. If the VT has been controlled and the patient has a pulse, start an IV infusion of lidocaine.
6. If the lidocaine is not successful, administer procainamide until any one of the following occurs:
   a. Total of 17 mg/kg has been given
   b. The PVCs stop or the dysrhythmia has converted
   c. The patient becomes hypotensive
   d. The QRS becomes 50% wider than before administration of procainamide
7. Start a procainamide infusion if the procainamide has controlled the VT and the patient has a pulse.
8. Reassess the patient. If neither lidocaine nor procainamide control the VT, administer bretylium.
9. If bretylium has controlled the VT and the patient has a pulse, start a continuous bretylium infusion.
10. Continue to assess and monitor the patient. If the patient has a pulse, but shows signs of poor cardiac output, begin the following treatment:
    a. Perform synchronized cardioversion if the heart rate is greater than 150
    b. If cardioversion is unsuccessful, administer lidocaine if maximum dose has not been given
    c. Continue cardioversion attempts. Repeat lidocaine every 5 to 10 minutes until a **total** of 3 mg/kg has been given
    d. If lidocaine is not successful, procainamide or bretylium tosylate may be used, as administered in the treatment of PVCs
11. If the patient does not have a pulse or loses the pulse at any time during treatment, begin CPR and follow the treatment guidelines for ventricular fibrillation.
12. Reassess the patient. If the dysrhythmia has converted to another rhythm, reassess the patient; if necessary, treat the new dysrhythmia.

Torsades de pointes

Because torsades de pointes may result from prolonged QT intervals, the standard treatment for ventricular tachycardia should **not** be used. Lidocaine, procainamide, and quinidine **all** may prolong QT intervals.

1. Assess the patient. If the patient has a pulse and is medically stable, continue to observe the patient. If the patient shows any signs of poor cardiac output, begin treatment.
2. Provide oxygen.
3. Begin IV fluids. Reassess the patient.
4. An artificial pacemaker (temporary or permanent) should be initiated as soon as possible, if the patient is unstable.
5. Magnesium sulfate may be used. Reassess the patient.
6. Isoproterenol may be used. Reassess the patient.
7. Consider unsynchronized cardioversion if patient does not convert to a more normal rhythm.
8. If the patient does not have a pulse or loses the pulse at any time during treatment, begin CPR and follow the treatment guidelines for ventricular fibrillation.
9. Reassess the patient. If the dysrhythmia has converted to another rhythm, reassess the patient; if necessary, treat the new dysrhythmia.

Ventricular fibrillation

1. Assess the patient. Remember: some types of artifact can mimic ventricular fibrillation. If the dysrhythmia is V-fib, treatment must be started immediately.
2. Begin CPR. Continue CPR **except** during defibrillation.
3. Defibrillate. Initially, three consecutive defibrillation attempts of 200, 200 to 300, and 360 joules should be used; defibrillate at 360 joules during the remaining treatment. Reassess the patient **before** and **after** each defibrillation attempt.
4. Administer 100% oxygen by bag-valve mask. Intubate the patient as soon as possible.
5. Begin IV fluids. Reassess the patient.
6. Defibrillate at 360 joules. Reassess the patient.
7. Administer epinephrine. Repeat every 3 to 5 minutes. Reassess the patient after **any** medication has been administered.
8. Defibrillate at 360 joules within 60 seconds of administering epinephrine.
9. Administer lidocaine. May repeat in 3 to 5 minutes.
10. Defibrillate at 360 joules after the administration of every medication.
11. If necessary, administer bretylium tosylate. May repeat in 5 minutes.
12. Administer procainamide if bretylium has not been effective.
13. Use magnesium sulfate in torsades de pointes or in severe V-fib that does not respond to defibrillation and usual medication administration.
14. Once the patient has a pulse, start an infusion drip of whatever medication was successful in ending the V-fib, using the treatment guidelines for PVCs.
15. Assess the patient for a change in rhythm after each dose of medication and before and after each defibrillation attempt. When the rhythm changes, reassess the patient; then treat the new dysrhythmia, if necessary.

Idioventricular and Agonal dysrhythmia

1. Assess the patient. Treatment must be started immediately.
2. If pulseless, treat as pulseless electrical activity (PEA).
3. If patient has a pulse, treat as bradycardia.

Ventricular standstill

1. Assess the patient. Treatment must be started immediately.
2. Treat as asystole.

Asystole

1. Assess the patient. Treatment must be started immediately.
2. Begin CPR.
3. Confirm asystole in two different monitor Leads (for example, Lead II and MCL I).
4. If unable to distinguish between fine ventricular fibrillation and asystole, treat as V-fib. If the dysrhythmia is identified as asystole, continue with the following guidelines:
   a. Reassess the patient
   b. Administer 100% oxygen by bag-valve mask; the patient should be intubated as soon as possible
   c. Begin IV fluids; reassess the patient
   d. Administer epinephrine; may repeat in 3 to 5 minutes
   e. Initiate an artificial pacemaker (temporary or permanent) as soon as possible
   f. Atropine may be administered IV; repeat in 3 to 5 minutes
5. Reassess the patient after each medication. If the cardiac dysrhythmia changes, treat the new dysrhythmia, if necessary.

"Funny Looking" Beats

Escape beats

1. Assess the patient. Escape beats by themselves do not require treatment.
2. If the escape beat is a new occurrence, observe the patient closely for a change in the cardiac rhythm.
3. If the patient is medically unstable or showing signs of poor cardiac output, treat the underlying rhythm.
4. Continue to reassess and monitor the patient.

Aberrantly conducted beats

1. Assess the patient. Aberrantly conducted beats (complexes) by themselves do not require treatment.
2. If the aberrantly conducted complex is a new occurrence, observe the patient closely for a change in the cardiac rhythm.
3. If the patient is medically unstable or showing signs of poor cardiac output, treat the underlying rhythm.
4. Continue to assess and monitor the patient.

Pulseless electrical activity

PEA includes electromechanical dissociation, idioventricular rhythms, and bradyasystole dysrhythmias.

1. Assess the patient. Treatment must be started immediately.
2. Begin CPR.
3. Provide 100% oxygen by bag-valve mask. Intubate as soon as possible.
4. Start IV fluids. Reassess the patient.
5. Consider possible causes:
   a. Hypovolemia—give fluid replacement; reassess the patient
   b. Hypoxia—increase ventilations and oxygen; reassess the patient
   c. Cardiac tamponade—physician performs pericardiocentesis; reassess the patient
   d. Tension pneumothorax—perform needle decompression; reassess the patient

Pulseless electrical activity, continued

6. Administer epinephrine. Repeat in 3 to 5 minutes. Reassess the patient.
7. If dysrhythmia is bradycardic, administer atropine. Repeat every 3 to 5 minutes until the maximum dose is given.
8. Reassess the patient. If the dysrhythmia has converted to another rhythm, reassess the patient; if necessary, treat the new dysrhythmia.

Pacemaker rhythms

1. Assess the patient. If medically unstable, treat the underlying rhythm.
2. If the pacemaker is malfunctioning (not pacing), the pacemaker must be replaced or repaired. A temporary pacemaker may be used until the permanent pacemaker is replaced.
3. Provide oxygen.
4. Start IV fluids.
5. Reassure the patient by giving frequent explanations of the procedures being performed, and by acting in a calm manner.
6. Continue to reassess and monitor the patient.

Dysrhythmia Interpretation Practice

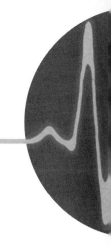

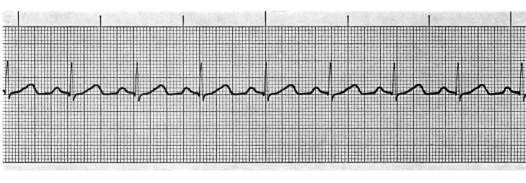

1. MEASURE: PR interval _____ Rhythm _____

                QRS complex _____ Heart rate _____

     INTERPRETATION: _____

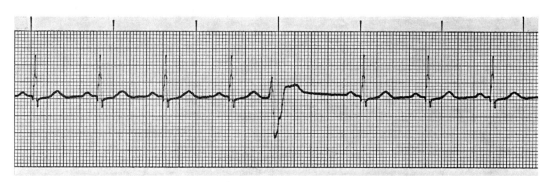

2. MEASURE: PR interval _____ Rhythm _____

                QRS complex _____ Heart rate _____

     INTERPRETATION: _____

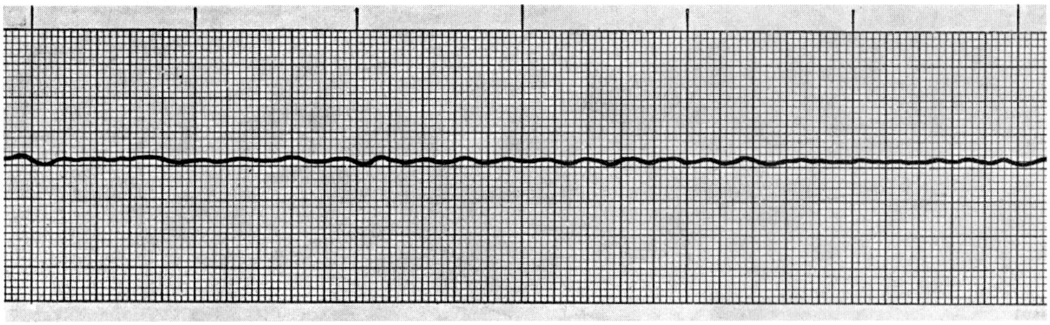

3. MEASURE: PR interval _____   Rhythm _____

                QRS complex _____   Heart rate _____

      INTERPRETATION: _____

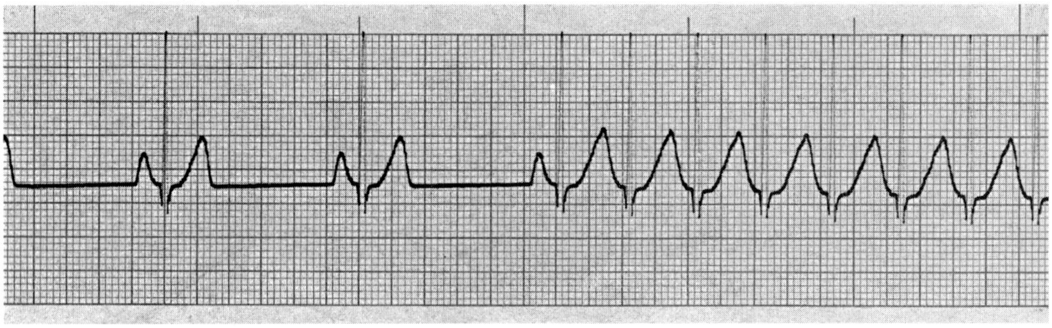

4. MEASURE: PR interval _____   Rhythm _____

                QRS complex _____   Heart rate _____

      INTERPRETATION: _____

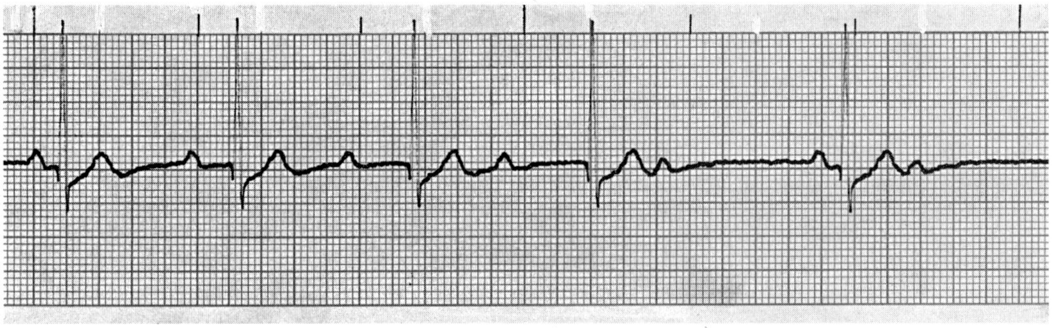

5. MEASURE: PR interval _____   Rhythm _____

                QRS complex _____   Heart rate _____

      INTERPRETATION: _____

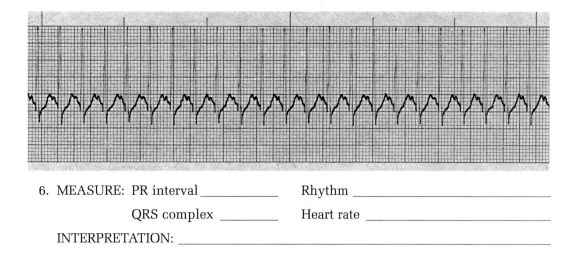

6. MEASURE: PR interval _____   Rhythm _____

                QRS complex _____   Heart rate _____

INTERPRETATION: _____

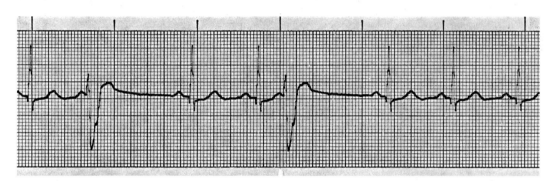

7. MEASURE: PR interval _____   Rhythm _____

                QRS complex _____   Heart rate _____

INTERPRETATION: _____

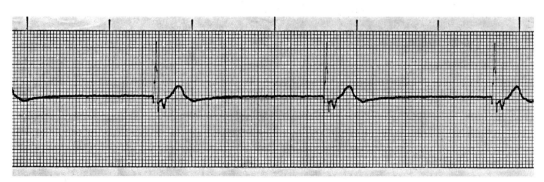

8. MEASURE: PR interval _____   Rhythm _____

                QRS complex _____   Heart rate _____

INTERPRETATION: _____

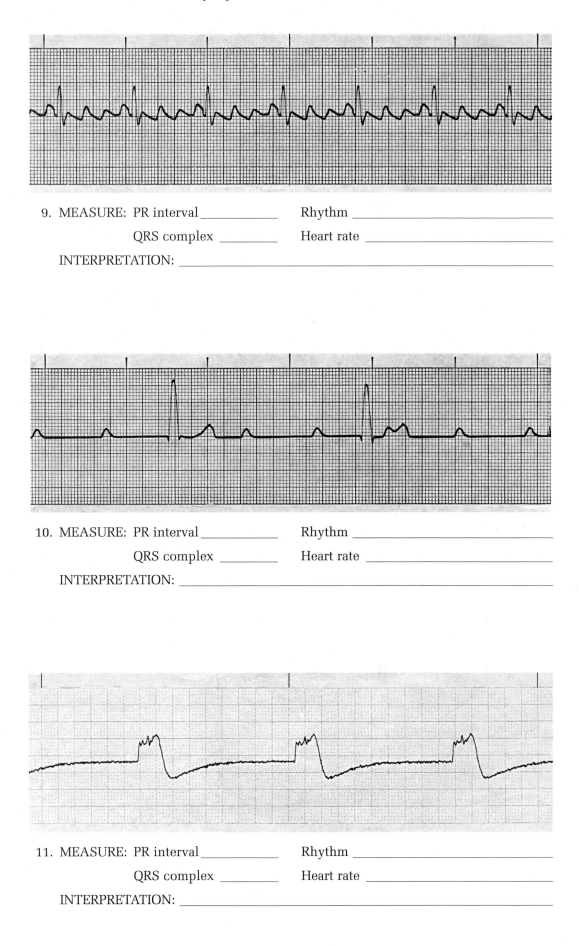

9. MEASURE: PR interval _____   Rhythm _____

                QRS complex _____   Heart rate _____

INTERPRETATION: _____

10. MEASURE: PR interval _____   Rhythm _____

                QRS complex _____   Heart rate _____

INTERPRETATION: _____

11. MEASURE: PR interval _____   Rhythm _____

                QRS complex _____   Heart rate _____

INTERPRETATION: _____

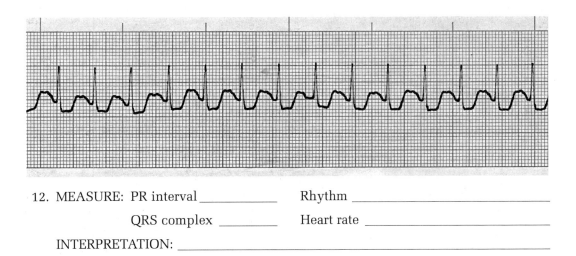

12. MEASURE: PR interval _____   Rhythm _____

QRS complex _____   Heart rate _____

INTERPRETATION: _____

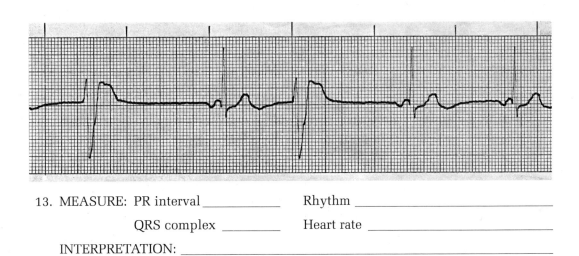

13. MEASURE: PR interval _____   Rhythm _____

QRS complex _____   Heart rate _____

INTERPRETATION: _____

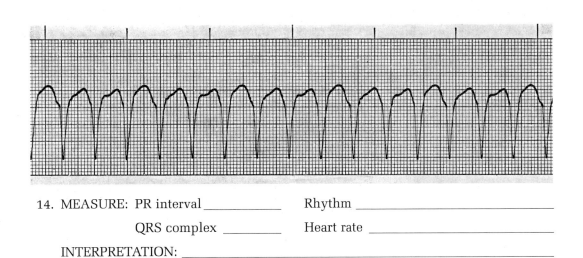

14. MEASURE: PR interval _____   Rhythm _____

QRS complex _____   Heart rate _____

INTERPRETATION: _____

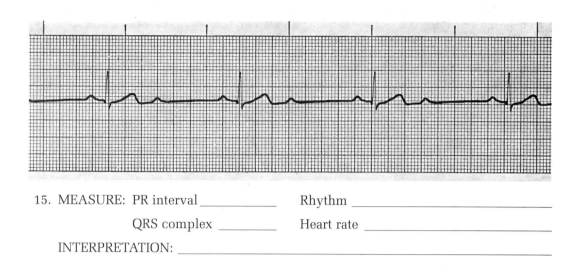

15. MEASURE: PR interval _____   Rhythm _____

QRS complex _____   Heart rate _____

INTERPRETATION: _____

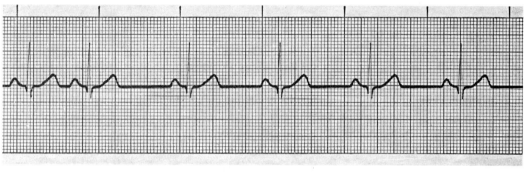

16. MEASURE: PR interval _____   Rhythm _____

QRS complex _____   Heart rate _____

INTERPRETATION: _____

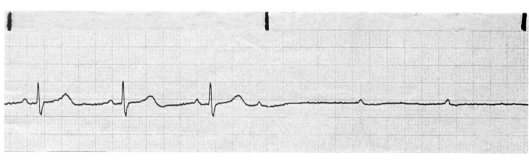

17. MEASURE: PR interval _____   Rhythm _____

QRS complex _____   Heart rate _____

INTERPRETATION: _____

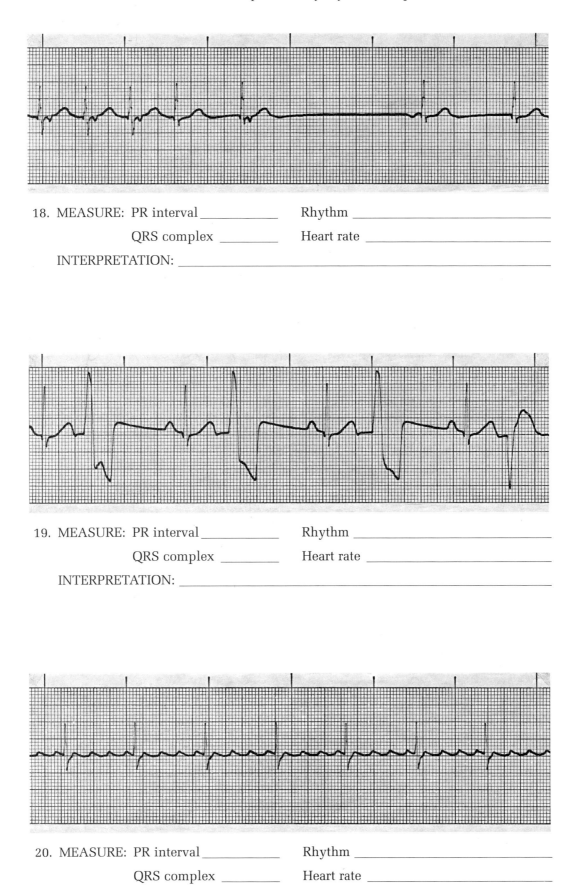

18. MEASURE: PR interval _____   Rhythm _____

                      QRS complex _____   Heart rate _____

        INTERPRETATION: _____

19. MEASURE: PR interval _____   Rhythm _____

                      QRS complex _____   Heart rate _____

        INTERPRETATION: _____

20. MEASURE: PR interval _____   Rhythm _____

                      QRS complex _____   Heart rate _____

        INTERPRETATION: _____

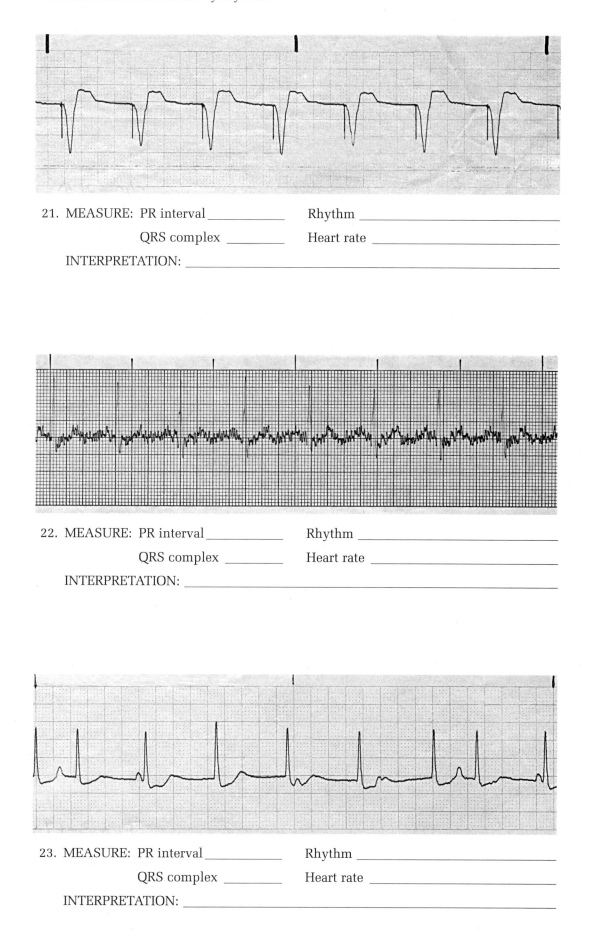

21. MEASURE: PR interval _____   Rhythm _____

QRS complex _____   Heart rate _____

INTERPRETATION: _____

22. MEASURE: PR interval _____   Rhythm _____

QRS complex _____   Heart rate _____

INTERPRETATION: _____

23. MEASURE: PR interval _____   Rhythm _____

QRS complex _____   Heart rate _____

INTERPRETATION: _____

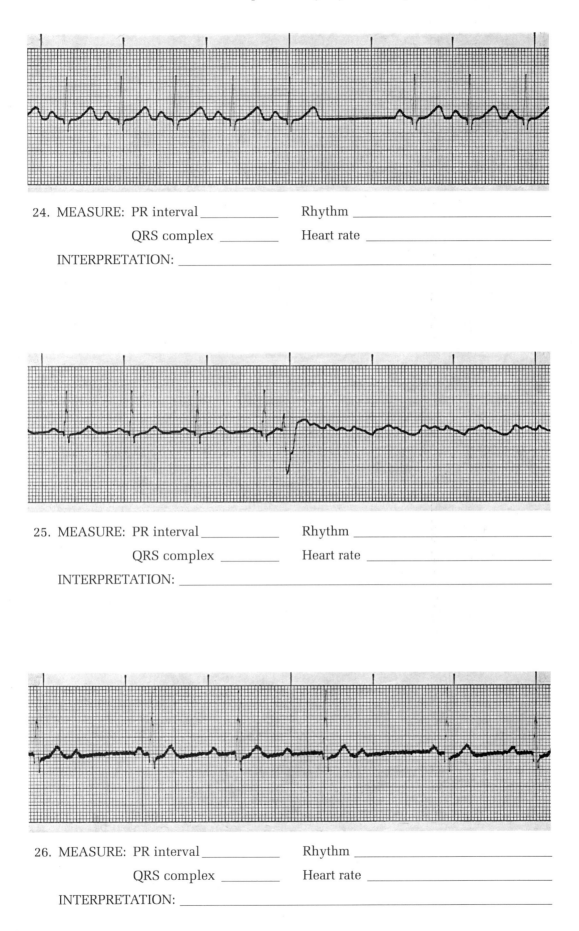

24. MEASURE: PR interval_____   Rhythm _____

    QRS complex _____   Heart rate _____

    INTERPRETATION: _____

25. MEASURE: PR interval_____   Rhythm _____

    QRS complex _____   Heart rate _____

    INTERPRETATION: _____

26. MEASURE: PR interval_____   Rhythm _____

    QRS complex _____   Heart rate _____

    INTERPRETATION: _____

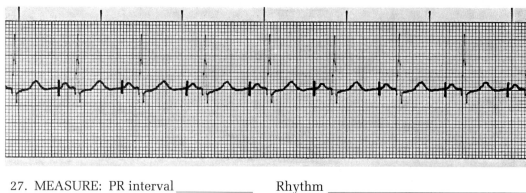

27. MEASURE: PR interval_____   Rhythm _____

    QRS complex _____   Heart rate _____

    INTERPRETATION: _____

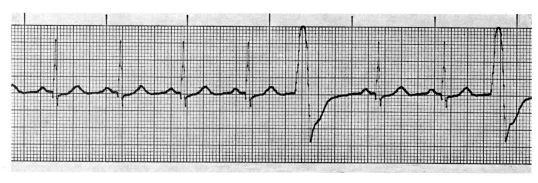

28. MEASURE: PR interval_____   Rhythm _____

    QRS complex _____   Heart rate _____

    INTERPRETATION: _____

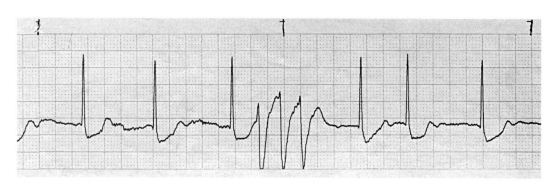

29. MEASURE: PR interval_____   Rhythm _____

    QRS complex _____   Heart rate _____

    INTERPRETATION: _____

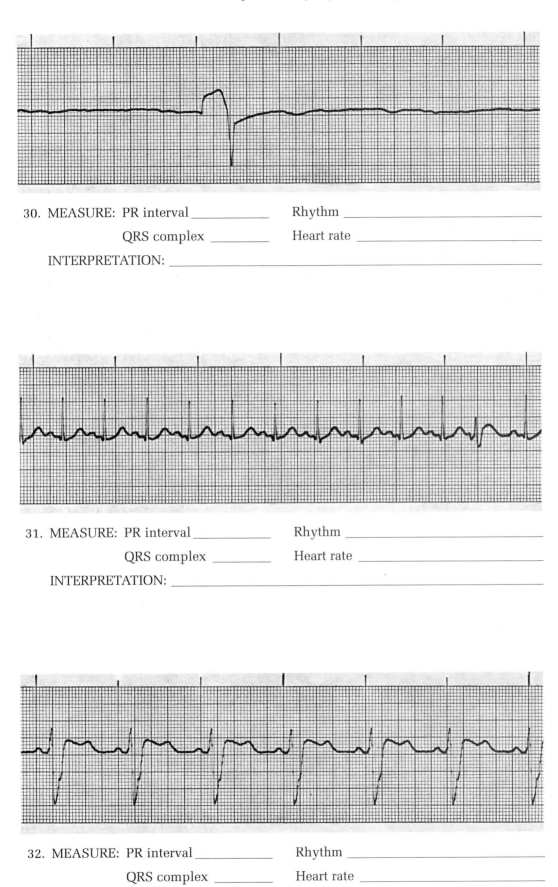

30. MEASURE: PR interval _____   Rhythm _____

                   QRS complex _____   Heart rate _____

     INTERPRETATION: _____

31. MEASURE: PR interval _____   Rhythm _____

                   QRS complex _____   Heart rate _____

     INTERPRETATION: _____

32. MEASURE: PR interval _____   Rhythm _____

                   QRS complex _____   Heart rate _____

     INTERPRETATION: _____

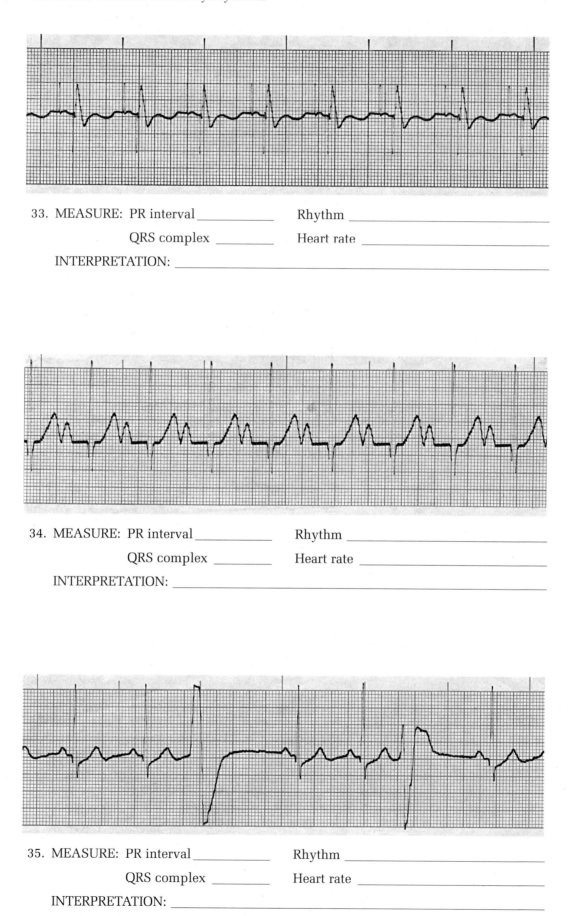

33. MEASURE: PR interval_____   Rhythm _____

QRS complex _____   Heart rate _____

INTERPRETATION: _____

34. MEASURE: PR interval_____   Rhythm _____

QRS complex _____   Heart rate _____

INTERPRETATION: _____

35. MEASURE: PR interval_____   Rhythm _____

QRS complex _____   Heart rate _____

INTERPRETATION: _____

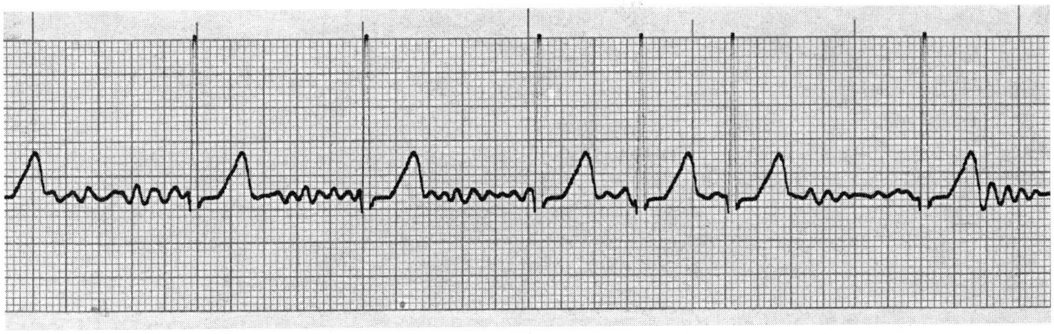

36. MEASURE: PR interval _____   Rhythm _____

               QRS complex _____   Heart rate _____

INTERPRETATION: _____

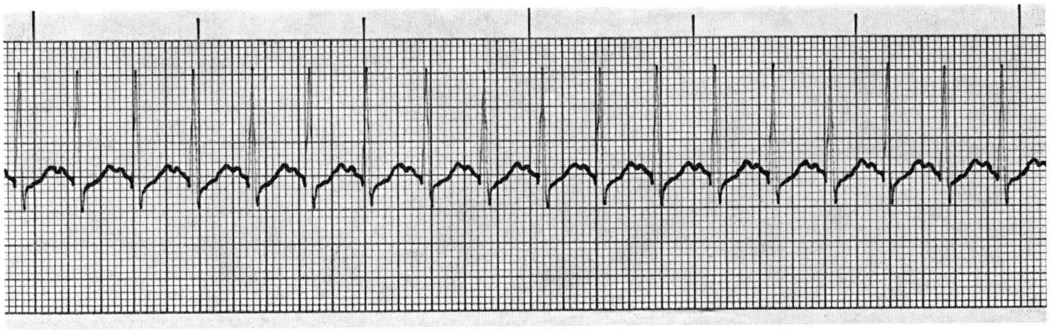

37. MEASURE: PR interval _____   Rhythm _____

               QRS complex _____   Heart rate _____

INTERPRETATION: _____

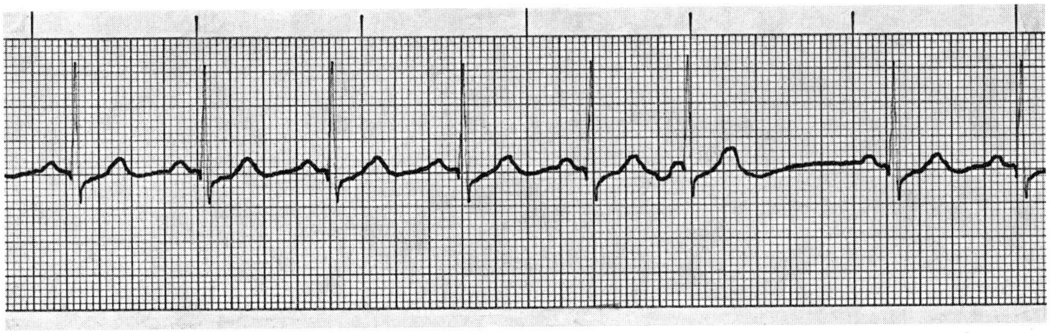

38. MEASURE: PR interval _____   Rhythm _____

               QRS complex _____   Heart rate _____

INTERPRETATION: _____

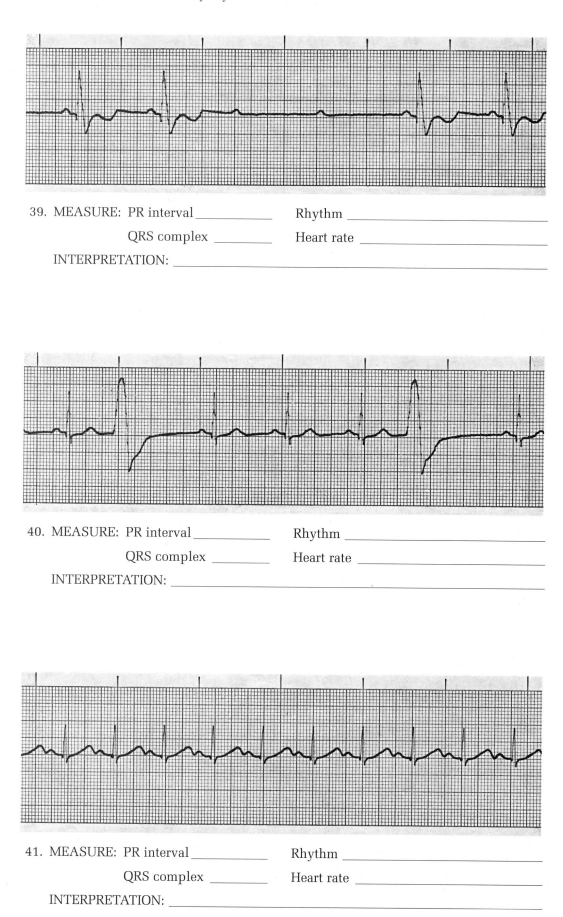

39. MEASURE: PR interval _____   Rhythm _____

              QRS complex _____   Heart rate _____

      INTERPRETATION: _____

40. MEASURE: PR interval _____   Rhythm _____

              QRS complex _____   Heart rate _____

      INTERPRETATION: _____

41. MEASURE: PR interval _____   Rhythm _____

              QRS complex _____   Heart rate _____

      INTERPRETATION: _____

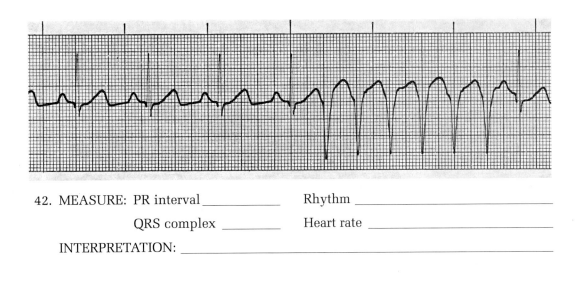

42. MEASURE: PR interval _____   Rhythm _____

QRS complex _____   Heart rate _____

INTERPRETATION: _____

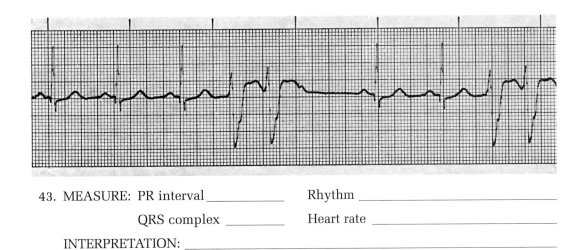

43. MEASURE: PR interval _____   Rhythm _____

QRS complex _____   Heart rate _____

INTERPRETATION: _____

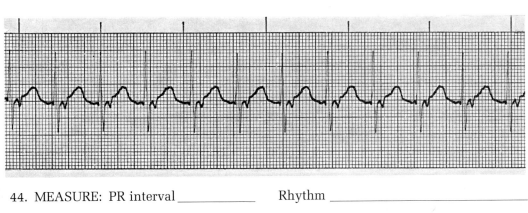

44. MEASURE: PR interval _____   Rhythm _____

QRS complex _____   Heart rate _____

INTERPRETATION: _____

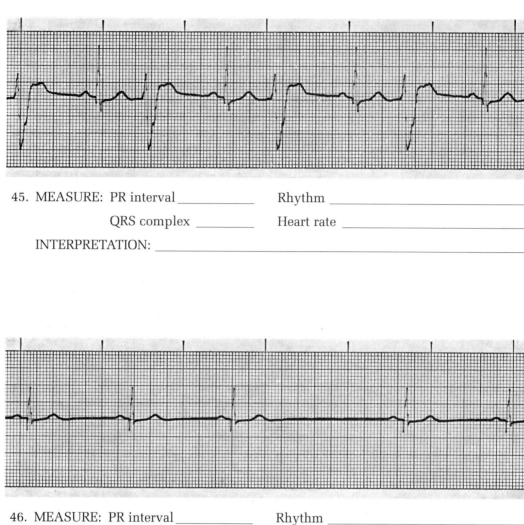

45. MEASURE: PR interval _____   Rhythm _____

              QRS complex _____   Heart rate _____

     INTERPRETATION: _____

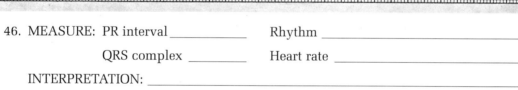

46. MEASURE: PR interval _____   Rhythm _____

              QRS complex _____   Heart rate _____

     INTERPRETATION: _____

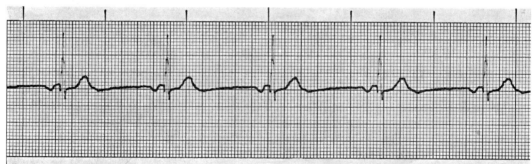

47. MEASURE: PR interval _____   Rhythm _____

              QRS complex _____   Heart rate _____

     INTERPRETATION: _____

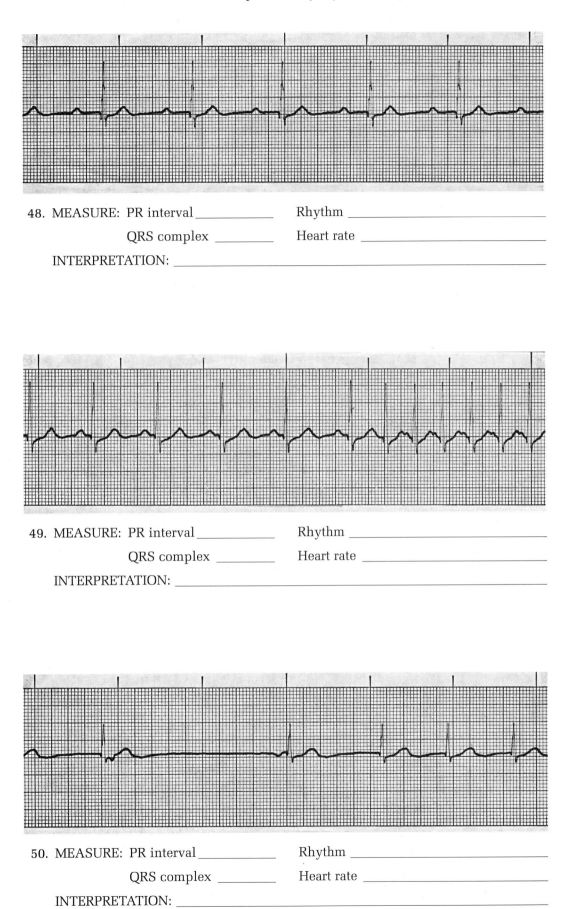

48. MEASURE: PR interval _____   Rhythm _____

                QRS complex _____   Heart rate _____

INTERPRETATION: _____

49. MEASURE: PR interval _____   Rhythm _____

                QRS complex _____   Heart rate _____

INTERPRETATION: _____

50. MEASURE: PR interval _____   Rhythm _____

                QRS complex _____   Heart rate _____

INTERPRETATION: _____

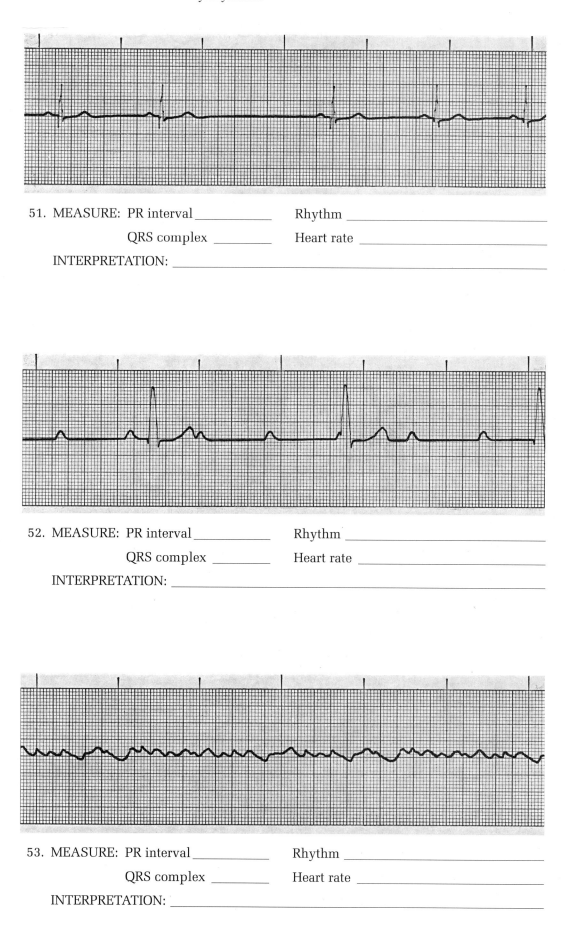

51. MEASURE: PR interval _____   Rhythm _____

              QRS complex _____   Heart rate _____

INTERPRETATION: _____

52. MEASURE: PR interval _____   Rhythm _____

              QRS complex _____   Heart rate _____

INTERPRETATION: _____

53. MEASURE: PR interval _____   Rhythm _____

              QRS complex _____   Heart rate _____

INTERPRETATION: _____

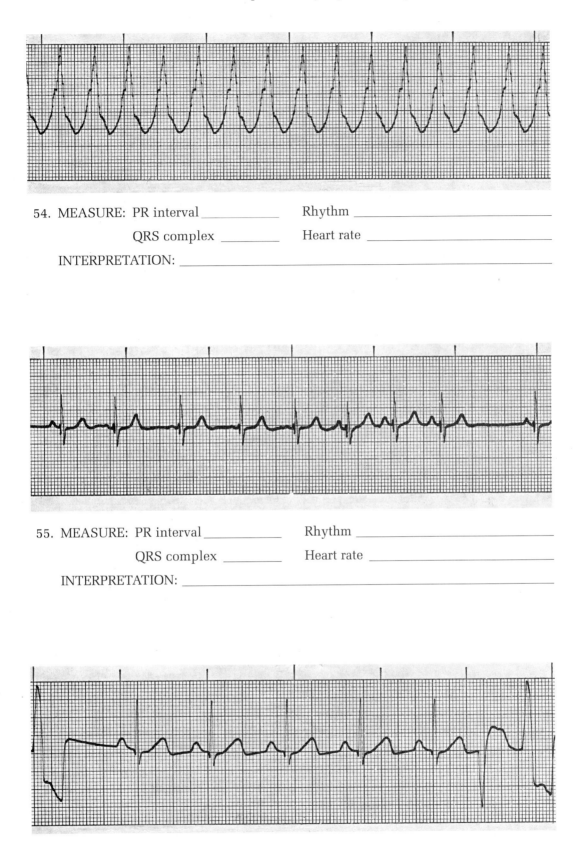

54. MEASURE: PR interval _____   Rhythm _____

QRS complex _____   Heart rate _____

INTERPRETATION: _____

55. MEASURE: PR interval _____   Rhythm _____

QRS complex _____   Heart rate _____

INTERPRETATION: _____

56. MEASURE: PR interval _____   Rhythm _____

QRS complex _____   Heart rate _____

INTERPRETATION: _____

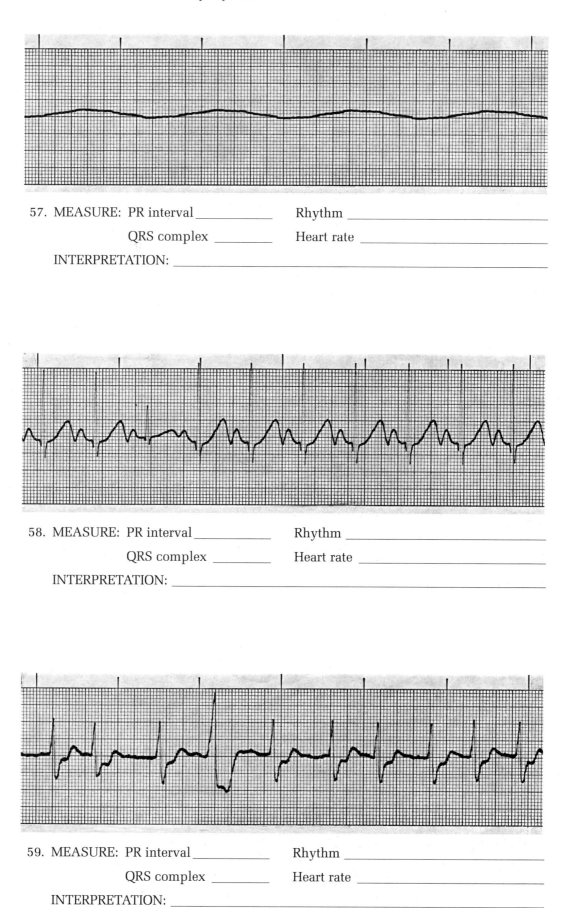

57. MEASURE: PR interval _____   Rhythm _____

QRS complex _____   Heart rate _____

INTERPRETATION: _____

58. MEASURE: PR interval _____   Rhythm _____

QRS complex _____   Heart rate _____

INTERPRETATION: _____

59. MEASURE: PR interval _____   Rhythm _____

QRS complex _____   Heart rate _____

INTERPRETATION: _____

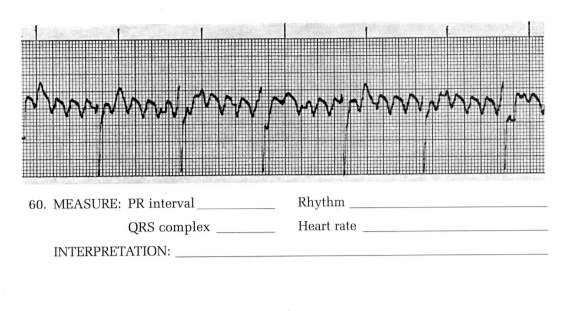

60. MEASURE: PR interval _____   Rhythm _____

QRS complex _____   Heart rate _____

INTERPRETATION: _____

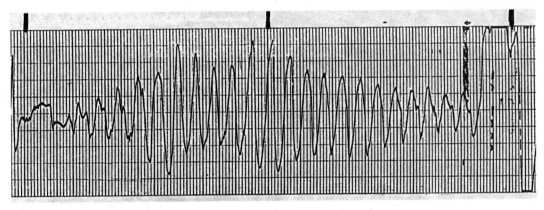

61. MEASURE: PR interval _____   Rhythm _____

QRS complex _____   Heart rate _____

INTERPRETATION: _____

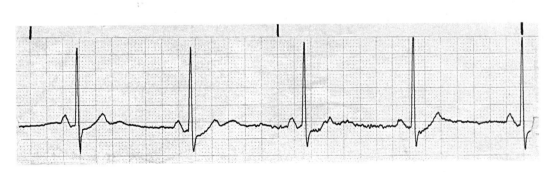

62. MEASURE: PR interval _____   Rhythm _____

QRS complex _____   Heart rate _____

INTERPRETATION: _____

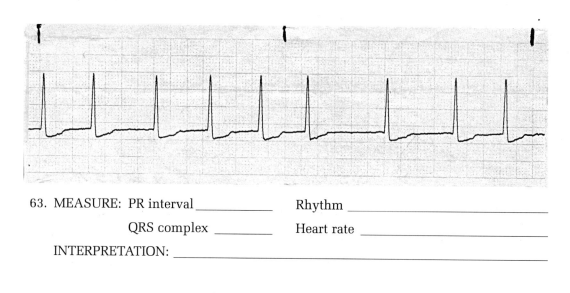

63. MEASURE: PR interval _____   Rhythm _____

    QRS complex _____   Heart rate _____

    INTERPRETATION: _____

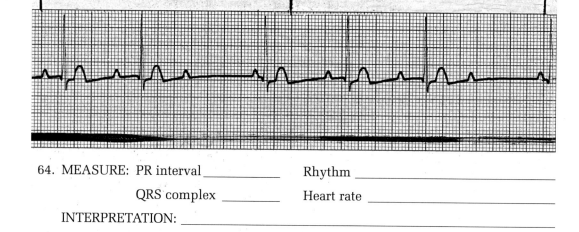

64. MEASURE: PR interval _____   Rhythm _____

    QRS complex _____   Heart rate _____

    INTERPRETATION: _____

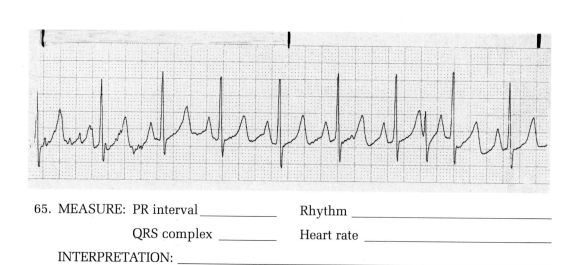

65. MEASURE: PR interval _____   Rhythm _____

    QRS complex _____   Heart rate _____

    INTERPRETATION: _____

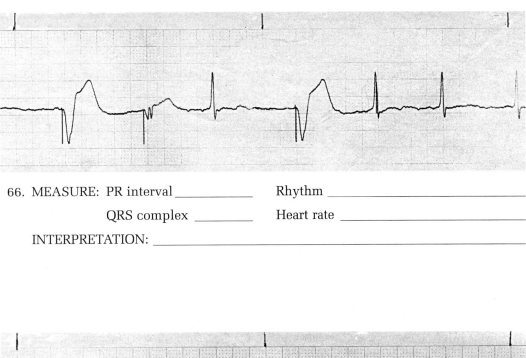

66. MEASURE: PR interval _____   Rhythm _____

               QRS complex _____   Heart rate _____

INTERPRETATION: _____

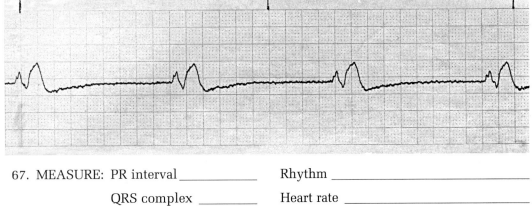

67. MEASURE: PR interval _____   Rhythm _____

               QRS complex _____   Heart rate _____

INTERPRETATION: _____

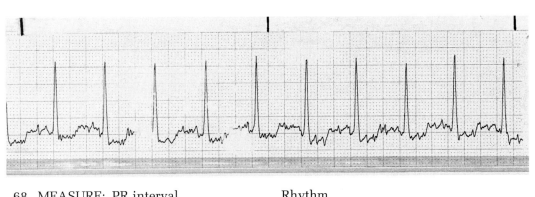

68. MEASURE: PR interval _____   Rhythm _____

               QRS complex _____   Heart rate _____

INTERPRETATION: _____

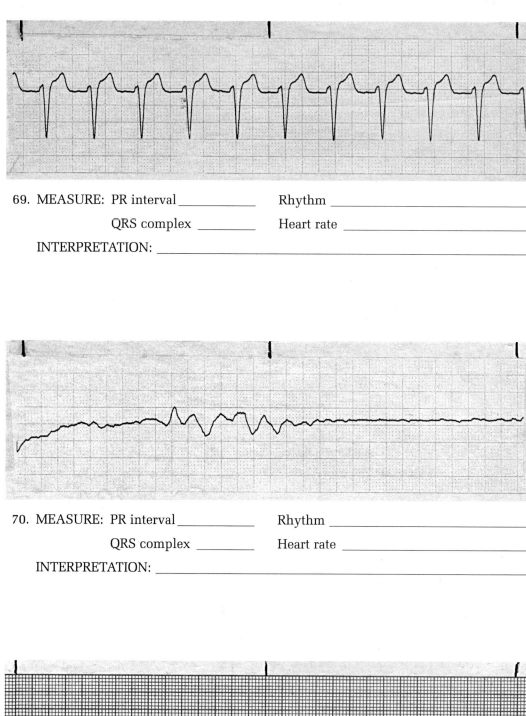

69. MEASURE: PR interval _____   Rhythm _____

    QRS complex _____   Heart rate _____

INTERPRETATION: _____

70. MEASURE: PR interval _____   Rhythm _____

    QRS complex _____   Heart rate _____

INTERPRETATION: _____

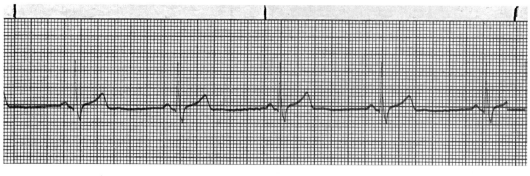

71. MEASURE: PR interval _____   Rhythm _____

    QRS complex _____   Heart rate _____

INTERPRETATION: _____

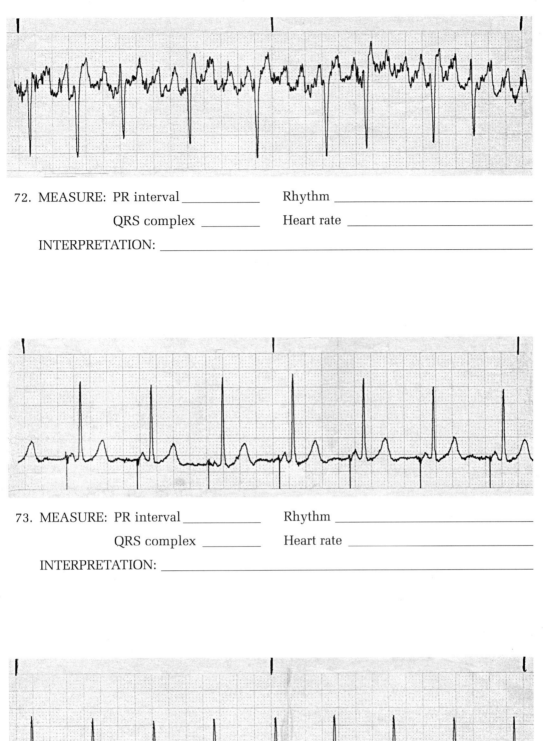

72. MEASURE: PR interval_____   Rhythm_____

    QRS complex_____   Heart rate_____

    INTERPRETATION:_____

73. MEASURE: PR interval_____   Rhythm_____

    QRS complex_____   Heart rate_____

    INTERPRETATION:_____

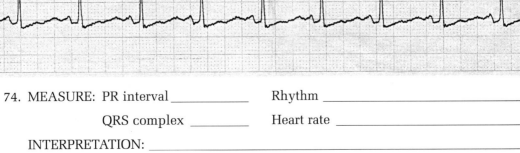

74. MEASURE: PR interval_____   Rhythm_____

    QRS complex_____   Heart rate_____

    INTERPRETATION:_____

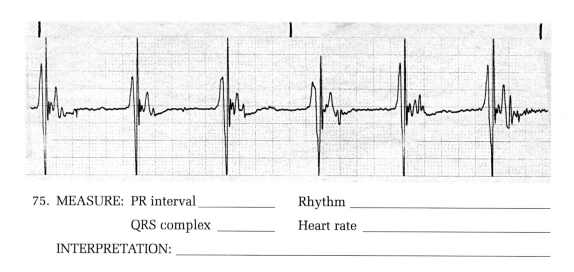

75. MEASURE: PR interval _____   Rhythm _____

              QRS complex _____   Heart rate _____

    INTERPRETATION: _____

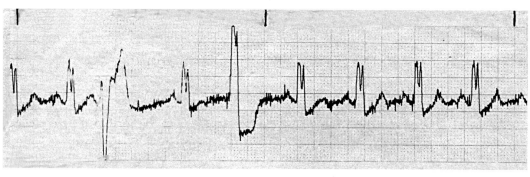

76. MEASURE: PR interval _____   Rhythm _____

              QRS complex _____   Heart rate _____

    INTERPRETATION: _____

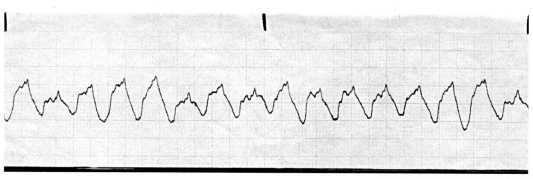

77. MEASURE: PR interval _____   Rhythm _____

              QRS complex _____   Heart rate _____

    INTERPRETATION: _____

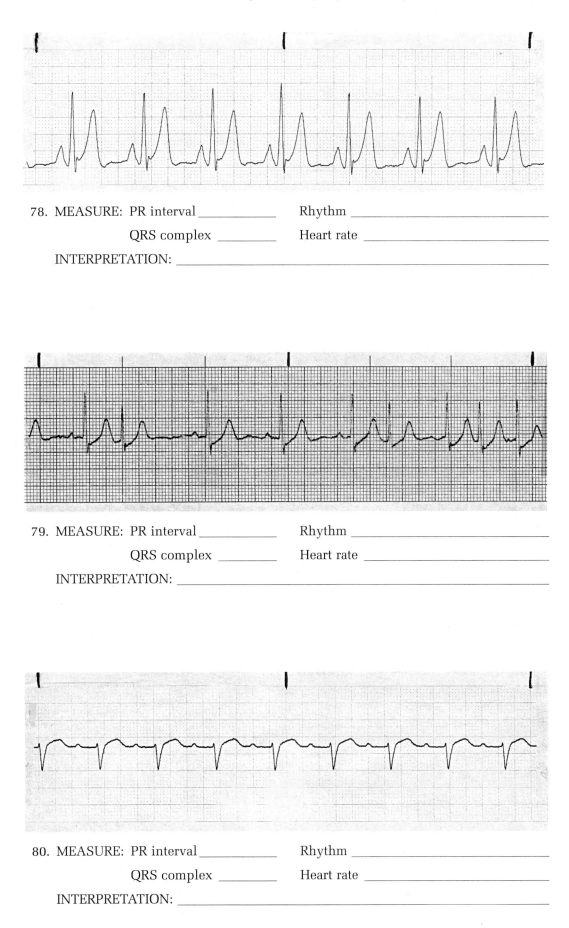

78. MEASURE: PR interval _____   Rhythm _____

    QRS complex _____   Heart rate _____

    INTERPRETATION: _____

79. MEASURE: PR interval _____   Rhythm _____

    QRS complex _____   Heart rate _____

    INTERPRETATION: _____

80. MEASURE: PR interval _____   Rhythm _____

    QRS complex _____   Heart rate _____

    INTERPRETATION: _____

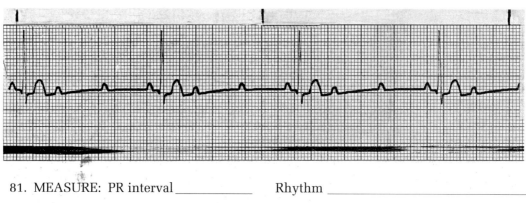

81. MEASURE: PR interval _____   Rhythm _____

    QRS complex _____   Heart rate _____

    INTERPRETATION: _____

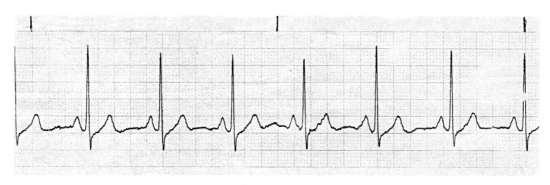

82. MEASURE: PR interval _____   Rhythm _____

    QRS complex _____   Heart rate _____

    INTERPRETATION: _____

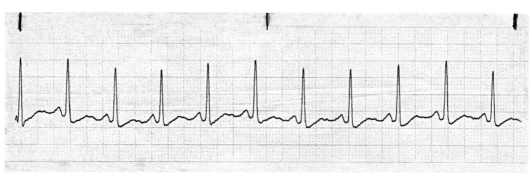

83. MEASURE: PR interval _____   Rhythm _____

    QRS complex _____   Heart rate _____

    INTERPRETATION: _____

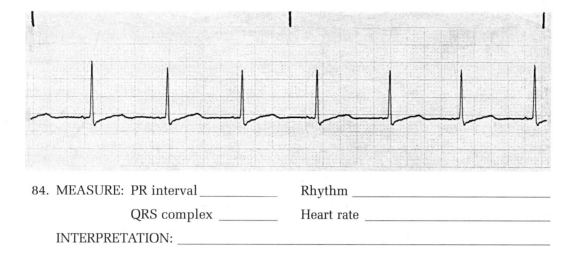

84. MEASURE: PR interval _____   Rhythm _____

                 QRS complex _____   Heart rate _____

INTERPRETATION: _____

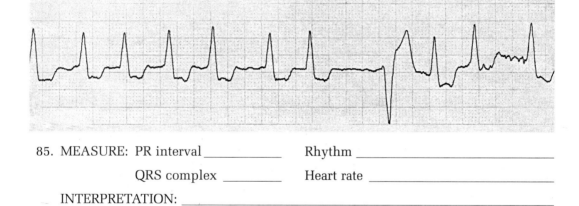

85. MEASURE: PR interval _____   Rhythm _____

                 QRS complex _____   Heart rate _____

INTERPRETATION: _____

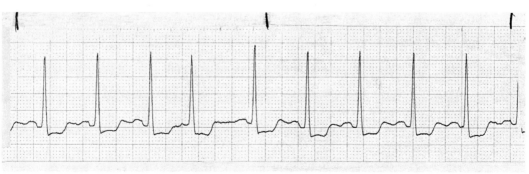

86. MEASURE: PR interval _____   Rhythm _____

                 QRS complex _____   Heart rate _____

INTERPRETATION: _____

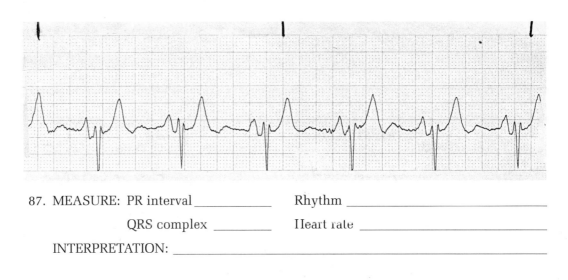

87. MEASURE: PR interval _____   Rhythm _____

             QRS complex _____   Heart rate _____

INTERPRETATION: _____

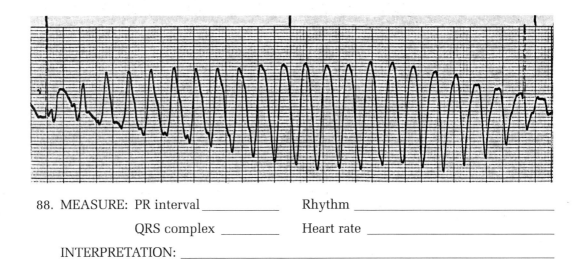

88. MEASURE: PR interval _____   Rhythm _____

             QRS complex _____   Heart rate _____

INTERPRETATION: _____

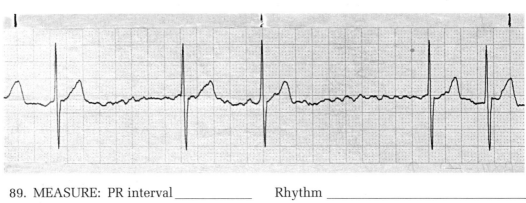

89. MEASURE: PR interval _____   Rhythm _____

             QRS complex _____   Heart rate _____

INTERPRETATION: _____

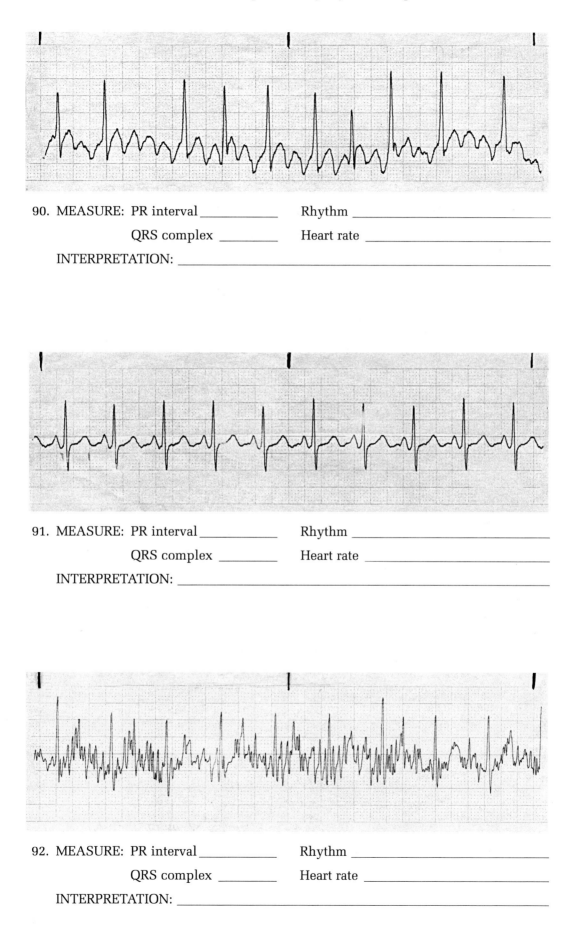

90. MEASURE: PR interval _____   Rhythm _____

                   QRS complex _____   Heart rate _____

     INTERPRETATION: _____

91. MEASURE: PR interval _____   Rhythm _____

                   QRS complex _____   Heart rate _____

     INTERPRETATION: _____

92. MEASURE: PR interval _____   Rhythm _____

                   QRS complex _____   Heart rate _____

     INTERPRETATION: _____

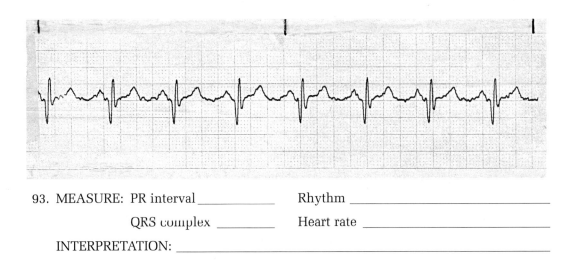

93. MEASURE: PR interval _____   Rhythm _____

QRS complex _____   Heart rate _____

INTERPRETATION: _____

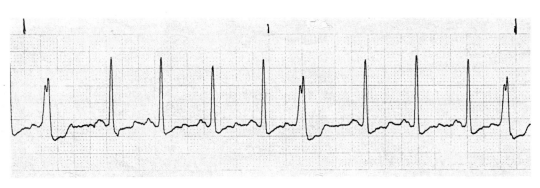

94. MEASURE: PR interval _____   Rhythm _____

QRS complex _____   Heart rate _____

INTERPRETATION: _____

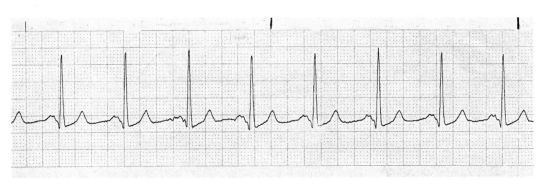

95. MEASURE: PR interval _____   Rhythm _____

QRS complex _____   Heart rate _____

INTERPRETATION: _____

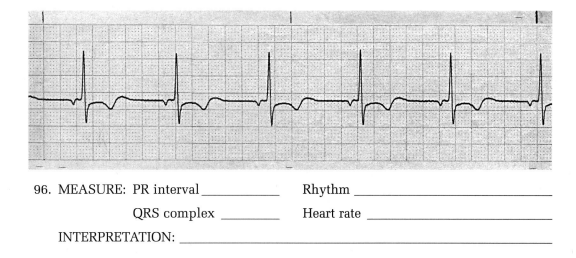

96. MEASURE: PR interval_____   Rhythm _____

QRS complex _____   Heart rate _____

INTERPRETATION: _____

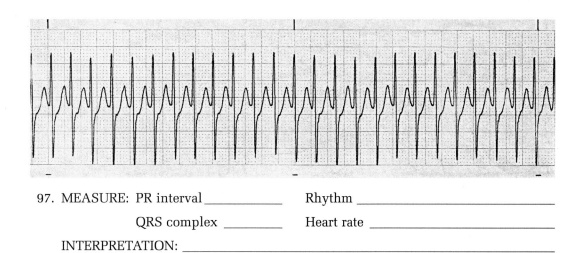

97. MEASURE: PR interval_____   Rhythm _____

QRS complex _____   Heart rate _____

INTERPRETATION: _____

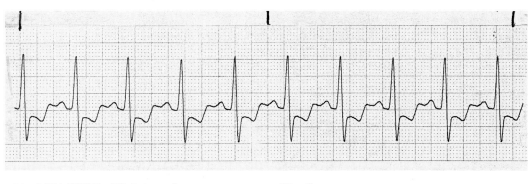

98. MEASURE: PR interval_____   Rhythm _____

QRS complex _____   Heart rate _____

INTERPRETATION: _____

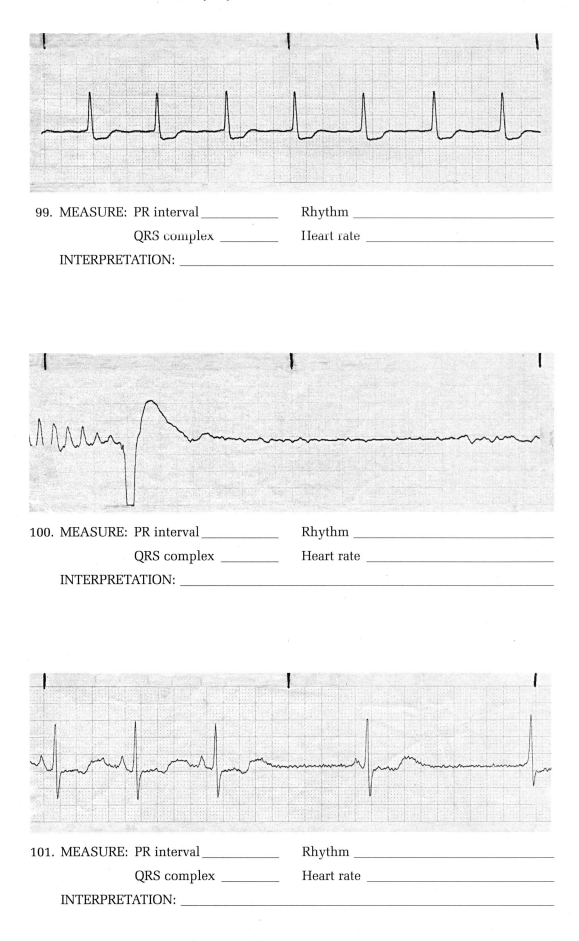

99. MEASURE: PR interval _____   Rhythm _____

                QRS complex _____   Heart rate _____

          INTERPRETATION: _____

100. MEASURE: PR interval _____   Rhythm _____

               QRS complex _____   Heart rate _____

          INTERPRETATION: _____

101. MEASURE: PR interval _____   Rhythm _____

               QRS complex _____   Heart rate _____

          INTERPRETATION: _____

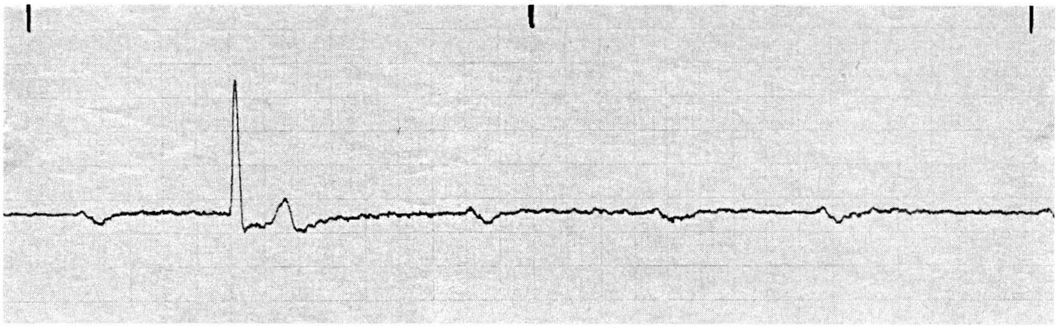

102. MEASURE: PR interval _____   Rhythm _____

QRS complex _____   Heart rate _____

INTERPRETATION: _____

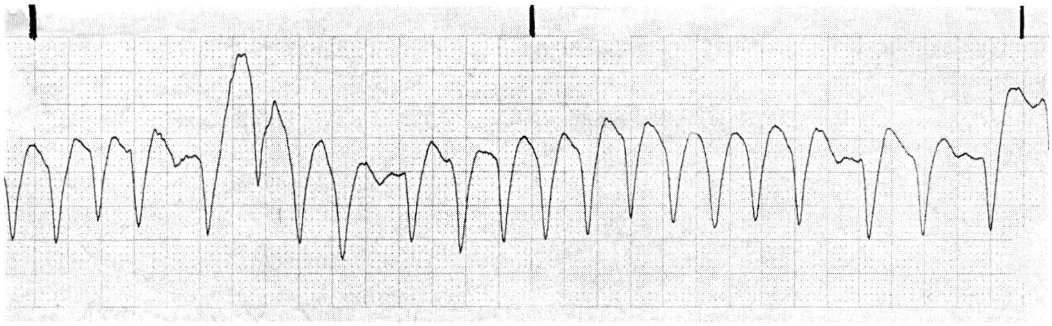

103. MEASURE: PR interval _____   Rhythm _____

QRS complex _____   Heart rate _____

INTERPRETATION: _____

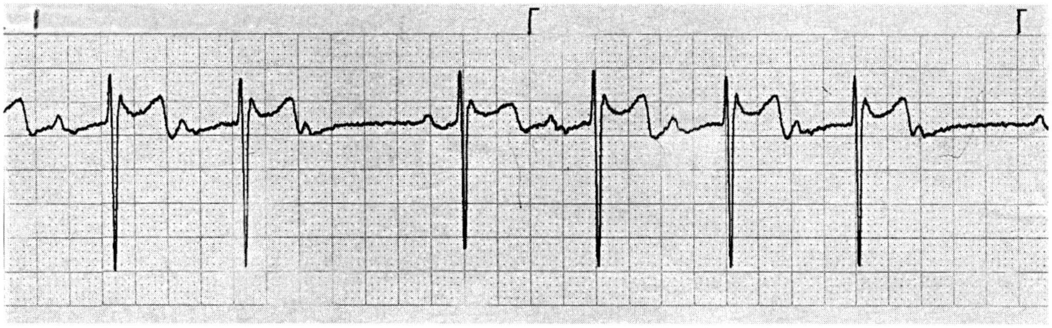

104. MEASURE: PR interval _____   Rhythm _____

QRS complex _____   Heart rate _____

INTERPRETATION: _____

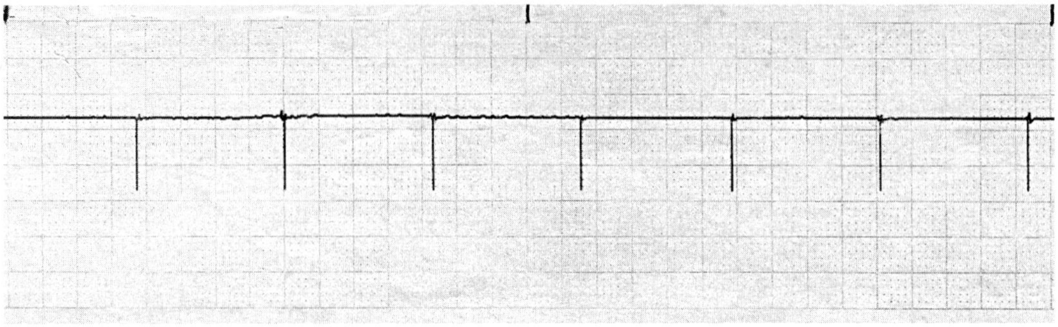

105. MEASURE: PR interval _____   Rhythm _____

QRS complex _____   Heart rate _____

INTERPRETATION: _____

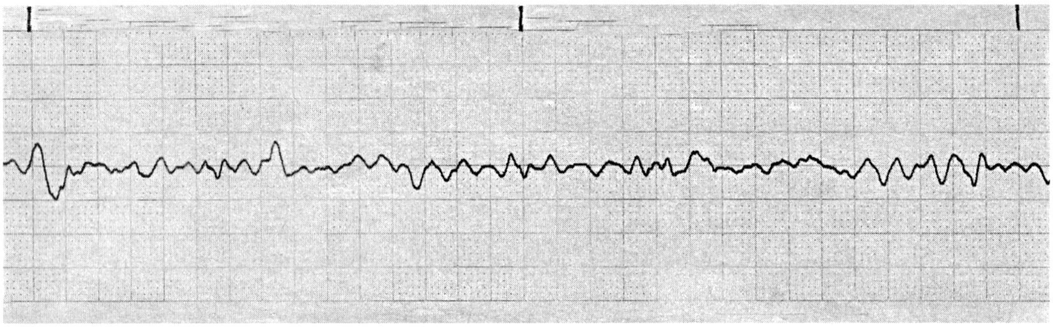

106. MEASURE: PR interval _____   Rhythm _____

QRS complex _____   Heart rate _____

INTERPRETATION: _____

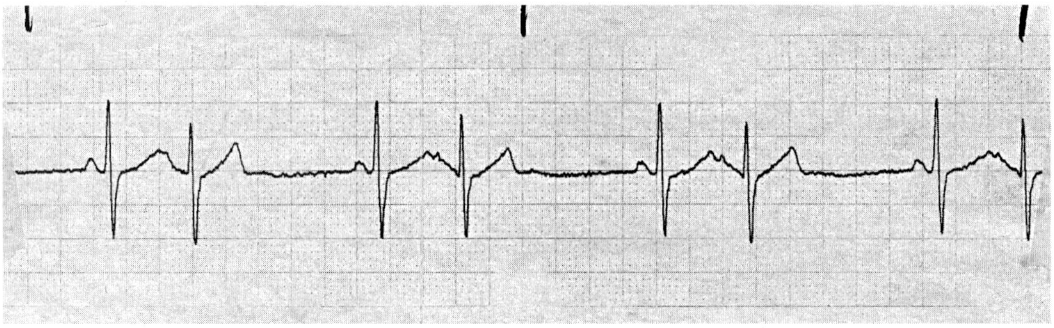

107. MEASURE: PR interval _____   Rhythm _____

QRS complex _____   Heart rate _____

INTERPRETATION: _____

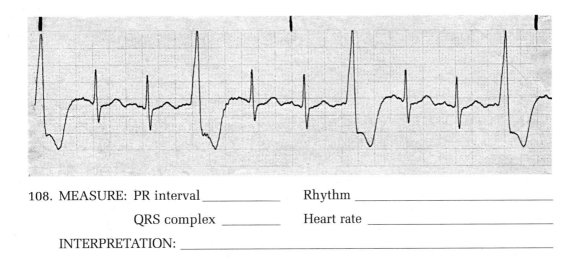

108. MEASURE: PR interval _____   Rhythm _____

QRS complex _____   Heart rate _____

INTERPRETATION: _____

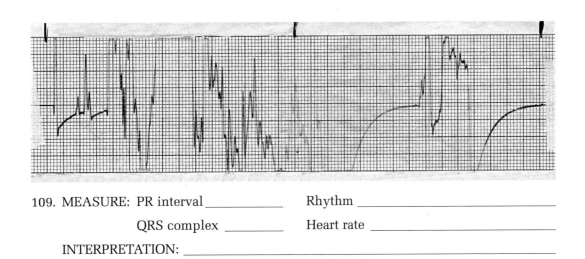

109. MEASURE: PR interval _____   Rhythm _____

QRS complex _____   Heart rate _____

INTERPRETATION: _____

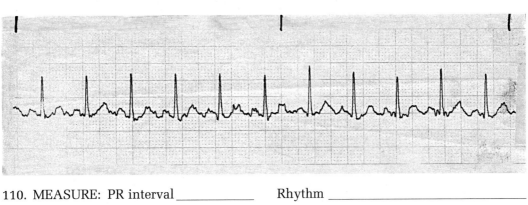

110. MEASURE: PR interval _____   Rhythm _____

QRS complex _____   Heart rate _____

INTERPRETATION: _____

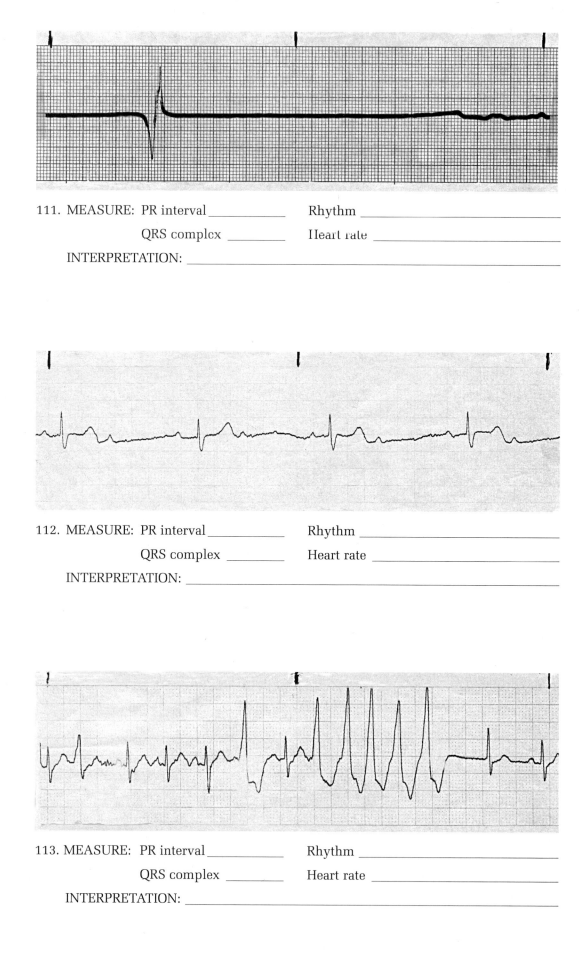

111. MEASURE: PR interval _____   Rhythm _____

     QRS complex _____   Heart rate _____

     INTERPRETATION: _____

112. MEASURE: PR interval _____   Rhythm _____

     QRS complex _____   Heart rate _____

     INTERPRETATION: _____

113. MEASURE: PR interval _____   Rhythm _____

     QRS complex _____   Heart rate _____

     INTERPRETATION: _____

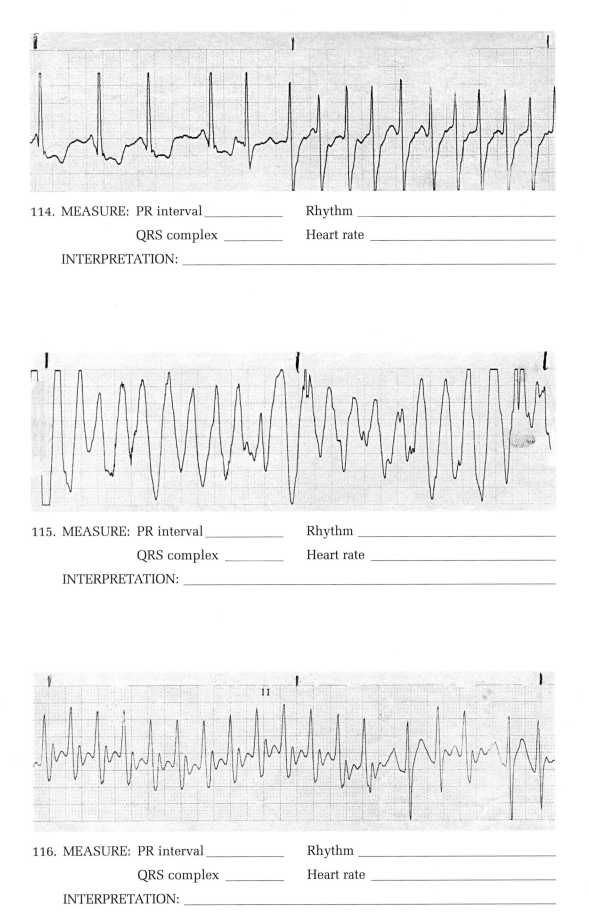

114. MEASURE: PR interval _____   Rhythm _____

                  QRS complex _____   Heart rate _____

     INTERPRETATION: _____

115. MEASURE: PR interval _____   Rhythm _____

                  QRS complex _____   Heart rate _____

     INTERPRETATION: _____

116. MEASURE: PR interval _____   Rhythm _____

                  QRS complex _____   Heart rate _____

     INTERPRETATION: _____

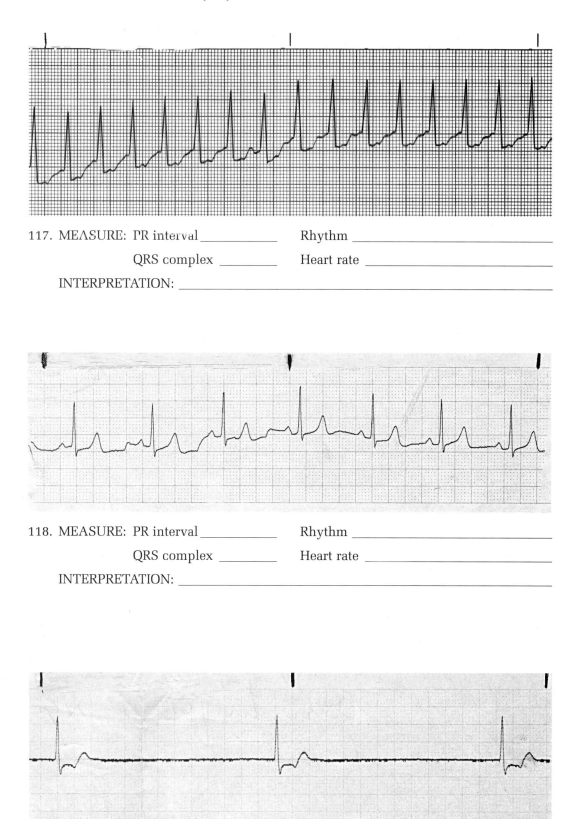

117. MEASURE: PR interval _____   Rhythm _____

     QRS complex _____   Heart rate _____

     INTERPRETATION: _____

118. MEASURE: PR interval _____   Rhythm _____

     QRS complex _____   Heart rate _____

     INTERPRETATION: _____

119. MEASURE: PR interval _____   Rhythm _____

     QRS complex _____   Heart rate _____

     INTERPRETATION: _____

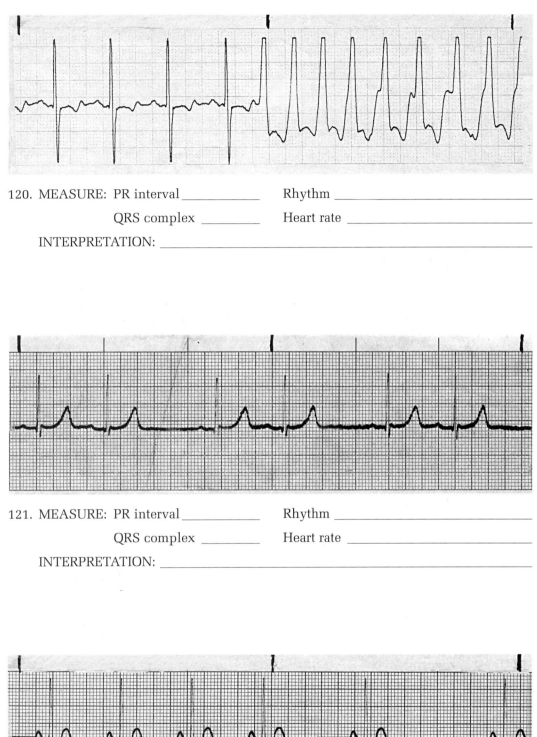

120. MEASURE: PR interval _____   Rhythm _____

QRS complex _____   Heart rate _____

INTERPRETATION: _____

121. MEASURE: PR interval _____   Rhythm _____

QRS complex _____   Heart rate _____

INTERPRETATION: _____

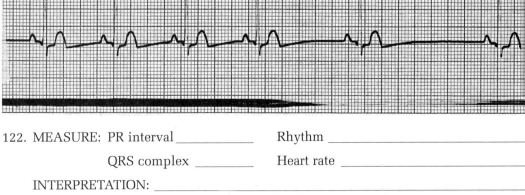

122. MEASURE: PR interval _____   Rhythm _____

QRS complex _____   Heart rate _____

INTERPRETATION: _____

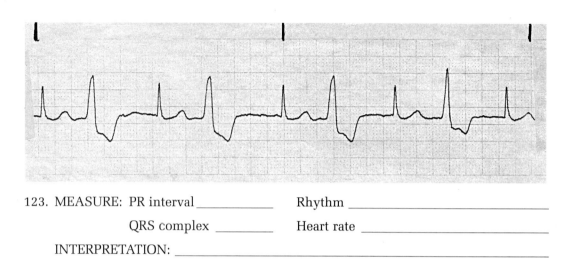

123. MEASURE: PR interval _____   Rhythm _____

QRS complex _____   Heart rate _____

INTERPRETATION: _____

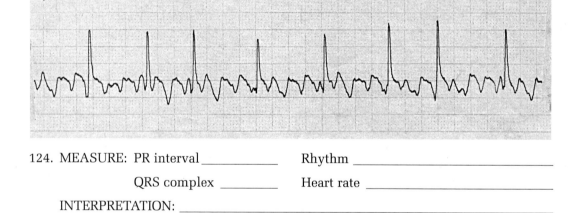

124. MEASURE: PR interval _____   Rhythm _____

QRS complex _____   Heart rate _____

INTERPRETATION: _____

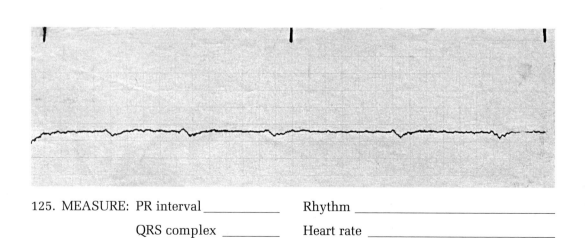

125. MEASURE: PR interval _____   Rhythm _____

QRS complex _____   Heart rate _____

INTERPRETATION: _____

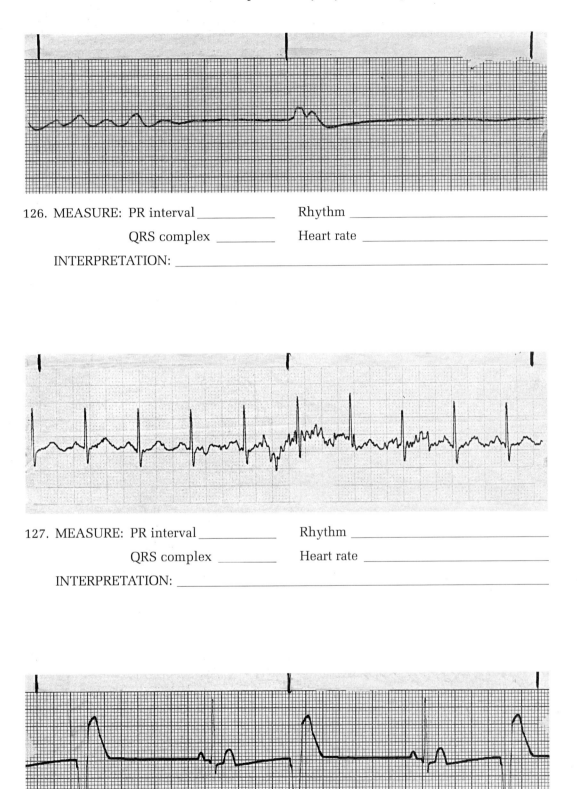

126. MEASURE: PR interval _____   Rhythm _____

              QRS complex _____   Heart rate _____

     INTERPRETATION: _____

127. MEASURE: PR interval _____   Rhythm _____

              QRS complex _____   Heart rate _____

     INTERPRETATION: _____

128. MEASURE: PR interval _____   Rhythm _____

              QRS complex _____   Heart rate _____

     INTERPRETATION: _____

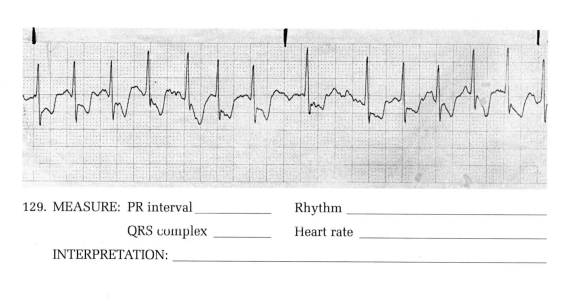

129. MEASURE: PR interval _____   Rhythm _____

QRS complex _____   Heart rate _____

INTERPRETATION: _____

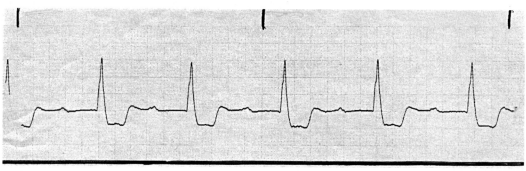

130. MEASURE: PR interval _____   Rhythm _____

QRS complex _____   Heart rate _____

INTERPRETATION: _____

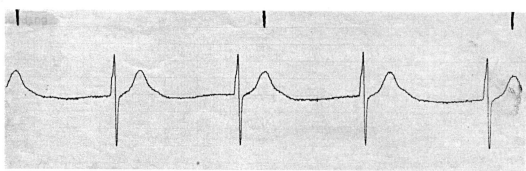

131. MEASURE: PR interval _____   Rhythm _____

QRS complex _____   Heart rate _____

INTERPRETATION: _____

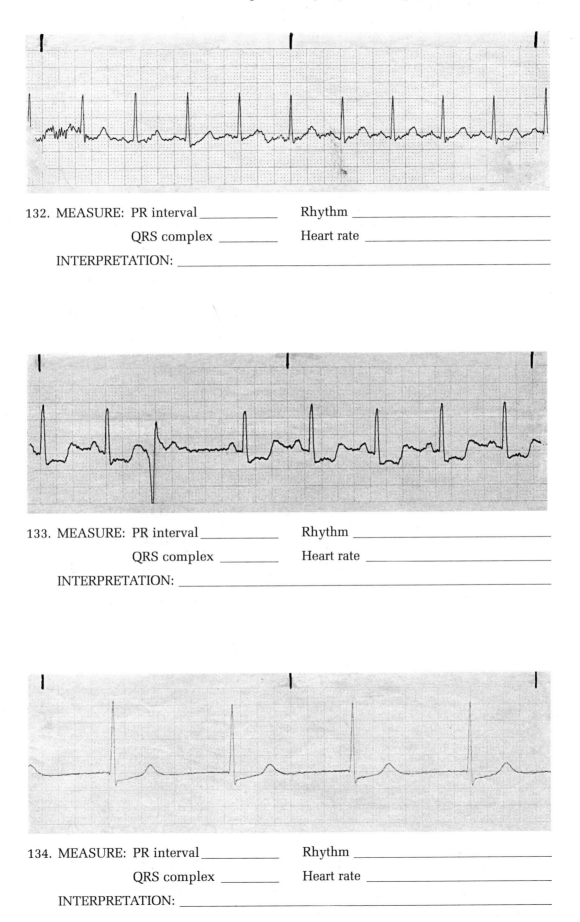

132. MEASURE: PR interval _____   Rhythm _____

QRS complex _____   Heart rate _____

INTERPRETATION: _____

133. MEASURE: PR interval _____   Rhythm _____

QRS complex _____   Heart rate _____

INTERPRETATION: _____

134. MEASURE: PR interval _____   Rhythm _____

QRS complex _____   Heart rate _____

INTERPRETATION: _____

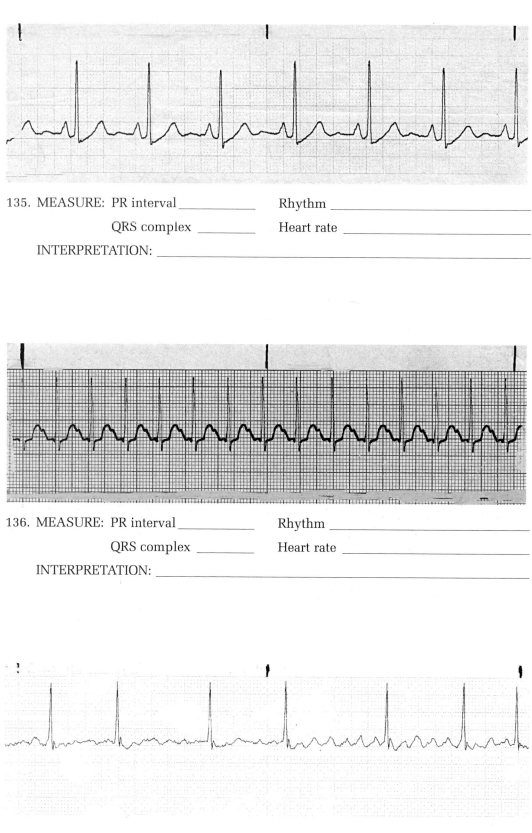

135. MEASURE: PR interval _____   Rhythm _____

               QRS complex _____   Heart rate _____

     INTERPRETATION: _____

136. MEASURE: PR interval _____   Rhythm _____

               QRS complex _____   Heart rate _____

     INTERPRETATION: _____

137. MEASURE: PR interval _____   Rhythm _____

               QRS complex _____   Heart rate _____

     INTERPRETATION: _____

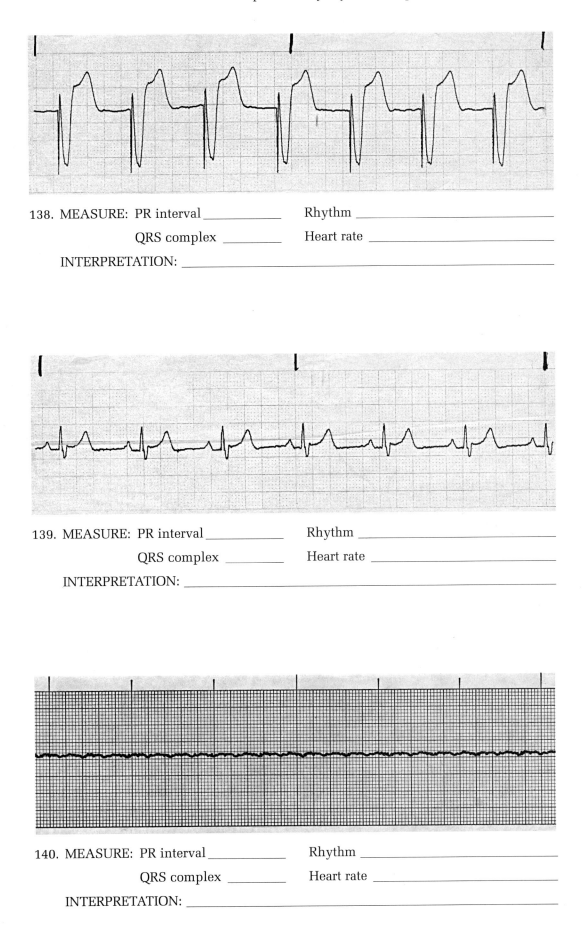

138. MEASURE: PR interval _____   Rhythm _____

QRS complex _____   Heart rate _____

INTERPRETATION: _____

139. MEASURE: PR interval _____   Rhythm _____

QRS complex _____   Heart rate _____

INTERPRETATION: _____

140. MEASURE: PR interval _____   Rhythm _____

QRS complex _____   Heart rate _____

INTERPRETATION: _____

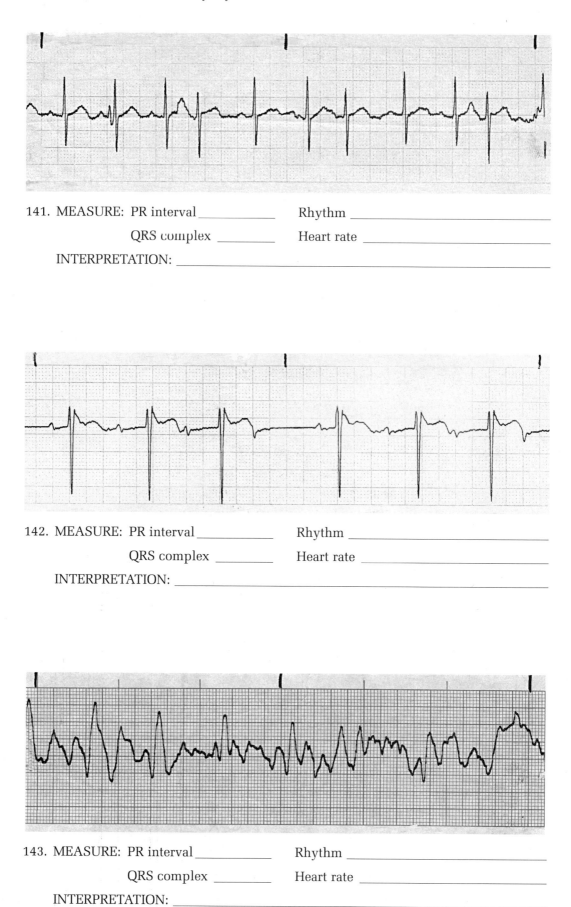

141. MEASURE: PR interval _____   Rhythm _____

QRS complex _____   Heart rate _____

INTERPRETATION: _____

142. MEASURE: PR interval _____   Rhythm _____

QRS complex _____   Heart rate _____

INTERPRETATION: _____

143. MEASURE: PR interval _____   Rhythm _____

QRS complex _____   Heart rate _____

INTERPRETATION: _____

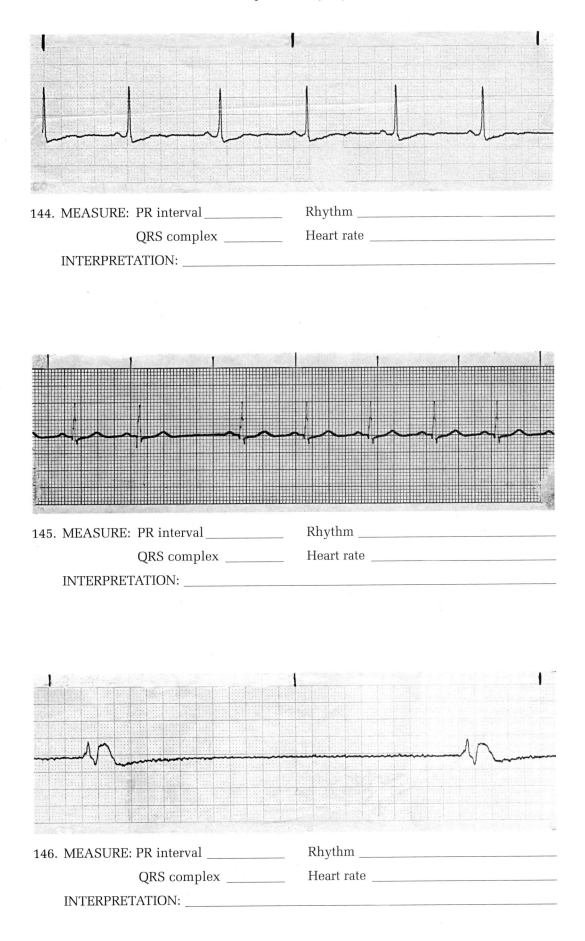

144. MEASURE: PR interval _____   Rhythm _____

QRS complex _____   Heart rate _____

INTERPRETATION: _____

145. MEASURE: PR interval _____   Rhythm _____

QRS complex _____   Heart rate _____

INTERPRETATION: _____

146. MEASURE: PR interval _____   Rhythm _____

QRS complex _____   Heart rate _____

INTERPRETATION: _____

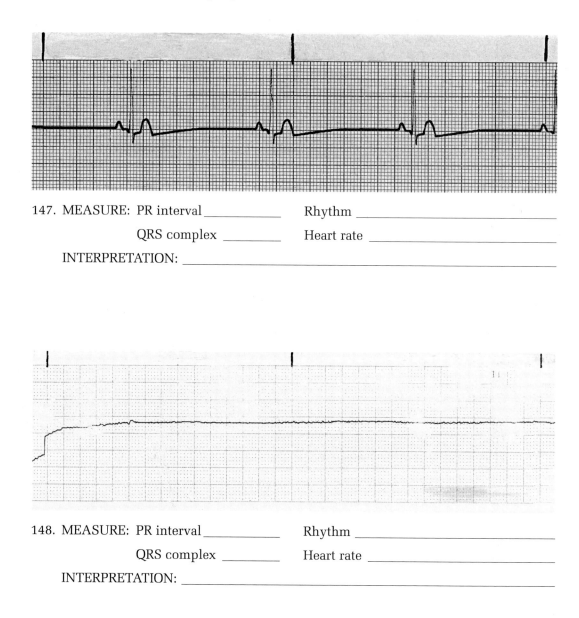

147. MEASURE: PR interval _____   Rhythm _____

                QRS complex _____   Heart rate _____

      INTERPRETATION: _____

148. MEASURE: PR interval _____   Rhythm _____

                QRS complex _____   Heart rate _____

      INTERPRETATION: _____

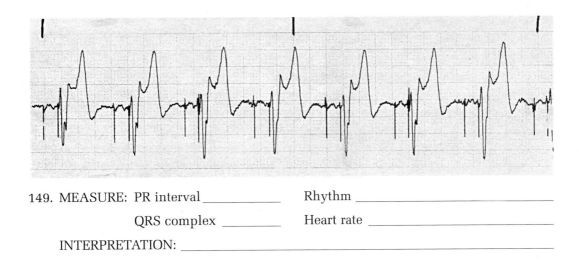

149. MEASURE: PR interval_____   Rhythm _____

QRS complex _____   Heart rate _____

INTERPRETATION: _____

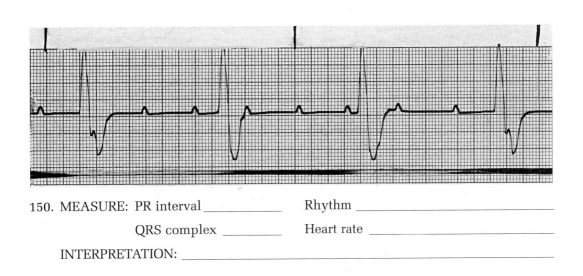

150. MEASURE: PR interval_____   Rhythm _____

QRS complex _____   Heart rate _____

INTERPRETATION: _____

Case Studies

This chapter uses case studies to help you "put it all together." Case studies are an excellent way to learn and remember new material. They increase your ability to relate signs and symptoms to patient care, and to recognize potential patient problems. Each case study is based on an actual patient situation.

To use the case studies, first identify the dysrhythmia and then determine the appropriate treatments based on that identification and on patient assessments. You are encouraged to use these case studies and to also make up additional situations. Just as interpreting rhythm strips becomes easier with practice, so will patient assessments and treatments.

Chapter Eleven

CASE STUDY 1

You are caring for a 76-year-old patient who complains that her heart is "racing." You assess the patient and find vital signs are blood pressure (BP) of 130/60, heart rate (HR) of 140, and a respiratory rate (RR) of 28. The monitor displays the rhythm shown in Fig. 11-1.

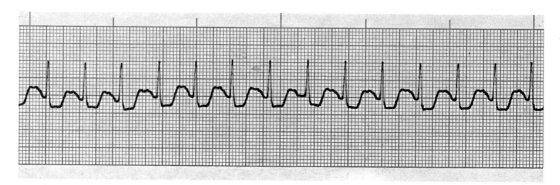

Fig. 11-1

1-A You identify the rhythm as _____.

You talk with the patient and find that she is anxious about some tests that are scheduled for the afternoon. You notice several empty coffee cups and many partially smoked cigarettes in an ashtray.

1-B Your next actions include:

1) _____

2) _____

3) _____

You notice that the patient looks less anxious. The monitor now displays the rhythm shown in Fig. 11-2.

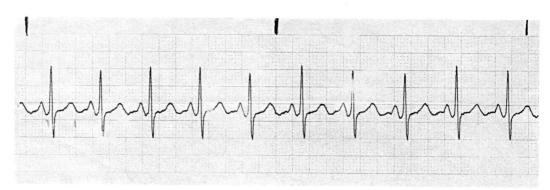

Fig. 11-2

1-C You identify the rhythm as _____.

You reassess the patient and find a BP of 128/68, a HR of 100, and a RR of 22. You continue monitoring the patient for any further dysrhythmias.

CASE STUDY 2

A patient is brought to your unit complaining of dizzy spells and passing out. The monitor displays the rhythm shown in Fig. 11-3.

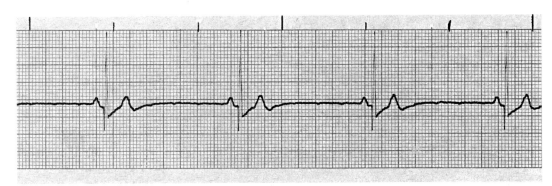

Fig. 11-3

2-A You identify the rhythm as _____.

You assess the patient and find signs of poor cardiac output including pale, cool skin; sweating; cyanosis of lips and nail beds. The patient is complaining of chest pain. Vital signs are: BP 80/45, HR 40, RR 24 and labored. You have standing orders to treat patients with life threatening dysrhythmias until the doctor arrives.

2-B Your initial actions are:

1) _____

2) _____

3) _____

4) _____

On reassessment, the patient has improved slightly and the vital signs are BP 86/48, HR 48, and RR 22.

2-C You repeat _____.

2-D You also initiate the use of a _____.

The patient shows signs of improvement. His skin is pink, warm, and dry. There is no cyanosis, and the patient denies chest pain. The BP is 100/63, HR 70, and RR 20 and even. The monitor displays the rhythm shown in Fig. 11-4.

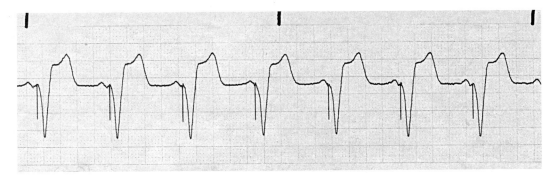

Fig. 11-4

2-E You identify this rhythm as _____.

2-F You should be sure the rhythm has 1) _____ capture, even if it is not 100%

2) _____.

The doctor arrives and preparations are started for a permanent pacemaker.

CASE STUDY 3

A new patient is admitted to your unit. During the assessment, you find the patient's vital signs are BP 120/80, HR 80, and RR 20. You place the patient on a monitor which displays the rhythm shown in Fig. 11-5.

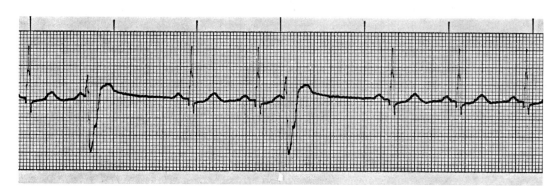

Fig. 11-5

3-A You identify the rhythm as _____.

You place a call to the physician. Before the physician can return your call, you see the rhythm on the monitor has changed to that shown in Fig. 11-6.

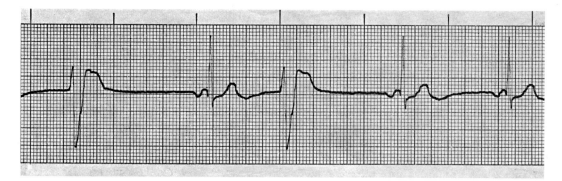

Fig. 11-6

3-B You identify the new rhythm as _____.

3-C You initiate the following treatments:

1) _____

2) _____

3) _____

You reassess the patient and find her vital signs to be BP 102/60, HR 50, and RR 26. The patient is pale, cool, clammy, anxious, and lethargic.

3-D You immediately _____. The patient's color improves and she is more alert. The BP is now 110/70, HR 80, RR 22. The monitor now displays the rhythm seen in Fig. 11-7.

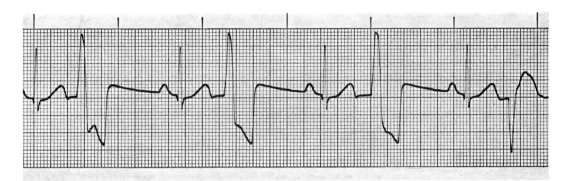

Fig. 11-7

3-E You identify the rhythm as _____.

3-F The physician has arrived and orders a bolus of 1) _____

followed by a continuous infusion of 2) _____.

You continue to monitor the patient for any change in the rhythm, especially for any of the "danger signs."

3-G These "danger signs" include:

1) _____

2) _____

3) _____

4) _____

5) _____

CASE STUDY 4

A patient is admitted to the emergency department. You assess the patient and find that he is pale, diaphoretic, and complaining of chest pain. His vital signs include a blood pressure of 100/50, a heart rate of 170, and respirations of 24.

You place the patient on a monitor, which shows the rhythm found in Fig. 11-8.

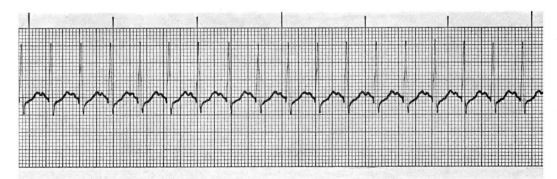

Fig. 11-8

4-A You recognize the dysrhythmia as _____.

4-B The physician initiates vagal maneuvers including 1)_____ and

2) _____. You find no change in the patient after reassessment.

4-C The doctor then orders the following treatments:

1) _____

2) _____

3) _____

4) _____

5) _____

You reassess the patient and find there is still no change in the patient's condition. The physician decides to cardiovert the patient.

4-D You prepare to cardiovert the patient by administering a sedative, being

sure the defibrillator is set for _____ cardioversion.

After the cardioversion, you assess the patient and find the monitor is now displaying the rhythm shown in Fig. 11-9.

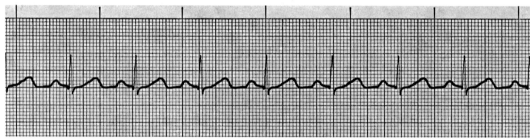

Fig. 11-9

4-E You identify the rhythm as _____.

The patient's vital signs now are BP 110/64, HR 70, RR 20. You continue to monitor the patient for any change in rhythm or condition.

CASE STUDY 5

A 27-year-old male is brought to the first-aid station, complaining of weakness and dizziness. After assessing the patient you find that he is diaphoretic, pale, and his vital signs are BP 138/66, HR 110, and RR 36. The patient has been jogging. He denies any pain. You place him on a monitor, which displays the rhythm seen in Fig. 11-10.

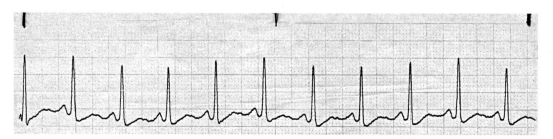

Fig. 11-10

5-A You identify the rhythm as _____.

5-B Your initial treatment of this patient includes:

  1) _____

  2) _____

  3) _____

  4) _____

After the patient has rested for twenty minutes, you reassess the patient. The monitor now shows the rhythm seen in Fig. 11-11.

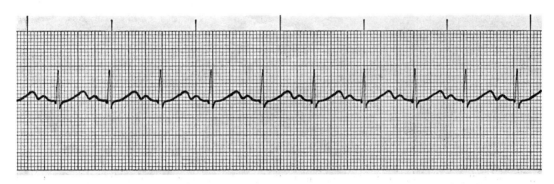

Fig. 11-11

5-C You identify the rhythm as _____.

5-D You expect to see the patient's symptoms:

  1) continue to improve

  2) worsen

  3) remain unchanged

CASE STUDY 6

A patient is admitted to your unit after being treated in the emergency department for an overdose. The monitor displays the rhythm shown in Fig. 11-12.

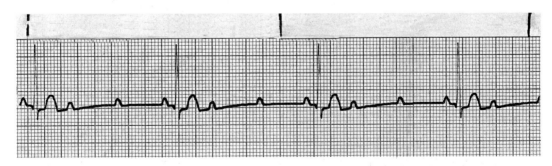

Fig. 11-12

6-A You identify the rhythm as _____.

You assess the patient and find he is clammy, hypotensive, and pale. Vital signs are BP 93/45, HR 40, and RR 18.

You call the physician. Anticipating his orders, you prepare the following medications and begin the following treatments.

6-B

1) _____

2) _____

3) _____

4) _____

You reassess the patient and find the vital signs are BP 94/55, HR 40, and RR 22. The monitor shows the patient's rhythm in Fig. 11-13.

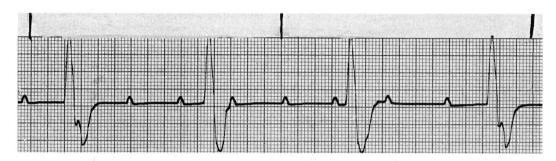

Fig. 11-13

6-C You identify this dysrhythmia as _____ .

6-D The physician arrives and initiates a _____ .

6-E The physician then orders the surgery crew to get ready to implant a _____

_____

CASE STUDY 7

You are watching the monitors in the unit and notice that one patient has an episode of R on T phenomenon. The monitor now shows the rhythm found in Fig. 11-14.

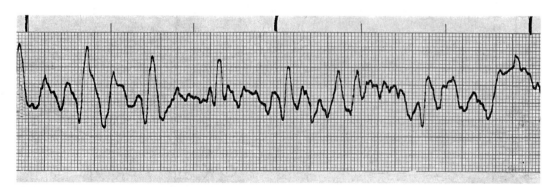

Fig. 11-14

7-A You identify the rhythm as _____ .

7-B You immediately rush to the patient's room and your first action is to _____

_____ .

You find the patient awake, alert, and talking on the telephone.

7-C Your next actions include:

1) _____

2) _____

3) _____

CASE STUDY 8

You are a member of the ambulance crew responding to a 911 call for an unresponsive male. When you arrive at the scene, you assess the patient while another crew member puts the patient on a monitor. You see the rhythm shown in Fig. 11-15.

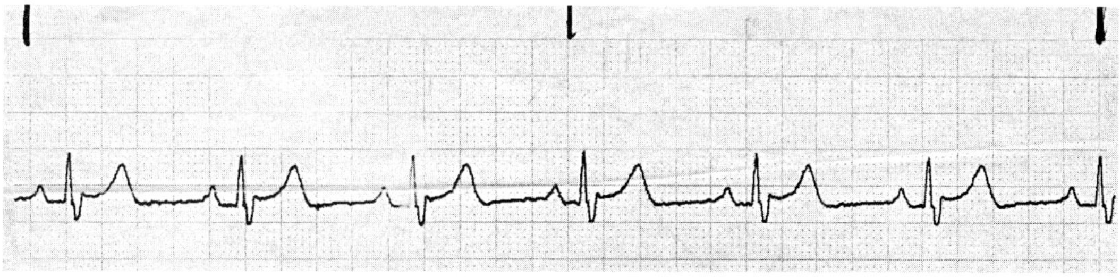

Fig. 11-15

8-A You identify the rhythm on the monitor as _____ .
However, you found no vital signs during your assessment.

8-B You correctly identify the dysrhythmia as _____ .

8-C You immediately begin the following treatment:

1) _____

2) _____

3) _____

4) _____

5) _____

6) _____

After transporting the patient to the nearest hospital, the emergency department physician reassesses the patient.

8-D The physician decides to perform a pericardiocentesis to relieve a _____

_____ .

8-E Other causes of PEA include:

1) _____

2) _____

3) _____

After the procedure, the patient's dysrhythmia converts to the rhythm shown in Fig. 11- 16.

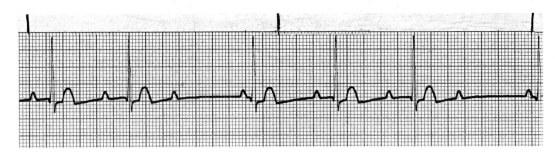

Fig. 11-16

8-F The rhythm is identified as _____.

The vital signs are now BP 90/60, HR 50 to 60, and RR 16.

8-G You continue to _____.

CASE STUDY 9

A patient's monitor on your unit suddenly shows the dysrhythmia seen in Fig. 11-17.

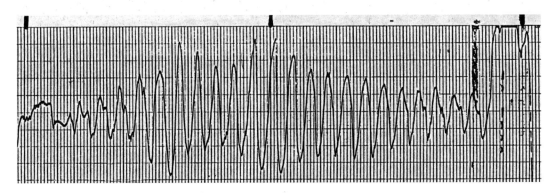

Fig. 11-17

9-A You identify the dysrhythmia as _____.

A careful assessment of the patient indicates signs of poor cardiac output.

9-B These include:

1) _____

2) _____

3) _____

4) _____

5) _____

6) _____

7) _____

8) _____

9-C Your initial treatment includes:

1) _____

2) _____

3) _____

4) _____

5) _____

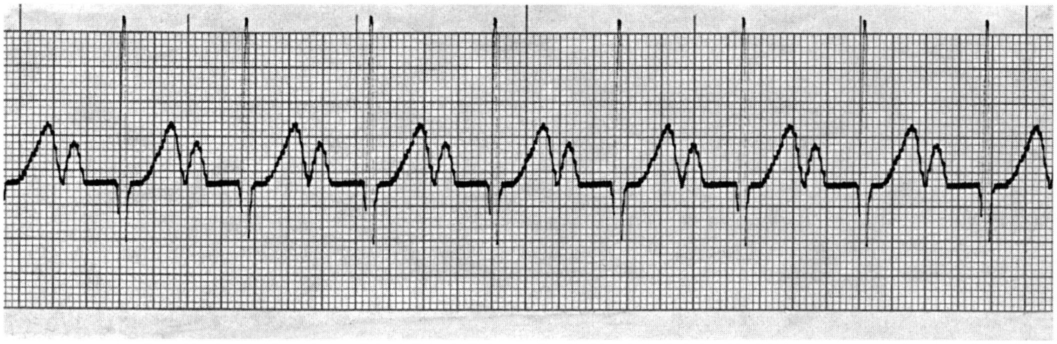

Fig. 11-18

9-D The patient converts to the rhythm shown in Fig. 11-18, which you iden-

tify as _____.

The patient no longer shows signs of poor cardiac output. You continue to monitor the patient.

CASE STUDY 10

A patient returns to the cardiac care unit (CCU) after a minor procedure. On assessment, the patient has vital signs of BP 115/88, HR 50, and RR 20. An IV is infusing and the monitor displays the rhythm found in Fig. 11-19.

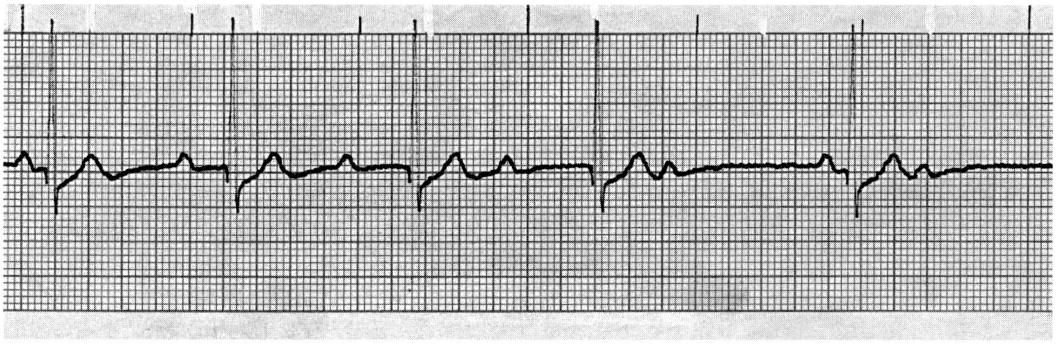

Fig. 11-19

10-A You identified the rhythm as _____.

10-B Your next actions are to:

1) _____

2) _____

After observing the patient for several hours, you see the rhythm shown in Fig. 11-20 on the monitor.

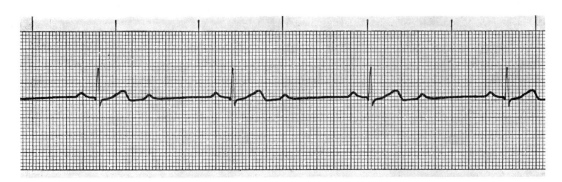

Fig. 11-20

10-C You identify the rhythm as _____ .

The patient's vital signs are now 98/60, HR 40, RR 22.

10-D You initiate the following steps:

    1) _____

    2) _____

    3) _____

    4) _____

You reassess the patient and find the vital signs are now BP 112/72, HR 100, and RR 20.

His new rhythm is shown in Fig. 11-21.

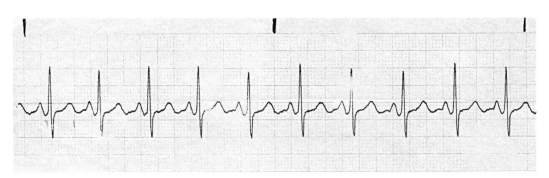

Fig. 11-21

10-E You identify the new rhythm as _____ .

You continue to monitor and observe the patient.

CASE STUDY 11

A 48-year-old man is brought to the emergency department, complaining of pressure in his chest, difficulty breathing, and nausea. On assessment, you find the patient is pale, cool, and diaphoretic. His vital signs are BP 98/60, HR 80, and RR 22.

11-A These are indications of poor _____ .

11-B You identify the rhythm shown in Fig. 11-22, as _____ .

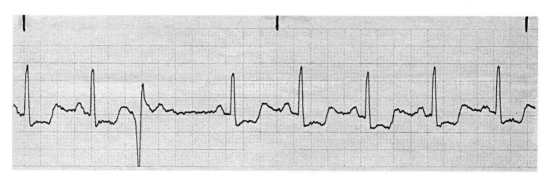

Fig. 11-22

11-C You immediately call the physician, who gives you orders to initiate:

1) _____

2) _____

3) _____

As you are completing these orders, the patient suddenly slumps over. You quickly assess the patient and find no vital signs. The monitor now shows the rhythm in Fig. 11-23.

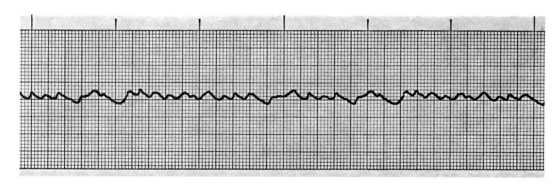

Fig. 11-23

11-D You identify the rhythm as _____ .

11-E You begin the following treatments:

1) _____

2) _____

3) _____

4) _____

5) _____

6) _____

7) _____

8) _____

9) _____

10) _____

11) _____

11-F The rhythm has changed to that shown in Fig. 11-24, which you identify

as _____.

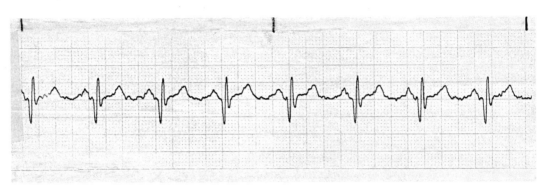

Fig. 11-24

On assessment, the patient has a BP of 96/56, a HR of 80, and a RR of 16.

You continue to monitor the patient as you transfer him to the cardiac care unit.

CASE STUDY 12

You come on duty and study the monitors. You observe the rhythm shown in Fig. 11-25 on one of the monitors.

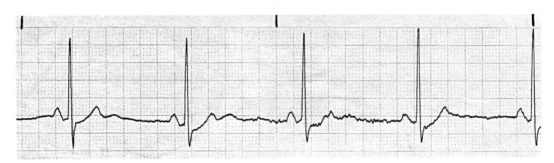

Fig. 11-25

12-A You identify the dysrhythmia as _____.

You go to the patient's room to assess the patient. He appears to be asleep. His respirations are deep and even at a rate of 16 and his HR is 50. He is in his early twenties. He has no signs of poor cardiac output.

12-B Your next actions are to:

1) _____.

2) _____.

CASE STUDY 13

A 56-year-old female is brought to the emergency department complaining of episodes of a "racing heart." Her vital signs are stable and she shows no signs of poor cardiac output.

When placed on a monitor, she has the rhythm shown in Fig. 11-26.

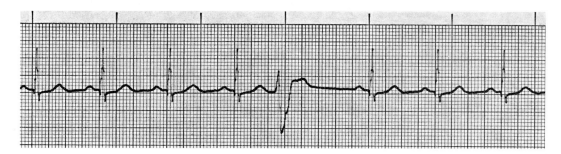

Fig. 11-26

13-A You identify the rhythm as _____.

As you continue your assessment, the patient suddenly complains of dizziness, trouble breathing, and chest pain. You notice she is pale and clammy and her vital signs are 90/50, HR 240, RR 28. The monitor now shows the rhythm in Fig. 11-27.

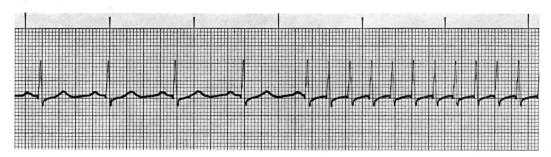

Fig. 11-27

13-B You identify this rhythm as_____.

13-C You notify the physician and immediately begin the following treatments:

    1) _____

    2) _____

    3) _____

    4) _____

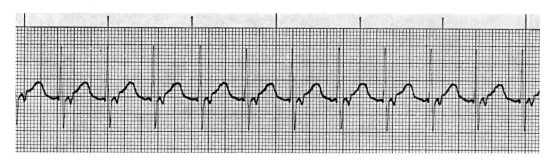

Fig. 11-28

13-D The patient now has the rhythm shown in Fig. 11-28, which you identify

as _____. Her vital signs are BP 106/60, HR 110, and RR 22. The patient continues to be observed and is transferred to the coronary care unit (CCU).

CASE STUDY 14

You respond with the ambulance crew to a call for a patient with chest pains. When you arrive, you find the patient is lying on the bed. He is pale and clammy, and has vital signs of BP 90/48, HR 50, and RR 28.

14-A These are indications of _____.

14-B You attach the monitor to the patient and identify the rhythm shown in Fig. 11-29 as _____.

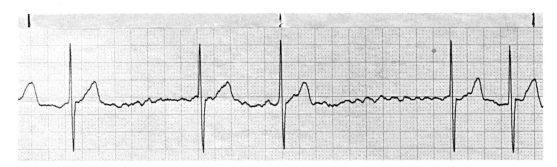

Fig. 11-29

14-C You radio the report to the hospital and receive the following orders:

1) _____

2) _____

3) _____

4) _____

5) _____

You continue to observe the patient while transporting him to the emergency department. On arrival, the patient is transferred to the emergency department's monitor, which shows the patient's rhythm has changed to that shown in Fig. 11-30.

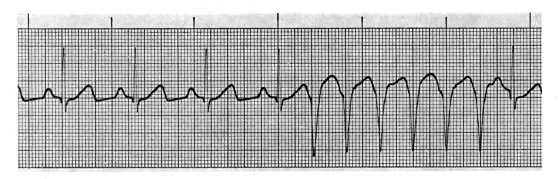

Fig. 11-30

14-D The rhythm is identified as _____.

The emergency room physician orders 1)_____

followed by a continuous 2) _____ to control the V tach.

The patient's skin is warm and dry. His vital signs are 110/70, HR 70, and RR 22. The physician transfers the patient to the coronary care unit.

CASE STUDY 15

A 45-year-old male is brought to the emergency department by his wife. The patient complains of indigestion lasting 2 to 3 hours, which is not relieved by antacids. He also complains that his shoulders feel heavy and his jaw aches. His wife states that he was sweating a lot earlier and vomited twice.

On your assessment you find vital signs of BP 136/75, HR of 70, and RR of 20.

15-A The monitor displays the rhythm shown in Fig. 11-31 which you identify

as _____ .

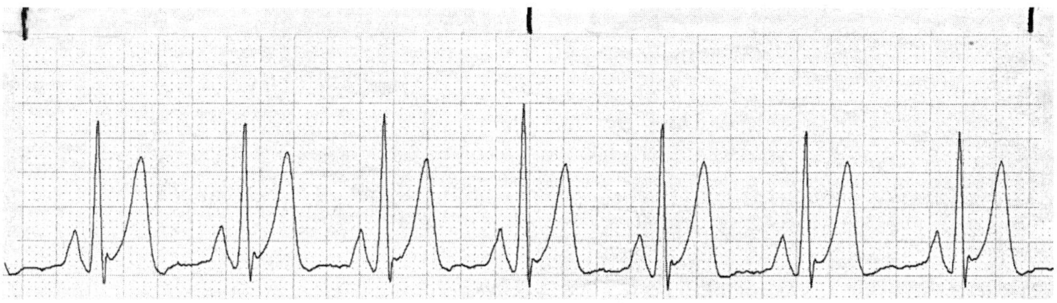

Fig. 11-31

15-B You follow the standing orders of your department and begin the following treatments:

1) _____

2) _____

3) _____

4) _____

You reassess the patient and find no change in the patient's condition or cardiac rhythm. The patient continues to complain of pain. You notify the physician who instructs you to continue the standing orders.

15-C You repeat the 1) _____ two times, without success.

You then administer a titrated dose of 2) _____ .

You reassess the patient. He continues to complain of pain. His vital signs are now 144/93, HR of 72, and RR of 20. You increase the oxygen to 4 L/min.

15-D While the EKG is being completed, you prepare to administer an intravenous infusion of nitroglycerin using an _____ _____ .

You reassess the patient after the infusion is started and find that the pain has decreased and vital signs are now BP 110/78, HR 82, and RR 20.

15-E The physician has determined that the patient is having an acute MI. After determining that there are no contraindications, the physician decides to

begin _____ .

Following the hospital's policy, you begin treatment by starting a continuous heparin infusion, administer a bolus of heparin, and giving two baby aspirin, while another nurse prepares the ordered medication.

15-F You make sure the "clot buster" medication is administered through an

_____ .

15-G You continue to _____ the patient and his cardiac rhythm.

The patient is transferred to the care of a cardiologist and is moved to the coronary care unit.

Answer Section

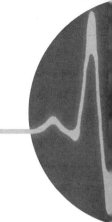

Chapter 1

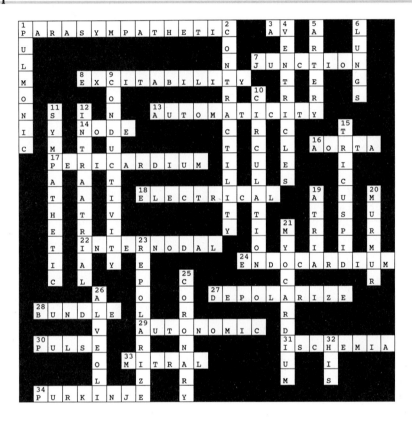

Chapter 2

Review question answers

1. True
2. False
3. True
4. True
5. Atria
6. 0.12, 0.20
7. Q wave, (or the R wave, if the Q wave is not present) to end of S wave
8. Repolarization of the ventricles
9. Equal to, or less than, one half the R to R interval of the same complex
10. Count the number of R waves in the 6-second rhythm strip and multiply by 10
11. a. 1) 300 divided by 3 equals 100
      2) 1500 divided by 15 equals 100

   b. 1) 300 divided by 7.5 equals 40
      2) 1500 divided by 37.5 equals 40
12. a. All are within normal limits of 0.12 to 0.20 second
   b. All PR intervals are equal
13. a. Within normal limits of less than 0.12 second
   b. All QRS complexes look alike
   c. A QRS complex after each P wave
   d. All R to R intervals are equal
14. Any 3 of the following:
   a. Electrode losing contact with the patient's skin
   b. Patient movement or shivering
   c. A broken cable or lead wire

14. Continued
    d. Improper grounding
    e. Patient or lead touching a metal object, such as a bed rail
15. Relative refractory period: the cardiac cells have repolarized to the point that some cells can again be stimulated to

depolarize, if the stimulus is strong enough

Absolute refractory period: the cardiac cells have not completed repolarization and cannot be stimulated to conduct an electrical impulse and contract (depolarize) again

Rhythm Strip Review Answers

1. PRI: 0.20
   QRS: 0.08
   QT: Normal
   Rhythm: Regular
   Heart rate: 30

2. PRI: Not measurable
   QRS: Not measurable
   QT: Not measurable
   Rhythm: Not measurable
   Heart rate: Not measurable

3. PRI: 0.20–0.24
   QRS: 0.04–0.06
   QT: Prolonged
   Rhythm: Regular
   Heart rate: 100

4. PRI: 0.12–0.14
   QRS: 0.06
   QT: Normal
   Rhythm: Regular
   Heart rate: 100

5. PRI: Not measurable
   QRS: Not measurable
   QT: Not measurable
   Rhythm: Not measurable
   Heart rate: Not measurable

6. PRI: 0.20
   QRS: 0.06
   QT: Normal
   Rhythm: Regular
   Heart rate: 70

7. PRI: Not measurable
   QRS: 0.04–0.08
   QT: Not measurable
   Rhythm: Regular
   Heart rate: 70

Chapter 3

Review Question Answers

1. True
2. True
3. False
4. False
5. True
6. 101, 150
7. Less than 0.12
8. Exactly 2 or more
9. b
10. a
11. a. Heart disease
    b. Myocardial infarction
    c. Drug toxicity
12. A varying number of flutter waves before each QRS complex

Rhythm Strip Review Answers

1. PRI: 0.16
   QRS: 0.06–0.08
   Interpretation: Normal Sinus Rhythm
   Rhythm: Regular
   Heart rate: 80

2. PRI: Not measurable
   QRS: 0.06–0.08
   Interpretation: Atrial flutter with a 3:1 Block
   Rhythm: Regular
   Heart rate: 90 (atrial flutter rate: 280)

3. PRI: 0.16–0.20
   QRS: 0.04–0.06
   Interpretation: Sinus tachycardia
   Rhythm: Regular
   Heart rate: 110

4. PRI: 0.20
   QRS: 0.06–0.08
   Interpretation: Sinus bradycardia with 1 PAC (4th complex)
   Rhythm: Irregular
   Heart rate: 50

5. PRI: 0.10–0.16
   QRS: 0.06–0.08
   Interpretation: Sinus rhythm to PAT (4th complex is a PAC)
   Rhythm: Irregular
   Heart rate: 100–160 (calculated with 3-second strip)

6. PRI: 0.20   Rhythm: Regular
   QRS: 0.06–0.08   Heart rate: 40
   Interpretation: Sinus bradycardia
7. PRI: 0.08–Not measurable   Rhythm: Irregular
   QRS: 0.06–0.08   Heart rate: 90
   Interpretation: Wandering atrial pacemaker
8. PRI: 0.14–0.16   Rhythm: Regular
   QRS: 0.08   Heart rate: 110
   Interpretation: Sinus tachycardia
9. PRI: Not measurable   Rhythm: Irregular
   QRS: 0.06–0.08   Heart rate: 70
   Interpretation: Controlled atrial fibrillation
10. PRI: Not measurable   Rhythm: Irregular
    QRS: 0.06–0.08   Heart rate: 80 (atrial flutter rate 280)
    Interpretation: Atrial flutter with varying block
11. PRI: Not measurable   Rhythm: Regular
    QRS: 0.04–0.06   Heart rate: 190
    Interpretation: Supraventricular tachycardia (with depressed ST segments)
12. PRI: 0.16–0.18   Rhythm: Irregular
    QRS: 0.04–0.06   Heart rate: 70
    Interpretation: Sinus arrhythmia
13. PRI: 0.16   Rhythm: Regular
    QRS: 0.06   Heart rate: 40
    Interpretation: Sinus bradycardia
14. PRI: Not measurable   Rhythm: Irregular
    QRS: 0.06–0.08   Heart rate: 90
    Interpretation: Controlled atrial fibrillation
15. PRI: 0.20   Rhythm: Irregular
    QRS: 0.04–0.06   Heart rate: 70
    Interpretation: Sinus arrest

Chapter 4

Review Question Answers

1. True
2. True
3. False
4. False
5. 40, 60
6. Less than 0.12
7. 101–150
8. 40–60
9. a. To appear behind or after
   b. To occur in a backward or reverse motion
10. A junctional complex that occurs earlier than the next expected complex of the underlying rhythm
11. a. Inverted
    b. Buried or hidden
    c. Retrograde
12. Compensatory

Rhythm Strip Review Answers

1. PRI: 0.16   Rhythm: Irregular
   QRS: 0.06–0.08   Heart rate: 80
   Interpretation: Sinus rhythm with one PJC (7th complex)
2. PRI: Not measurable   Rhythm: Regular
   QRS: 0.04–0.06   Heart rate: 30
   Interpretation: Junctional bradycardia (with retrograde P waves)
3. PRI: 0.16–0.18   Rhythm: Regular
   QRS: 0.04–0.06   Heart rate: 50
   Interpretation: Junctional rhythm (with inverted P waves)
4. PRI: Not measurable   Rhythm: Regular
   QRS: 0.04–0.06   Heart rate: 70
   Interpretation: Accelerated junctional rhythm
5. PRI: Not measurable   Rhythm: Regular
   QRS: 0.08   Heart rate: 110
   Interpretation: Junctional tachycardia (with retrograde P waves)

6. PRI: 0.14–Not measurable   Rhythm: Irregular
   QRS: 0.04–0.06   Heart rate: 50
   Interpretation: Wandering junctional pacemaker

Chapter 5

Review Question Answers

1. True
2. False
3. False
4. True
5. c
6. b
7. c
8. 0.20
9. Third-degree heart block
10. Longer, QRS complex
11. It has no pattern and may lead to third-degree heart block, or if the block is severe enough, the rate may be too bradycardic to maintain life
12. a. Underlying rhythm
    b. Ratio of P waves to each QRS complex
    c. Frequency, or how often the dysrhythmia occurs

Rhythm Strip Review Answers

1. PRI: 0.20–0.32   Rhythm: Irregular
   QRS: 0.04–0.08   Heart rate: 50 (atrial rate: 80)
   Interpretation: Mobitz I, with bradycardiac rate

2. PRI: 0.32–0.36   Rhythm: Regular
   QRS: 0.04–0.06   Heart rate: 60
   Interpretation: Sinus rhythm with first-degree block

3. PRI: 0.22–0.24   Rhythm: Regular
   QRS: 0.06   Heart rate: 40 (atrial rate: 80)
   Interpretation: Sinus bradycardia with Mobitz II (2:1 block) and first degree block

4. PRI: 0.16   Rhythm: Irregular
   QRS: 0.16   Heart rate: 40 (atrial rate: 60)
   Interpretation: Sinus bradycardia with Mobitz II (3:1 block) and BBB (with depressed ST segments and depressed T wave)

5. PRI: 0.20–0.32   Rhythm: Irregular
   QRS: 0.06–0.08   Heart rate: 50 (atrial rate: 80)
   Interpretation: Mobitz I with bradycardiac rate

6. PRI: 0.24   Rhythm: Regular
   QRS: 0.06   Heart rate: 20 (atrial rate: 50)
   Interpretation: Sinus bradycardia with Mobitz II (2:1 block) and a first-degree block

7. PRI: 0.18   Rhythm: Irregular
   QRS: 0.14–0.16   Heart rate: 30 (atrial rate: 60)
   Interpretation: Sinus bradycardia with Mobitz II (varying block) and BBB (with depressed ST segments and depressed T waves

8. PRI: 0.16–0.20   Rhythm: Regular
   QRS: 0.16–0.20   Heart rate: 60
   Interpretation: Sinus rhythm with bundle branch block (and elevated ST segments)

9. PRI: Not measurable (No true PRI)   Rhythm: Regular
   QRS: 0.14   Heart rate: 30 (atrial rate: 70)
   Interpretation: Third-degree heart block

10. PRI: 0.24–0.28   Rhythm: Regular
    QRS: 0.04   Heart rate: 70
    Interpretation: Sinus rhythm with first-degree block

11. PRI: 0.22–0.24   Rhythm: Regular
    QRS: 0.08   Heart rate: 20 (atrial rate: 60)
    Interpretation: Sinus bradycardia with Mobitz II (2:1 block) and first-degree block

12. PRI: Not measurable (No true PRI)   Rhythm: Regular
    QRS: 0.12   Heart rate: 30 (atrial rate: 50)
    Interpretation: Third-degree heart block

Chapter 6

Review Questions Answers

1. False
2. True
3. True
4. False
5. False
6. 20
7. The QRS complexes of Torsade de Pointes begin close to the baseline, and gradually increase and decrease in amplitude, in a twisting, repeating pattern. The QRS complexes of ventricular tachycardia remain more similar in height, without the twisting and turning motion.
8. a. Different ventricular sites and different appearances
   b. Two PVCs in a row
   c. Every other complex is a PVC, with at least three episodes in a row
9. Severe heart disease, electrical shock, drug toxicity
10. b
11. d
12. d

Rhythm Strip Review Answers

1. PRI: 0.20
   QRS: 0.06–0.16
   Rhythm: Irregular
   Heart rate: overall 110
           Sinus rhythm rate: 72;
           VT rate: 150
   Interpretation: Sinus rhythm with run of ventricular tachycardia

2. PRI: Not measurable
   QRS: Not measurable
   Rhythm: Not measurable
   Heart rate: 0
   Interpretation: Asystole

3. PRI: 0.16–0.20
   QRS: 0.06–0.20
   Rhythm: Irregular
   Heart rate: 80
   Interpretation: Sinus rhythm with unifocal PVCs, occurring in bigeminy

4. PRI: 0.16
   QRS: 0.06–0.26
   Rhythm: Irregular
   Heart rate: Sinus rhythm: 60 (V Fib: 0)
   Interpretation: Sinus rhythm with multifocal PVCs; R on T phenomenon, going into ventricular fibrillation

5. PRI: 0.20
   QRS: 0.06–0.34
   Rhythm: Irregular
   Heart rate: 70
   Interpretation: Sinus rhythm with multifocal PVCs, with one multifocal couplet

6. PRI: Not measurable
   QRS: Greater than 0.12
   Rhythm: Regular
   Heart rate: 310
   Interpretation: Torsades de Pointes

7. PRI: 0.12
   QRS: 0.04–0.14
   Rhythm: Irregular
   Heart rate: 60
   Interpretation: Junctional rhythm with one PVC

8. PRI: Not measurable
   QRS: Not measurable
   Rhythm: Not measurable
   Heart rate: 0
   Interpretation: Fine ventricular fibrillation

9. PRI: Not measurable
   QRS: 0.36–0.40
   Rhythm: Regular
   Heart rate: 30
   Interpretation: Idioventricular rhythm

10. PRI: Not measurable
    QRS: 0.16
    Rhythm: Regular
    Heart rate: 160
    Interpretation: Ventricular tachycardia

11. PRI: Not measurable
    QRS: 0.10–0.32
    Rhythm: Irregular
    Heart rate: 100
    Interpretation: Controlled atrial fibrillation with one PVC (with depressed ST segments)

12. PRI: 0.20
    QRS: 0.04–0.12
    Rhythm: Irregular
    Heart rate: 70
    Interpretation: Sinus rhythm with one multifocal PVC couplet

13. PRI: Not measurable
    QRS: Not measurable
    Rhythm: Not measurable
    Heart rate: 0
    Interpretation: Coarse ventricular fibrillation

14. PRI: Not measurable
    QRS: Not measurable
    Interpretation: Ventricular standstill

    Rhythm: Regular
    Heart rate: 0 (atrial rate: 50)

15. PRI: Not measurable
    QRS: 0.44
    Interpretation: Agonal rhythm

    Rhythm: Not measurable
    Heart rate: 10

Chapter 7

Review Question Answers

1. False
2. True
3. False
4. a. At a constant rate; usually 72–80 impulses per minute
   b. On demand; when the patient's heart rate falls below a predetermined rate; usually 70 beats per minute
5. a. A vertical line seen on the rhythm strip when the pacemaker fires
   b. The cardiac muscle's ability to respond to the pacemaker, indicated by a QRS complex after every pacer spike
6. Sequential
7. 100
8. Less than 0.12
9. a. Transvenous
   b. Transdermal (Transcutanous)
10. Pulseless Electrical Activity is the current term used to describe any dysrhythmia that shows the conduction of electrical impulses, without contraction of the cardiac muscle. The patient does not have a pulse, even though a rhythm is seen on the monitor screen

Rhythm Strip Review Answers

1. PRI: Not measured
   QRS: 0.06–0.08
   Rhythm: Regular
   Heart rate: 70
   Interpretation: Atrial pacemaker rhythm with 100% pacing and 100% capture
2. PRI: 0.20
   QRS: 0.06–0.08
   Rhythm: Regular
   Heart rate: 90
   Interpretation: Sinus rhythm with an aberrant beat (5th complex)
3. PRI: Not measured
   QRS: 0.10
   Rhythm: Regular
   Heart rate: 80
   Interpretation: Sequential pacemaker rhythm with 100% pacing and 100% capture
4. PRI: Not measured
   QRS: 0.10–0.12
   Rhythm: Regular
   Heart rate: 70
   Interpretation: Ventricular pacemaker rhythm with 100% pacing and 100% capture
5. PRI: 0.16–0.18
   QRS: 0.04–0.10
   Rhythm: Irregular
   Heart rate: 120
   Interpretation: Sinus tachycardia with one aberrant beat
6. PRI: Not measured
   QRS: 0.12
   Rhythm: Regular
   Heart rate: 70
   Interpretation: Sequential pacemaker rhythm with 100% pacing and 100% capture
7. PRI: Not measured
   QRS: 0.12–0.14
   Rhythm: Regular
   Heart rate: 70
   Interpretation: Ventricular pacemaker rhythm with 100% pacing and 100% capture
8. PRI: 0.20
   QRS: 0.04–0.08
   Rhythm: Regular
   Heart rate: 90
   Interpretation: Sinus rhythm with two aberrant beats (first and sixth complexes)
9. PRI: Not measured
   QRS: Not measurable
   Rhythm: Regular
   Heart rate: 0; Pacemaker rate: 70
   Interpretation: Pacemaker rhythm with 100% pacing and 0% capture
10. PRI: Not measured
    QRS: 0.04–0.06
    Rhythm: Regular
    Heart rate: 70
    Interpretation: Atrial pacemaker; 100% pacing, 100% capture
11. PRI: Not measured
    QRS: 0.06–0.22
    Rhythm: Irregular
    Heart rate: 60
    Interpretation: Junctional rhythm with 50% pacing and 66% capture
12. PRI: 0.16–0.20 (Sinus rhythm) to not measurable
    QRS: 0.14–0.16
    Rhythm: Irregular
    Heart rate: 50
    Interpretation: Sinus bradycardia with 60% pacing and 100% capture

Chapter 10

Rhythm Strip Review Answers

1. PRI: 0.20–0.22   Rhythm: Regular
   QRS: 0.06   Heart rate: 70
   Interpretation: Sinus rhythm with first-degree block

2. PRI: 0.16   Rhythm: Irregular
   QRS: 0.06–0.20   Heart rate: 80
   Interpretation: Sinus with 1 PVC

3. PRI: Not measurable   Rhythm: Not measurable
   QRS: Not measurable   Heart rate: Not measurable
   Interpretation: Fine ventricular fibrillation

4. PRI: 0.16   Rhythm: Irregular
   QRS: 0.04   Heart rate: 40 to 140 (each calculated by 3-second strip)
   Interpretation: Sinus brachycardia going into sinus tachycardia

5. PRI: 0.20–0.58   Rhythm: Irregular
   QRS: 0.06–0.08   Heart rate: 50 (atrial rate: 70)
   Interpretation: Mobitz I, with bradycardic rate

6. PRI: 0.08   Rhythm: Regular
   QRS: 0.04–0.06   Heart rate: 220
   Interpretation: Supraventricular tachycardia

7. PRI: 0.16–0.20   Rhythm: Irregular
   QRS: 0.06–0.16   Heart rate: 80
   Interpretation: Sinus rhythm with 2 unifocal PVCs

8. PRI: Not measurable   Rhythm: Regular
   QRS: 0.06   Heart rate: 30
   Interpretation: Junctional bradycardia (with retrograde P waves)

9. PRI: Not measurable   Rhythm: Regular
   QRS: 0.12   Heart rate: 70 (atrial flutter rate: 270)
   Interpretation: Atrial flutter with 4:1 block

10. PRI: Not measurable   Rhythm: Regular
    QRS: 0.12–0.14   Heart rate: 20 (atrial rate: 70)
    Interpretation: Third-degree heart block

11. PRI: Not measurable   Rhythm: Regular
    QRS: 0.36–0.40   Heart rate: 30
    Interpretation: Idioventricular rhythm

12. PRI: 0.14   Rhythm: Regular
    QRS: 0.04–0.06   Heart rate: 140
    Interpretation: Sinus tachycardia (with depressed ST segments)

13. PRI: 0.16 to not measurable   Rhythm: Irregular
    QRS: 0.06–0.20   Heart rate: 50
    Interpretation: Junctional rhythm with 2 unifocal PVCs

14. PRI: Not measurable   Rhythm: Regular
    QRS: 0.16–0.20   Heart rate: 150–160
    Interpretation: Ventricular tachycardia

15. PRI: 0.22–0.24   Rhythm: Regular
    QRS: 0.06   Heart rate: 40 (atrial rate: 70)
    Interpretation: Sinus bradycardia with first-degree block and Mobitz II (2:1 block)

16. PRI: 0.20   Rhythm: Irregular
    QRS: 0.06   Heart rate: 60
    Interpretation: Sinus rhythm with a PAC

17. PRI: 0.16   Rhythm: R to R regular; P to P irregular
    QRS: 0.08–0.10   Heart rate: 60 (first 3 seconds); atrial rate: 60
          Ventricular rate: 0 (2nd 3 seconds)
    Interpretation: Sinus rhythm going into ventricular standstill

18. PRI: 0.16 to not measurable   Rhythm: Irregular
    QRS: 0.04–0.06   Heart rate: 60–70
    Interpretation: Wandering junctional pacemaker

19. PRI: 0.20   Rhythm: Irregular
    QRS: 0.06–0.40   Heart rate: 80
    Interpretation: Sinus rhythm with multifocal PVCs in bigeminy

20. PRI: Not measurable   Rhythm: Regular
    QRS: 0.06–0.10   Heart rate: 70 (atrial flutter rate: 280)
    Interpretation: Atrial flutter with 4:1 block
21. PRI: Not measurable   Rhythm: Regular
    QRS: 0.16   Heart rate: 70
    Interpretation: Ventricular pacemaker rhythm with 100% pacing and 100% capture
22. PRI: Not measurable   Rhythm: Regular
    QRS: 0.06–0.08   Heart rate: 80
    Interpretation: Artifact (60-cycle interference)
23. PRI: 0.08 to not measurable   Rhythm: Irregular
    QRS: 0.06–0.08   Heart rate: 90
    Interpretation: Wandering atrial pacemaker
24. PRI: 0.20   Rhythm: Irregular
    QRS: 0.06–0.08   Heart rate: 80
    Interpretation: Sinus rhythm with sinus arrest
25. PRI: 0.16 to not measurable   Rhythm: Irregular
    QRS: 0.06 to not measurable   Heart rate: 100 (first 3 seconds)
                                                             0 (second 3 seconds)
    Interpretation: Sinus rhythm with a PVC (R on T phenomenon), going into ventricular fibrillation
26. PRI: 0.16–0.48   ,   Rhythm: Irregular
    QRS: 0.04–0.08   Heart rate: 50 (atrial rate: 70)
    Interpretation: Mobitz I, with slight artifact, and bradycardic rate
27. PRI: Not measured   Rhythm: Regular
    QRS: 0.04–0.06   Heart rate: 70
    Interpretation: Atrial pacemaker rhythm with 100% pacing and 100% capture
28. PRI: 0.20   Rhythm: Irregular
    QRS: 0.06–0.24   Heart rate: 80
    Interpretation: Sinus rhythm with unifocal PVCs
29. PRI: Not measurable   Rhythm: Irregular
    QRS: 0.06–0.24   Heart rate: 90
    Interpretation: Atrial fibrillation with R on T phenomenon and run of ventricular tachycardia
30. PRI: Not measurable   Rhythm: Not measurable
    QRS: 0.40   Heart rate: 10
    Interpretation: Agonal rhythm
31. PRI: 0.16–0.20   Rhythm: Irregular
    QRS: 0.04–0.14   Heart rate: 120
    Interpretation: Sinus tachycardia with an aberrantly conducted complex
32. PRI: 0.16–0.18   Rhythm: Regular
    QRS: 0.18–0.20   Heart rate: 70
    Interpretation: Sinus rhythm with BBB
33. PRI: Not measurable   Rhythm: Regular
    QRS: 0.16   Heart rate: 80
    Interpretation: Sequential pacemaker rhythm with 100% pacing and 100% capture
34. PRI: 0.32   Rhythm: Regular
    QRS: 0.08   Heart rate: 80
    Interpretation: Sinus rhythm with first-degree heart block
35. PRI: 0.16–0.18   Rhythm: Irregular
    QRS: 0.06–0.40   Heart rate: 70
    Interpretation: Sinus rhythm with multifocal PVCs
36. PRI: Not measurable   Rhythm: Irregular
    QRS: 0.04   Heart rate: 60
    Interpretation: Controlled atrial fibrillation
37. PRI: 0.08–0.10   Rhythm: Regular
    QRS: 0.06–0.08   Heart rate: 170
    Interpretation: Supraventricular tachycardia
38. PRI: 0.16–0.20   Rhythm: Irregular
    QRS: 0.06–0.08   Heart rate: 80
    Interpretation: Sinus rhythm with a PJC
39. PRI: 0.16   Rhythm: Irregular
    QRS: 0.16–0.20   Heart rate: 40 (atrial rate: 60)
    Interpretation: Sinus bradycardia with Mobitz II (3:1 block) and BBB

40. PRI: 0.16   Rhythm: Irregular
    QRS: 0.04–0.44   Heart rate: 70
    Interpretation: Sinus rhythm with unifocal PVCs
41. PRI: 0.20   Rhythm: Regular
    QRS: 0.06–0.08   Heart rate: 100
    Interpretation: Normal sinus rhythm
42. PRI: 0.22   Rhythm: Irregular
    QRS: 0.06–0.16   Heart rate: 80–140 (each calculated by 3-second strip)
    Interpretation: Sinus rhythm with a run of ventricular tachycardia
43. PRI: 0.18–0.20   Rhythm: Irregular
    QRS: 0.06–0.20   Heart rate: 90
    Interpretation: Sinus rhythm with two episodes of unifocal PVC couplets
44. PRI: Not measurable   Rhythm: Regular
    QRS: 0.06–0.08   Heart rate: 110
    Interpretation: Junctional tachycardia (with retrograde P waves)
45. PRI: 0.16–0.18   Rhythm: Irregular
    QRS: 0.06–0.20   Heart rate: 80
    Interpretation: Sinus rhythm with unifocal PVCs in bigeminy
46. PRI: 0.16–0.18   Rhythm: Irregular
    QRS: 0.06   Heart rate: 50
    Interpretation: Sinus bradycardia with sinus arrest
47. PRI: 0.16–0.18   Rhythm: Regular
    QRS: 0.04–0.06   Heart rate: 50
    Interpretation: Junctional rhythm (with inverted P waves)
48. PRI: 0.32–0.36   Rhythm: Regular
    QRS: 0.06   Heart rate: 50
    Interpretation: Sinus bradycardia with first-degree block
49. PRI: 0.16 to not measurable   Rhythm: Irregular
    QRS: 0.04–0.06   Heart rate: 79–187 (calculated by division)
    Interpretation: Sinus rhythm changing to PAT
50. PRI: Not measurable   Rhythm: Irregular
    QRS: 0.06   Heart rate: 50
    Interpretation: Wandering junctional pacemaker
51. PRI: 0.12–0.16   Rhythm: Irregular
    QRS: 0.04–0.06   Heart rate: 50
    Interpretation: Sinus arrhythmia
52. PRI: Not measurable   Rhythm: Regular
    QRS: 0.14   Heart rate: 20 (atrial rate: 70)
    Interpretation: Third-degree heart block
53. PRI: Not measurable   Rhythm: Not measurable
    QRS: Not measurable   Heart rate: 0
    Interpretation: Coarse ventricular fibrillation
54. PRI: Not measurable   Rhythm: Regular
    QRS: 0.20–0.24   Heart rate: 140
    Interpretation: Ventricular tachycardia
55. PRI: 0.12 to not measurable   Rhythm: Irregular
    QRS: 0.06   Heart rate: 90
    Interpretation: Wandering atrial pacemaker
56. PRI: 0.20   Rhythm: Irregular
    QRS: 0.06–0.36   Heart rate: 80
    Interpretation: Sinus rhythm with multifocal PVCs and one multifocal couplet
57. PRI: Not measurable   Rhythm: Not measurable
    QRS: Not measurable   Heart rate: 0
    Interpretation: Asystole
58. PRI: 0.20–0.22   Rhythm: Regular
    QRS: 0.06   Heart rate: 100
    Interpretation: Sinus rhythm with one aberrantly conduction complex and intermittent first-degree block

59. PRI: Not measurable   Rhythm: Irregular
    QRS: 0.12–0.32   Heart rate: 100
    Interpretation: Atrial fibrillation with one PVC
60. PRI: Not measurable   Rhythm: Regular
    QRS: 0.08   Heart rate: 60 (atrial flutter rate: 270–300)
    Interpretation: Atrial flutter with regular ventricular response
61. PRI: Not measurable   Rhythm: Regular
    QRS: Not measurable   Heart rate: 240
    Interpretation: Torsades de Pointes
62. PRI: 0.16–0.20   Rhythm: Regular
    QRS: 0.08–0.10   Heart rate: 50
    Interpretation: Sinus bradycardia with artifact
63. PRI: Not measurable   Rhythm: Irregular
    QRS: 0.06–0.08   Heart rate: 90
    Interpretation: Controlled atrial fibrillation
64. PRI: 0.14–0.30   Rhythm: Irregular
    QRS: 0.06   Heart rate: 50 (atrial heart rate: 80)
    Interpretation: Mobitz I, with bradycardic rate
65. PRI: 0.16–0.20   Rhythm: Irregular
    QRS: 0.06–0.08   Heart rate: 90–100
    Interpretation: Sinus rhythm with one aberrantly conducted complex and artifact
66. PRI: Not measurable   Rhythm: Irregular
    QRS: 0.06–0.22   Heart rate: 50
    Interpretation: Ventricular pacemaker rhythm with 40% pacing and 66% capture and
    artifact
67. PRI: Not measurable   Rhythm: Regular
    QRS: 0.36–0.40   Heart rate: 40
    Interpretation: Idioventricular rhythm
68. PRI: Not measurable   Rhythm: Regular
    QRS: 0.08–0.10   Heart rate: 100
    Interpretation: Artifact
69. PRI: Not measurable   Rhythm: Regular
    QRS: 0.08   Heart rate: 100–110
    Interpretation: Junctional tachycardia
70. PRI: Not measurable   Rhythm: Not measurable
    QRS: Not measurable   Heart rate: 0
    Interpretation: Ventricular fibrillation (fine VF to coarse VF to fine VF)
71. PRI: 0.16   Rhythm: Regular
    QRS: 0.08–0.12   Heart rate: 50
    Interpretation: Sinus bradycardia
72. PRI: Not measurable   Rhythm: Irregular
    QRS: 0.04–0.08   Heart rate: 90; (atrial flutter rate:
                                          varies up to 250)
    Interpretation: Atrial flutter with variable block and artifact
73. PRI: Not measured   Rhythm: Regular
    QRS: 0.04–0.06   Heart rate: 70
    Interpretation: Atrial pacemaker rhythm with 100% pacing and 100% capture
74. PRI: 0.14–0.20   Rhythm: Regular
    QRS: 0.04–0.08   Heart rate: 90
    Interpretation: Normal sinus rhythm with artifact
75. PRI: Not measurable   Rhythm: Regular
    QRS: 0.16   Heart rate: 60
    Interpretation: Junctional rhythm with BBB and artifact
76. PRI: difficult to measure   Rhythm: Irregular
    QRS: 0.10–0.36   Heart rate: 90
    Interpretation: Sinus rhythm with bundle branch block, two multifocal PVCs and
    60 cycle interference
77. PRI: Not measurable   Rhythm: Regular
    QRS: 0.26–0.28   Heart rate: ventricular rate: 160
    Interpretation: Ventricular tachycardia

78. PRI: 0.16   Rhythm: Regular
    QRS: 0.08   Heart rate: 70
    Interpretation: Normal sinus rhythm with elevated T wave
79. PRI: 0.16–0.20   Rhythm: Irregular
    QRS: 0.04–0.08   Heart rate: 90
    Interpretation: Wandering atrial pacemaker rhythm
80. PRI: 0.28   Rhythm: Regular
    QRS: 0.08–0.10   Heart rate: 90
    Interpretation: Sinus rhythm with first degree block
81. PRI: 0.16   Rhythm: Regular
    QRS: 0.04   Heart rate: ventricular rate: 40
                                                   atrial rate: 110
    Interpretation: Sinus bradycardia with Mobitz II block (3:1 ratio)
82. PRI: 0.16   Rhythm: Regular
    QRS: 0.06–0.08   Heart rate: 70
    Interpretation: Normal sinus rhythm
83. PRI: 0.12–0.14   Rhythm: Regular
    QRS: 0.04–0.06   Heart rate: 110
    Interpretation: Sinus tachycardia
84. PRI: Not measurable   Rhythm: Regular
    QRS: 0.06   Heart rate: 70
    Interpretation: Accelerated junctional rhythm
85. PRI: Not measurable   Rhythm: Irregular
    QRS: 0.12–0.36   Heart rate: 100–110
    Interpretation: Atrial fibrillation with rapid ventricular response, depressed ST segments
    and one PVC
86. PRI: 0.20   Rhythm: Irregular
    QRS: 0.06–0.10   Heart rate: 90
    Interpretation: Sinus rhythm with depressed ST segments and one PAC
87. PRI: 0.16   Rhythm: Regular
    QRS: 0.08   Heart rate: 60
    Interpretation: Sinus rhythm with elevated T waves
88. PRI: Not measurable   Rhythm: Regular
    QRS: Not measurable   Heart rate: ventricular rate: 230
    Interpretation: Torsades de Pointes
89. PRI: Not measurable   Rhythm: Irregular
    QRS: 0.08   Heart rate: 50
    Interpretation: Atrial fibrillation with slow ventricular response
90. PRI: Not measurable   Rhythm: Irregular
    QRS: 0.04–0.06   Heart rate: 100; atrial flutter rate:
                                       varies up to 230
    Interpretation: Atrial flutter with varying block; also with wandering baseline
91. PRI: 0.12–0.14   Rhythm: Regular
    QRS: 0.08–0.10   Heart rate: 100
    Interpretation: Normal sinus rhythm
92. PRI: Not measurable   Rhythm: Regular
    QRS: Not measurable   Heart rate: 90–100
    Interpretation: Artifact
93. PRI: 0.12–0.16   Rhythm: Regular
    QRS: 0.12–0.14   Heart rate: 80
    Interpretation: Sinus rhythm with bundle branch block
94. PRI: 0.16   Rhythm: Irregular
    QRS: 0.06–0.16   Heart rate: 100
    Interpretation: Sinus rhythm with three aberrantly conducted PACs
95. PRI: 0.14–0.16   Rhythm: Regular
    QRS: 0.08–0.10   Heart rate: 80
    Interpretation: Normal sinus rhythm
96. PRI: 0.14   Rhythm: Regular
    QRS: 0.08   Heart rate: 50
    Interpretation: Junctional rhythm

97. PRI: Not measurable   Rhythm: Regular
      QRS: 0.06–0.08   Heart rate: 250
      Interpretation: Supraventricular tachycardia

98. PRI: 0.20   Rhythm: Regular
      QRS: 0.12–0.14   Heart rate: 100
      Interpretation: Sinus rhythm with depressed ST segments

99. PRI: Not measurable   Rhythm: Regular
      QRS: 0.08   Heart rate: 70
      Interpretation: Accelerated junctional rhythm

100. PRI: Not measurable   Rhythm: Irregular
      QRS: Not measurable   Heart rate: ventricular rate: unable to measure to 0;
                                              atrial rate: 0
      Interpretation: Ventricular tachycardia (possible torsades de pointes) going into fine ventricular fibrillation

101. PRI: 0.14–0.20 when present   Rhythm: Irregular
      QRS: 0.10–0.12   Heart rate: 50
      Interpretation: Wandering atrial pacemaker rhythm with bradycardic rate

102. PRI: Not measurable   Rhythm: atrial: regular
      QRS: 0.10   Heart rate: ventricular rate: 10
                                              atrial rate: 40–50
      Interpretation: Ventricular standstill with one escape beat

103. PRI: Not measurable   Rhythm: Irregular
      QRS: 0.14–0.16   Heart rate: ventricular rate: 210;
      Interpretation: Ventricular tachycardia

104. PRI: 0.20–0.40   Rhythm: Irregular
      QRS: 0.08   Heart rate: ventricular rate: 60;
                                              atrial rate: 80
      Interpretation: Mobitz I heart block

105. PRI: Not measurable   Rhythm: Regular
      QRS: Not measurable   Heart rate: 0
      Interpretation: Pacemaker rhythm with 100% pacing and 0% capture

106. PRI: Not measurable   Rhythm: Not measurable
      QRS: Not measurable   Heart rate: 0
      Interpretation: Coarse ventricular fibrillation

107. PRI: 0.10   Rhythm: Irregular
      QRS: 0.08–0.10   Heart rate: 80
      Interpretation: Sinus rhythm with PACs

108. PRI: 0.16   Rhythm: Regular
      QRS: 0.08–0.24   Heart rate: 100
      Interpretation: Sinus rhythm with unifocal PVCs in trigeminy

109. PRI: Not measurable   Rhythm: Not measurable
      QRS: Not measurable   Heart rate: Not measurable
      Interpretation: Loose lease or patient movement

110. PRI: 0.12–0.16   Rhythm: Regular
      QRS: 0.04–0.06   Heart rate: 110
      Interpretation: Sinus tachycardia

111. PRI: Not measurable   Rhythm: Not measurable
      QRS: 0.26   Heart rate: ventricular rate: 10;
      Interpretation: Agonal rhythm going into asystole

112. PRI: 0.24   Rhythm: Regular
      QRS: 0.10   Heart rate: ventricular rate: 40;
                                              atrial rate: 80
      Interpretation: Sinus bradycardia with a Mobitz II, (2 : 1 block) and a first-degree block

113. PRI: 0.16   Rhythm: Irregular
      QRS: 0.08–0.24   Heart rate: Overall rate is 140
      Interpretation: Sinus rhythm with unifocal PVCs and a run of ventricular tachycardia, and a junctional escape beat

114. PRI: 0.12–0.16   Rhythm: Irregular
      QRS: 0.06–0.14   Heart rate: 150 overall
                                           Sinus rate: 100; PAT rate: 200
      Interpretation: Sinus rhythm changing to PAT

115. PRI: Not measurable
     QRS: Not measurable
     Interpretation: Ventricular tachycardia

     Rhythm: Regular
     Heart rate: ventricular rate: 220

116. PRI: 0.10–Not measurable
     QRS: 0.08–0.16
     Interpretation: Supraventricular tachycardia

     Rhythm: Irregular
     Heart rate: 180

117. PRI: Not measurable
     QRS: 0.06–0.08
     Interpretation: Sinus tachycardia

     Rhythm: Regular
     Heart rate: 150

118. PRI: 0.12–0.16
     QRS: 0.04–0.06
     Interpretation: Sinus rhythm with wandering baseline

     Rhythm: Regular
     Heart rate: 70

119. PRI: Not measurable
     QRS: 0.06–0.08
     Interpretation: Junctional bradycardia

     Rhythm: Regular
     Heart rate: 30

120. PRI: 0.14–0.20
     QRS: 0.08–0.22

     Rhythm: Irregular overall
     Heart rate: 80 (sinus rhythm)
     160 (VTach)

     Interpretation: Sinus rhythm with R on T phenomenon, followed by ventricular tachycardia

121. PRI: 0.20
     QRS: 0.04–0.06
     Interpretation: Sinus rhythm with three abberantly conducted PACs

     Rhythm: Irregular
     Heart rate: 60

122. PRI: 0.14–0.16
     QRS: 0.04–0.06
     Interpretation: Sinus arrhythmia

     Rhythm: Irregular
     Heart rate: 60

123. PRI: Not measurable
     QRS: 0.08–0.18
     Interpretation: Junctional rhythm with unifocal PVCs in bigeminy

     Rhythm: Irregular
     Heart rate: 90

124. PRI: Not measurable
     QRS: 0.08 to unmeasurable

     Rhythm: Irregular
     Heart rate: ventricular rate: 80;
     atrial flutter rate: 250–270

     Interpretation: Atrial flutter with variable block

125. PRI: Not measurable
     QRS: Not measurable

     Rhythm: Irregular
     Heart rate: ventricular rate: 0;
     atrial rate: 50

     Interpretation: Ventricular standstill

126. PRI: Not measurable
     QRS: Not measurable

     Rhythm: Not measurable
     Heart rate: Ventricular: 10

     Interpretation: Coarse ventricular fibrillation, going into agonal rhythm, followed by asystole

127. PRI: 0.12 to not measurable
     QRS: 0.06–0.08
     Interpretation: Sinus rhythm with artifact, possible patient movement

     Rhythm: Regular
     Heart rate: 90

128. PRI: 0.14–0.16
     QRS: 0.06–0.16
     Interpretation: Sinus bradycardia with unifocal PVCs

     Rhythm: Irregular
     Heart rate: 50

129. PRI: 0.16, not measurable
     QRS: 0.06–0.08
     Interpretation: Sinus rhythm with 1 PJC

     Rhythm: Irregular
     Heart rate: 80

130. PRI: 0.40–0.48
     QRS: 0.12–0.16
     Interpretation: Sinus bradycardia with first-degree block and depressed ST segments
     (possible BBB)

     Rhythm: Regular
     Heart rate: 50

131. PRI: Not measurable
     QRS: 0.10
     Interpretation: Junctional rhythm

     Rhythm: Regular
     Heart rate: 40

132. PRI: Difficult to measure to 0.16
     QRS: 0.06
     Interpretation: Sinus rhythm with artifact

     Rhythm: Regular
     Heart rate: 90–100

133. PRI: 0.16–0.18
     QRS: 0.06–0.16
     Interpretation: Sinus rhythm with depressed ST segments and one PVC

     Rhythm: Irregular
     Heart rate: 80

134. PRI: Not measurable   Rhythm: Regular
     QRS: 0.06–0.08   Heart rate: 40
     Interpretation: Junctional rhythm
135. PRI: 0.16   Rhythm: Regular
     QRS: 0.04–0.06   Heart rate: 70
     Interpretation: Normal sinus rhythm
136. PRI: Not measurable   Rhythm: Regular
     QRS: 0.04–0.06   Heart rate: 150
     Interpretation: Sinus tachycardia
137. PRI: Not measurable   Rhythm: Irregular
     QRS: 0.06–0.08   Heart rate: 70 overall;
                                                flutter rate: 300
     Interpretation: Atrial fibrillation going into atrial flutter with a variable block
138. PRI: Not measurable   Rhythm: Regular
     QRS: 0.14–0.18   Heart rate: 70
     Interpretation: Ventricular pacemaker rhythm with 100% pacing and 100% capture
139. PRI: 0.18–0.20   Rhythm: Regular
     QRS: 0.10   Heart rate: 70
     Interpretation: Sinus rhythm with elevated T waves
140. PRI: Not measurable   Rhythm: Not measurable
     QRS: Not measurable   Heart rate: Not measurable
     Interpretation: Fine ventricular fibrillation
141. PRI: 0.18–Not measurable   Rhythm: Irregular
     QRS: 0.06–0.08   Heart rate: 100–110
     Interpretation: Wandering atrial pacemaker
142. PRI: 0.20–0.40   Rhythm: Irregular
     QRS: 0.06–0.8   Heart rate: 60; atrial rate: 80
     Interpretation: Mobitz I heart block
143. PRI: Not measurable   Rhythm: Not measurable
     QRS: Not measurable   Heart rate: Not measurable
     Interpretation: Coarse ventricular fibrillation
144. PRI: 0.16–0.18   Rhythm: Regular
     QRS: 0.06–0.08   Heart rate: 60
     Interpretation: Normal sinus rhythm
145. PRI: 0.16   Rhythm: Irregular
     QRS: 0.06   Heart rate: 70
     Interpretation: Sinus rhythm with sinus arrest
146. PRI: Not measurable   Rhythm: Not measurable
     QRS: 0.18–0.20   Heart rate: 20
     Interpretation: Agonal rhythm with 60 cycle interference
147. PRI: 0.14–0.16   Rhythm: Regular
     QRS: 0.06   Heart rate: 30–40
     Interpretation: Sinus bradycardia
148. PRI: Not measurable   Rhythm: Not measurable
     QRS: Not measurable   Heart rate: 0
     Interpretation: Asystole
149. PRI: Not measurable   Rhythm: Regular
     QRS: 0.10   Heart rate: 70
     Interpretation: Sequential pacemaker rhythm with 100% pacing and 100%
     capture
150. PRI: Not measurable   Rhythm: Regular
     QRS: 0.28–0.32   Heart rate: ventricular rate: 40
                                                           atrial rate: 90–100

     Interpretation: Third-degree heart block

Chapter 11

Case study 1

1–A Sinus tachycardia

1–B 1) Notify the physician
    2) Reassure the patient and listen to her fears. Inform her of the possibility that anxiety, caffeine, and nicotine can cause a rapid heart beat and palpitations
    3) Continue to monitor the patient

1–C Normal sinus rhythm

Case study 2

2–A Sinus bradycardia

2–B 1) Provide oxygen.
    2) Establish intravenous access.
    3) Notify the physician.
    4) Administer atropine.

2–C Repeat atropine IV until the maximum dose has been given.

2–D Temporary, external, transdermal, or transcutaneous pacemaker

2–E Ventricular pacemaker rhythm, or paced rhythm

2–F 1) 100 percent
    2) Paced

Case study 3

3–A Sinus rhythm with PVCs

3–B Junctional rhythm with PVCs

3–C 1) Provide oxygen.
    2) Start an IV of normal saline or lactated Ringer's.
    3) Administer atropine IV.

3–D Repeat atropine IV until the maximum dose has been given or the rate is increased.

3–E Sinus rhythm with PVCs in bigeminy

3–F 1) Lidocaine
    2) Lidocaine

3–G 1) More than 6 PVCs in one minute
    2) Multifocal PVCs
    3) Couplets
    4) R-on-T phenomenon
    5) Runs of ventricular tachycardia

Case study 4

4–A Supraventricular tachycardia

4–B 1) Valsalva's (bearing down)
    2) Carotid massage

4–C 1) Provide oxygen.
    2) Start IV of normal saline or lactated Ringer's.
    3) Administer adenosine IV rapidly.
    4) Reassess the patient.
    5) Repeat adenosine IV rapidly, if necessary.

4–D Synchronized

4–E Normal sinus rhythm

Case study 5

5–A Sinus tachycardia

5–B 1) Place patient in a position of rest.
    2). Provide oxygen.
    3) Offer cool fluids to drink, or start an IV of normal saline or lactated Ringer's.
    4) Continue monitoring the patient.

5–C Normal sinus rhythm

5–D Continue to improve

Case study 6

6–A Mobitz Type II; 3:1 block

6–B 1) Provide oxygen.
    2) Start an IV of normal saline or lactated Ringer's.
    3) Administer atropine IV.
    4) Prepare for a temporary, external, transdermal, or transcutaneous pacemaker.

6–C   Third degree heart block.

6–D   Temporary, external, transdermal, or transcutaneous pacemaker.

6–E   Permanent pacemaker

Case study 7

7–A   Ventricular fibrillation

7–B   Assess the patient.

7–C   1) Check the telemetry leads and electrodes; change any electrode that is dry and recon-
nect any leads that are loose.
2) Inform the physician about the R-on-T phenomenon.
3) Continue observing the patient.

Case study 8

8–A   Normal sinus rhythm

8–B   Pulseless electrical activity (PEA)

8–C   1) Begin CPR.
2) Provide 100% oxygen by bag-valve-mask and intubate as soon as possible.
3) Start an IV of normal saline or lactated Ringer's.
4) Administer epinephrine IV push; repeat as necessary according to protocol.
5) Reassess patient
6) Give atropine IV if dysrhythmia is bradycardic (less than 60 electrical impulses/min);
repeat according to protocol until the maximum dose has been given.

8–D   Cardiac tamponade.

8–E   1) Hypovolemia, for which you would give fluids.
2) Hypoxia, for which you would increase ventilations and oxygen
3) Tension pneumothorax, for which you would perform needle decompressions.

8–F   Mobitz Type I (Wenkebach, second-degree type I)

8–G   Observe the patient for any change in the dysrhythmia or in cardiac output.

Case study 9

9–A   Torsades de Pointes

9–B   1) Cold, sweaty skin
2) Hypotension (low blood pressure)
3) Pallor (pale, grayish skin)
4) Cyanosis (bluish tint to lips, nailbeds and skin)
5) Dyspnea (difficulty breathing)
6) Dizziness
7) Nausea or vomiting
8) Lethargy (decrease in level of consciousness)

9–C   1) Provide oxygen.
2) Start an IV of normal saline or lactated Ringer's.
3) Administer isoproterenol IV.
4) Reassess the patient.
5) Administer magnesium sulfate IV.

9–D   Sinus rhythm with first degree heart block

Case study 10

10–A   Mobitz I, (Wenchenbach, second-degree type I) with bradycardia

10–B   1) Assess the patient.
2) Continue to monitor the patient.

10–C   Mobitz II, (second-degree type II) with bradycardia

10–D   1) Reassess the patient.
2) Provide oxygen.
3) Administer atropine IV.
4) Continue to observe and assess the patient while you prepare the external pacemaker
for use, if necessary.

10–E   Normal sinus rhythm

Case study 11

11–A   Cardiac output

11–B   Sinus rhythm with first degree heart block and a PVC

11–C 1) Provide oxygen.
   2) Start an IV of normal saline or lactated Ringer's.
   3) Give nitroglycerin sublingually (under the tongue).
11–D Ventricular fibrillation
11–E 1) Begin CPR.
   2) Administer 100% oxygen via bag-valve-mask and intubate as soon as possible.
   3) Start an IV if not already established.
   4) Defibrillate. Multiple defibrillation attempts may be necessary throughout treatment. Initially, three consecutive shocks at 200, 200–300, and 360 joules should be used. Then, defibrillate at 360 joules during the remaining treatment.
   5) Reassess the patient before and after each defibrillation or medication.
   6) Administer IV epinephrine; repeat according to protocol. Defibrillate at 360 joules within 30–60 seconds of giving epinephrine.
   7) Administer lidocaine IV; repeat per protocol until the maximum dose has been given.
   8) If necessary, administer bretylium tosylate IV; repeat according to protocol.
   9) Give magnesium sulfate in Torsades de pointes or severe ventricular fibrillation unresponsive to defibrillation and epinephrine.
   10) Give procainamide IV until the maximum dose has been given.
   11) Once the patient has a pulse, start an infusion drip of the medication that was successful in ending the ventricular fibrillation. Use the guidelines for PVCs.
11–F Sinus rhythm with bundle branch block

Case study 12

12–A Sinus bradycardia
12–B 1) Do nothing. It is normal for young adults to have a bradycardic rate during sleep.
   2) Continue to observe the patient and monitor for any changes.

Case study 13

13–A Sinus rhythm with PVC
13–B Paroxysmal atrial tachycardia (PAT)
13–C 1) Provide oxygen.
   2) Start an IV of normal saline or lactated Ringer's.
   3) Administer adenosine rapid IV push.
   4) Reassess the patient and repeat adenosine rapid IV if necessary and according to protocol.
13–D Junctional tachycardia

Case study 14

14–A Poor cardiac output
14–B Intermittant atrial flutter with varying block
14–C 1) Provide oxygen.
   2) Start an IV of normal saline or lactated Ringer's.
   3) Administer atropine, IV push
   4) Continue to observe and monitor the patient.
   5) Transport to the emergency department.
14–D Sinus rhythm with run of ventricular tachycardia
14–E 1) Lidocaine IV push
   2) Lidocaine infusion

Case study 15

15–A Sinus rhythm with elevated T waves
15–B 1) Provide oxygen.
   2) Start an IV of normal saline or lactated Ringer's.
   3) Order an EKG.
   4) Administer sublingual nitroglycerin.
15–C 1) Nitroglycerin tablet
   2) Morphine sulfate
15–D Infusion pump
15–E Thrombolytic therapy
15–F Infusion pump
15–G Assess or monitor

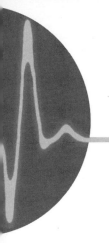

Glossary

Aberrant Different than normal; may refer to individual complexes or entire rhythm

Aberrantly conducted complexes Single complexes that appear different than the underlying rhythm because they do not follow the same conduction pathway

Absolute refractory period Time in the cardiac cycle when the myocardial cells have not completed repolarization and cannot conduct an electrical impulse; seen from Q wave to the first third of the T wave

Accelerated junctional rhythm Dysrhythmia that occurs when all the electrical impulses originate from a single site within the atrioventricular junctional area at a rate between 61 and 100 impulses per minute

Adenosine Drug that decreases heart rate by depressing SA node and AV node activity; may used in paroxysmal atrial tachycardia and supraventricular tachycardia

Agonal rhythm Dying heart; ventricular rate less than 20; *see* idioventricular rhythm

Amplitude Height of a wave or complex measured in millivolts (mV)

Aorta Largest artery in the body

Aortic valve Located between the left ventricle and the aorta

Arrhythmia Absence of cardiac rhythm; also frequently used to mean dysrhythmia

Artifact Abnormality in an EKG tracing that does not originate in the heart, such as static electricity, patient movement, or loose leads

Asystole Absence of electrical activity in the cardiac muscle; also called cardiac standstill

Atria Upper chambers of the heart

Atrial fibrillation (A fib) Dysrhythmia that originates from many atrial sites; the atria are making ineffective quivering movements, not actual contractions; only the ventricles are contracting

Atrial flutter Dysrhythmia in which flutter waves are formed instead of P waves

Atrial rhythm Any rhythm that originates from a pacemaker cell within the atria

Atrioventricular node (AV node) Acts as a backup pacemaker of the heart

Atrium One of the upper chambers of the heart

Atropine sulfate Drug that increases the heart rate and ability of the cardiac cells to conduct an electrical impulse; used in bradycardic rhythms

Automatic implantable cardioverter defibrillator (AICD) Surgically implanted overdrive pacer/defibrillator that can identify and treat some rapid lethal dysrhythmias, such as ventricular tachycardia

Automaticity Ability of cardiac pacemaker cells to generate an electrical impulse

Autonomic nervous system Nerves that maintain the heart and blood vessels in a normal state; divided into the sympathetic and parasympathetic systems

Atrioventricular dissociation (AV disassociation) Occurs when the atria and ventricles function independently, as in third degree heart block

Bag-valve mask Device that is used to assist with artificial ventilation and in the delivery of 100% oxygen to patients

Baseline Imaginary line on the rhythm strip from which all waves and deflections are measured; also known as isoelectric line

Beta Blockers Drugs used to treat hypertension and ventricular dysrhythmias

Bigeminy Dysrhythmia in which every other complex is premature; a minimum of three occurrences is needed to identify a dysrhythmia as bigeminy

Biphasic Any S-shaped wave that lies both above and below the baseline of the rhythm strip

Blood pressure Measurement of pressure within the blood vessels

Bradycardia Cardiac dysrhythmia that has a slower than normal heart rate; usually less than 60 impulses per minute

Bretylium tosylate Drug that decreases cardiac muscle irritability; decreases the occurrence of ectopic complexes (PVCs, VT)

Bundle branches (BB) Part of the conduction system of the heart; located below the bundle of His, leading to Purkinje's fibers; divided into left and right bundle branches

Bundle branch block (BBB) Dysrhythmia in which the electrical impulse is blocked at a bundle branch; the QRS complex has a notched appearance and is usually greater than 0.12 second

Bundle of His Part of the conduction system of the heart; located below the AV node and above the bundle branches

CC Measure of liquids; 1000 CC = 1 liter

Calcium chloride Drug used to increase cardiac muscle contractility

Caliper Instrument used to measure R to R and P to P intervals on a rhythm strip

Capture Ability of cardiac muscle to respond to an electrical stimulus from a mechanical pacemaker and conduct the electrical impulse throughout the cardiac muscle

Cardiac arrest Lack of both electrical and mechanical activity in the heart; blood is not being pumped throughout the body and the patient does not have a pulse

Cardiac cycle Period from the beginning of one cardiac contraction to the beginning of another; usually includes a P wave, PR interval, QRS complex, and T wave

Cardiac irritability Ability of cardiac cells to respond to an electrical impulse; used interchangeably with excitability

Cardiac output The amount of blood pumped by the left ventricle in one minute

Cardiac tamponade The presence of blood or excess fluid in the pericardial sac that decreases the heart's ability to contract and expand effectively

Cardiovascular Pertaining to the heart and blood vessels

Cardioversion Procedure that uses controlled electrical currents to correct dysrhythmias such as ventricular tachycardia

Cardiovert Process of cardioversion

Circulatory system Body system that includes the heart, lungs, blood vessels, and blood

Compensatory pause Pause that follows a premature beat, allowing the underlying rhythm to begin again at its normal rate; may be either complete or incomplete pause

Complex Segment of the rhythm strip that refers to any wave or group of waves; such as the Q, R, and S waves

Component Any part of a cardiac cycle seen on the monitor or rhythm strip; includes the P wave, the PR interval, the QRS complex, the ST segment, the T wave, and/or the QT interval

Conduct Transmit; send; carry an electrical impulse from cell to cell

Conduction system Series of cardiac cells that transmit an electrical impulse throughout the heart muscle in a sequential manner, from the SA node to the ventricular muscle

Conductivity Ability of cardiac cells to conduct electrical impulses

Contractility Ability of cardiac cells to shorten, causing cardiac contraction

Contraction Tightening or squeezing action of a muscle; the contraction of the cardiac muscle pumps blood throughout the body

Coronary Pertaining to the heart; is also used to mean a heart attack

Coronary arteries Arteries that supply oxygenated blood to the heart muscle

Coronary artery disease (CAD) Progressive blockage of one or more coronary arteries, resulting in lack of oxygen to the heart muscle

Coronary occlusion Obstruction or extreme narrowing of the coronary arteries; blockage

Couplet Two premature complexes occurring in a row

Cyanosis Bluish or grayish color of the skin, mucous membranes, and nail beds; caused by lack of oxygen in the tissue

Defibrillation Procedure that uses electrical current to correct ventricular fibrillation or pulseless ventricular tachycardia; may be called unsynchronized cardioversion

Deflection Movement of a wave or complex away from the baseline on a rhythm strip or monitor

Depolarization Conduction of an electrical impulse through the heart muscle; normally causes a cardiac contraction

Depressed wave Wave that is below the baseline

Digitalis glycoside Drug used to decrease heart rate and strengthen the force of cardiac contractions

Diltiazem hydrochloride Drug used to decrease heart rate

Dobutamine hydrochloride Drug used to increase the force of cardiac contraction

Dopamine hydrochloride Drug used to maintain or increase blood pressure

Dysrhythmia Abnormal cardiac rate or rhythm; frequently used interchangeably with arrhythmia

Ectopic complex Complex initiated from a site other than the SA node

Electrical impulse Electrical stimulus generated by pacemaker cells in the myocardium, which causes depolarization of the myocardial cells; normally initiated by the SA node

Electrocardiogram (EKG, ECG) A graphic record of electrical impulses of the heart

Electrode Conduction pad that connects the patient to a telemetry monitor or an EKG machine; also the tip of the pacemaker wire

Electromechanical dissociation (EMD) A term used to describe pulseless electrical activity; dysrhythmia in which there is no cardiac muscle contraction in response to electrical stimulus; patient has no pulse

Electrophysiology Study of the ability of cells and tissue to use electrical currents

Endocardium Lining of the heart

Epicardium Thin, protective membrane that covers the outside of the heart

Epinephrine hydrochloride Drug that increases the irritability, conductivity, and contractility of cardiac muscle; increases the rate and force of cardiac contractions

Escape beat Complex initiated from a site other than the SA node; usually is the heart's attempt to maintain a normal rate or rhythm

Excitability Ability of cardiac cells to respond to an electrical impulse; used interchangeably with irritability

Fibrillation Uncontrolled, uncoordinated, and ineffective quivering movements of cardiac muscle

First-degree heart block Dysrhythmia caused by a delay in the conduction system between the atria and the bundle of His; PR intervals measure greater than 0.20 second

Flutter wave (F Wave) Wave formed instead of a P wave during a rapid, flutter dysrhythmia

Foci Two or more pacemaker sites

Focus Single site of origin of an electrical impulse

Furosemide Drug used to remove excess fluid from tissues

Generate Initiate; begin an electrical impulse

Gram (gm) Measurement of weight used in the metric system; frequently used in drug dosages; 1 gram = 1000 milligrams

Ground electrode Electrode used to help prevent artifact

Hypertension Blood pressure measurement above normal

Hypotension Blood pressure measurement below normal

Hypovolemia Decreased amount of blood in the heart chambers and blood vessels

Hypoxia Decreased amount of oxygen in the body tissues or organs

Idioventricular rhythm Dysrhythmia in which the atria, AV junction, bundle of His, and bundle branches are no longer functioning; only the ventricular muscle is attempting to function

Infarction Death of tissue; as in myocardial infarction

Inherent Normal, natural, or inborn; for example, the inherent rate of the atria is 60 to 100 beats per minute

Initiate Generate or start an electrical impulse

Internodal pathways Multiple electrical conduction pathways between the SA node and the AV node

Interval Period of time used to measure the distance between waves or complexes on the rhythm strip, such as PR interval or P to P interval

Intraatrial Pathways Multiple electrical conduction pathways between the right and left atrium

Intravenous (IV) Administration of medication or fluids into a vein

Irritability Ability of cardiac cells to respond to an electrical impulse; used interchangeably with excitability

Ischemia Lack of oxygen in tissue cells due to decreased blood supply

Isoelectric line See *baseline*

Isoproterenol hydrochloride Drug used to increase the force of myocardial contraction and blood pressure

Junctional bradycardia Junctional dysrhythmia in which the heart rate is less than 40 impulses per minute

Junctional rhythm Dysrhythmia occurring when the electrical impulses are generated by a site in the AV junctional area; inherent rate is 40–60 impulses per minute

Junctional tachycardia Junctional dysrhythmia with a heart rate between 101 and 150 impulses per minute

Lead Identifies different types of electrode placement, such as Lead I or Lead II

Lead wire Wires that connect the electrodes to a monitor or telemetry unit; also wires leading from a pacemaker generator to the myocardium

Lethal Death producing

Lidocaine hydrochloride Drug that decreases cardiac muscle irritability, as well as ectopic beats (PVCs and VT)

Loss of capture QRS complex does not follow a pacemaker spike; myocardium does not respond to electrical stimulus and does not contract

Magnesium sulfate Drug used in treatment of torsades de pointes

Medically unstable Patient's condition in which the following symptoms of poor cardiac output occur: chest pain, difficulty breathing, pale or dusky color, sudden change in blood pressure, or change in the level of consciousness

Microgram (mcg) Measurement of weight used in the metric system; used in drug dosages; 1 mcg = 0.001 milligrams; 1000 mcg = 1 milligram

Milligram (mg) Measurement of weight used in the metric system; frequently used in drug dosages; 1 mg = 0.001 gm; 1000 mg = 1 gm

Millimeter (mm) Measurement of distance used in the metric system; 1 mm is equal to one small square on rhythm strip graph paper; 1 mm = 0.04 second

Millivolt (mV) Measurement of amplitude; 0.1 mV equals one small square on the rhythm strip

Mitral valve Located between the left atria and the left ventricle

Mobitz I Progressive heart block that occurs when the atrial impulse is interrupted at the AV junction; also called Wenckebach or second-degree heart block, type I

Mobitz II Intermittent interruption in the electrical conduction system at the AV junction that occurs suddenly and without warning; also called second-degree heart block, type II

Morphine sulfate Narcotic drug used to relieve pain in myocardial infarctions and pulmonary edema

Multifocal Complexes that originate from different pacemaker sites and look different from each other; usually refers to ventricular complexes

Murmur Abnormal sound made by blood flowing through a valve that is not functioning correctly

Myocardial infarction Death of part of the cardiac muscle caused by a blockage in one or more of the cardiac arteries; also called MI, heart attack, or coronary

Myocardium Cardiac muscle

Nitroglycerin Drug used to relieve cardiac chest pain by increasing flow of oxygenated blood to cardiac tissue; drug used to treat hypertension

Nodal Term that has been used to mean AV junctional area

Normal sinus rhythm (NSR) Normal cardiac rhythm; electrical impulses are generated by the SA node; 60 to 100 impulses per minute

Oxygen (O_2) Gas necessary for cell life; drug used to increase oxygen available to tissue cells; decreases shortness of breath and pain caused by ischemia

Pacemaker Cardiac cells that initiate an electrical impulse, causing cardiac contraction; the SA node is the normal pacemaker of the heart; also refers to an artificial or mechanical pacemaker

Pacemaker cells Any cardiac cell that is capable of initiating an electrical impulse

Pacer Abbreviated term for artificial pacemaker

Pacer spike A vertical line seen on the rhythm strip that represents the electrical impulse from a mechanical pacemaker

Pacing Use of mechanically generated electrical impulses that follow the electrical conduction system of the heart and usually stimulate the cardiac muscle to contract; also refers to the percent of complexes initiated by a mechanical pacemaker

Palpitations Sensation of being able to feel own heart beating or "skipping beats"; frequently associated with rapid heart rates or premature complexes

Parasympathetic nervous system Nerves that decrease the rate of cardiac contractions, usually after stress or emergencies, allowing the body to restore energy

Paroxysmal Sudden onset of a rapid cardiac rhythm

Paroxysmal atrial tachycardia (PAT) Dysrhythmia with a sudden onset; the electrical impulses are generated at a rate greater than 151 impulses per minute

Pericardial sac Tough, double walled, fibrous sac that contains the heart

Permanent pacemaker Mechanical pacemaker that is surgically implanted under the patient's skin

Polarization Cardiac ready state; the cells are ready to receive an electrical impulse

Potassium (K) Chemical found in the body that aids in the conduction of electricity through the cells

Premature atrial contraction (PAC) Atrial complex that occurs earlier than the next expected complex of the underlying rhythm

Premature junctional contraction (PJC) Complex initiated from the junctional area that occurs earlier than the next expected complex of the underlying rhythm

Premature ventricular contraction (PVC) Complex initiated from an area below the AV junction and occurs earlier than the next expected complex of the underlying rhythm

PR interval (PRI) Time required for an electrical impulse to travel through the atria and AV junction; measured from the beginning of the P wave to the beginning of the QRS complex

Procainamide hydrochloride Drug that decreases cardiac muscle irritability and ectopic beats (PVCs, and VT)

P to P interval Measurement of time between one P wave to the following P wave

Pulmonary Pertaining to the lungs

Pulmonic valve Valve between the right ventricle and the pulmonary artery

Pulse Wave of pressure caused by the pumping action of the left ventricle that can be counted; usually defined as heart beats per minute

Pulseless electrical activity (PEA) Dysrhythmia that occurs when there is electrical activity in the heart, but the cardiac muscle does not contract in response to the electrical stimulus; the patient does not have a pulse

Purkinje's fibers Muscular fibers found in the ventricles; part of the electrical conduction system of the heart

P wave Small wave before the QRS that represents the depolarization of both right and left atria

QRS complex Group of one Q, R, and S wave that represents the depolarization of both right and left ventricles

QT interval Time required for an electrical impulse to travel through the ventricles and then for the ventricles to repolarize;

measured from beginning of Q wave to end of T wave

Quadrigeminy Dysrhythmia in which every fourth complex is premature; must have a minimum of three occurrences to be identified

Quinidine sulfate Drug that decreases cardiac irritability and ectopic beats (premature atrial or junctional contractions)

Refractory period Time between the end of a contraction and the return of the cardiac cells to the ready state; divided into absolute and relative refractory periods

Relative refractory period Time during the cardiac cycle when cardiac cells have repolarized to the point that some cells can be stimulated to contract again, if the stimulus is strong enough

Repolarization Cardiac recovery phase; the cells are returning to the ready state

Responsiveness Term used in assessment of patient condition, such as responsive to painful stimulation or lack of responsiveness; used interchangeably with consciousness

Retrograde In reverse, behind, or in a backward direction

R on T phenomenon Occurs when the R wave of a premature ventricular contraction falls on the T wave of the preceding complex; can lead to a lethal dysrhythmia

Run of ventricular tachycardia (run of VT) Group of three or more premature ventricular contractions in a row; usually has a duration of less than 30 seconds

Septum Thick, muscular wall that separates the right and left sides of the heart

Sinoatrial node (SA node) Located in the upper right atrium; normal pacemaker of the heart

Sinus arrest Dysrhythmia that occurs when the SA node fails to initiate an electrical impulse; therefore, the atrium does not depolarize

Sinus arrhythmia Dysrhythmia that occurs when the heart rate changes with respirations; meets all criteria of normal sinus rhythm except it is NOT regular

Sinus bradycardia Dysrhythmia that occurs when all electrical impulses originate from the SA node, but at a rate slower than 60 impulses per minute

Sinus exit block Dysrhythmia that occurs when the SA node initiates an electrical impulse that is blocked and not conducted to the atria; pause ended by an escape beat

Sinus rhythm Any cardiac rhythm that originates from the SA node; heart rate between 60–100 impulses per minute

Sinus tachycardia Dysrhythmia that occurs when all electrical impulses originate from the SA node, but at a rate of 101 to 150 impulses per minute

Sodium (NA) Chemical found in the body that aids in the conduction of electricity through the cells

Sodium bicarbonate Drug that is sometimes used in the treatment of cardiac arrest

Spike See *pacer spike*

Stroke volume The amount of blood pumped by the left ventricle with each contraction or beat; usually about 70 cc

Supraventricular tachycardia (SVT) Dysrhythmia that has all the characteristics of paroxysmal atrial tachycardia, but the onset is not seen; general term describing any rapid dysrhythmia (heart rate greater than 151) originating from above the bundle of His

Sympathetic nervous system Nerves that prepare the body to react in times of stress or emergencies by increasing the heart rate and force of cardiac contractions

Symptomatic Showing signs of poor cardiac output; See *medically unstable*

Synchronized cardioversion Procedure used to correct unstable rapid dysrhythmias using electrical current timed to discharge or "fire" only on the R wave, avoiding the relative refractory period

Tachycardia Dysrhythmia in which the heart rate is faster than normal; usually greater than 101 beats per minute

Telemetry System of electrodes, leads, monitors, and graph paper that receives and displays cardiac electrical impulses

Third-degree heart block Dysrhythmia in which both the atria and the ventricles are beating independently; functioning as two separate hearts

Thrombolytic therapy Drugs used to dissolve clots in coronary arteries; may reduce number of deaths from myocardial infarctions

Torsades de pointes Dysrhythmia that resembles VT; has increasing and decreasing amplitude along the baseline; usually occurs in rhythms with a prolonged QT interval

Transmit Conduct or carry electrical impulses through the cardiac muscle; usually using normal conduction pathways

Tricuspid valve Located between the right atria and right ventricle

Trigeminy Dysrhythmia in which every third complex is premature; must have a minimum of 3 occurrences to be identified as trigeminy

T wave Represents repolarization of the ventricles

Underlying rhythm Basic cardiac rhythm in which dysrhythmias and/or premature contractions can be identified

Unifocal Complexes that originate from a single pacemaker site and look alike; usually refers to ventricular complexes

Valsalva maneuver Forceful bearing down, as if trying to have a bowel movement; sometimes used to treat paroxysmal atrial tachycardia

Valves Flap-like structures in the heart that open and close in response to the pumping action of the myocardium; prevent the backflow of blood

Vena cava Superior and Inferior; largest veins in the body

Venous Pertaining to or referring to veins

Ventricles Lower right and left chambers of the heart

Ventricular fibrillation (V fib) Dysrhythmia that originates from many ventricular sites; the ventricles make ineffective, quivering movements, not actual contractions; the patient does not have a pulse

Ventricular muscle Layer of specialized tissue containing pacemaker cells; the muscle of the left ventricle is thicker since it pumps blood throughout the entire body

Ventricular rate Number of times the left ventricle contracts in one minute; inherent rate is 60 to 100; should equal the pulse rate

Ventricular standstill Dysrhythmia that occurs when no ventricular activity exists, only atrial complexes; the patient does not have a pulse

Ventricular tachycardia (VT) Dysrhythmia that contains more than three premature ventricular contractions in a row; duration of more than 30 seconds; also called sustained ventricular tachycardia

Verapamil hydrochloride Drug used in treatment of PAT and SVT to slow heart rate

Voltage Measurement of electrical force

Wandering atrial pacemaker Dysrhythmia originating from at least three different sites above the bundle of His

Wandering junctional pacemaker Dysrhythmia that originates from at least three different sites within the AV junctional area

Wenckebach Second-degree heart block, type I; See *Mobitz I*

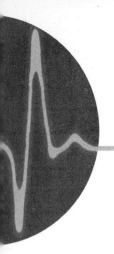

Abbreviation List

A Fib	Atrial fibrillation
AICD	Automatic implanted cardioversion defibrillator
AV	Atrioventricular
BB	Bundle branch
BBB	Bundle branch block
BP	Blood pressure
Brady	Bradycardia
CAD	Coronary artery disease
CC	Cubic centimeter
CO	Cardiac output
CPR	Cardiopulmonary resuscitation
CVA	Cerebral vascular accident
ECG, EKG	Electrocardiogram
EMD	Electromechanical Dissociation
F Wave	Flutter wave
FLBs	Funny looking beats
gm	Gram
HR	Heart rate
Hr	Hour
IV	Intravenous
K	Potassium
kg	Kilogram
L	Liter
mcg	Microgram
mg	Milligram

MI	Myocardial infarction
min	Minute
ml	Milliliter
mm	Millimeter
mV	Millivolt
Na	Sodium
NSR	Normal sinus rhythm
O2	Oxygen
PAC	Premature atrial contraction
PAT	Paroxysmal atrial tachycardia
PEA	Pulseless electrical activity
PJC	Premature junctional contraction
PRI	PR interval
PVC	Premature ventricular contraction
QT	Interval between beginning of Q wave and end of T wave
RR	Respitatory rate
SA	Sinoatrial
SV	Stroke volume
SVT	Supraventricular tachycardia
Tach	Tachycardia
VF	Ventricular fibrillation
V Fib	Ventricular fibrillation
VR	Ventricular rate
VT, V Tach	Ventricular tachycardia

Background References

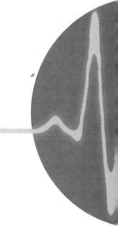

These books and materials were used as background and reference information sources.

1. American Heart Association: 1996 Handbook of emergency cardiac care for healthcare providers, St. Louis, Mosby–Year Book, 1996.

2. American Heart Association: Guidelines for cardiopulmonary resuscitation and emergency cardiac care: *The Journal of the American Medical Association*, volume 268, number 16, pages 2171-2302, 1992.

3. Anthony CP and Thibodeau GA: Structure and function of the body, ed 7, St. Louis, 1984, Mosby–Year Book.

4. Berne RM and Levy M: Cardiovascular physiology, ed 5, St. Louis, 1986, Mosby–Year Book.

5. Brown KR and Jacobson S: Mastering dysrhythmias: a problem-solving guide, Philadelphia, 1988, FA Davis.

6. Conover: Understanding electrocardiography: arrhythmias and the 12-lead ECG, ed 6, St. Louis, 1992, Mosby–Year Book.

7. Dubin D: Rapid interpretation of EKGs: a programmed course, ed 3, Tampa, Fla., 1987, Cover Publishing.

8. Gray H: Anatomy of the human body: 30th American edition, Philadelphia, 1985, Lea and Febiger.

9. Gussella C and Dorsey B: Cardiovascular nursing: body mind tapestry, Montgomery, Ala., American Association of Critical Care Nurses.

10. Hollingshead WH and Roose C: Textbook of anatomy, Philadelphia, 1985, Harper and Row.

11. Huang SH: Coronary care nursing, ed 2, Philadelphia, 1989, WB Saunders.

12. Huzar RJ: Basic dysrhythmias: interpretation and management, ed 2, St. Louis, 1994, Mosby–Year Book.

13. Mandele WJ: Cardiac arrhythmias: their mechanisms, diagnosis, and management, ed 2, Philadelphia, 1987, JB Lippincott.

14. Miller R and Wilson J: Manual of prehospital emergency medicine, St. Louis, 1992, Mosby–Year Book.

15. Physician's Desk Reference, ed 50: Sifton DW, editor, Montvale NJ, 1996, Medical Economics Production Company.

16. Skidmore-Roth L: Mosby's nursing drug reference, St. Louis, 1994, Mosby–Year Book.

17. Solomon EP: Introduction to human anatomy and physiology, Philadelphia, 1992, WB Saunders.

18. Vinsant MIS: Common sense approach to coronary care: a program, ed 4, St. Louis, 1984, Mosby–Year Book.

19. Walraven G: Basic arrhythmias, ed 3, Englewood Cliffs, N.J., 1992, Prentice Hall.

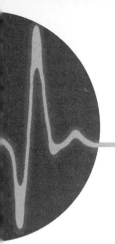

Index

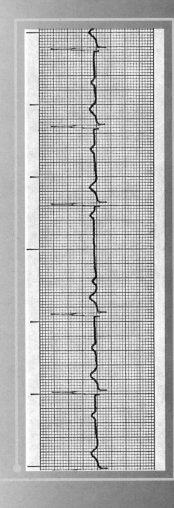

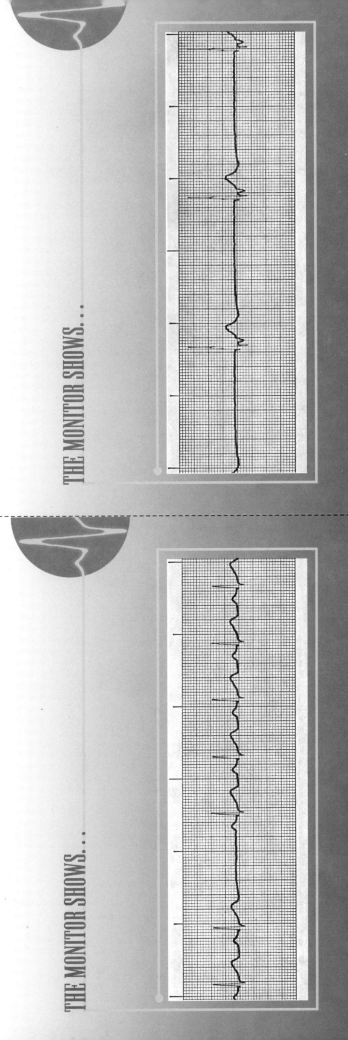

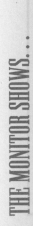

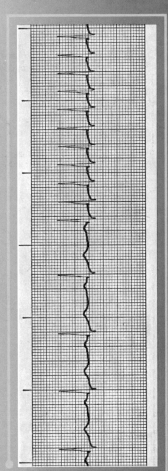

RHYTHM IDENTIFICATION

JUNCTIONAL BRADYCARDIA
retrograde P waves;
heart rate: 30

RHYTHM IDENTIFICATION

SINUS EXIT BLOCK
pause equal to exactly two or more complete cardiac cycles;
heart rate: 70

RHYTHM IDENTIFICATION

MOBITZ I (Wenckebach, Second Degree, Type I)
progressively longer PR intervals, followed by a dropped QRS, pattern is then repeated;
heart rate: 50
atrial rate: 60

RHYTHM IDENTIFICATION

PAROXYSMAL ATRIAL TACHYCARDIA (PAT)
beginning of the PAT must be seen and HR must be greater than 151
normal sinus→ → → PAT
heart rate: 80→ → heart rate: 220

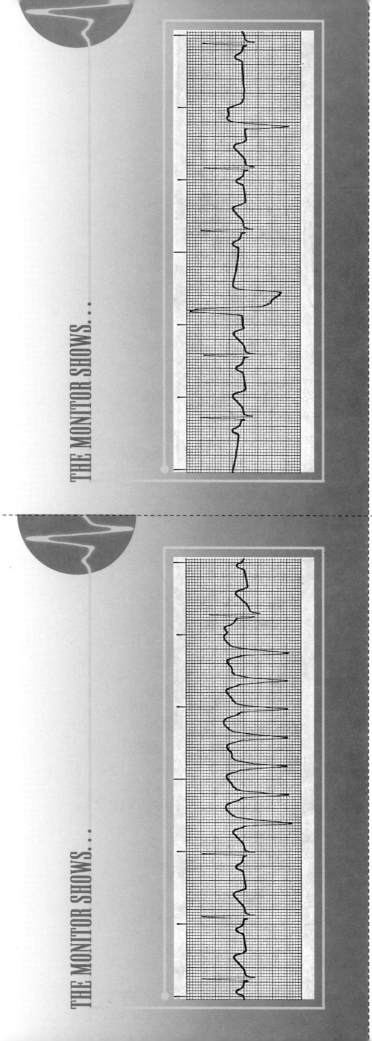

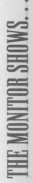

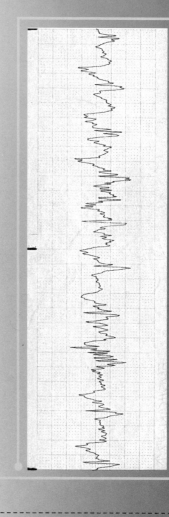

MULTIFOCAL PVCs in a sinus rhythm; complex occurs earlier than expected; originates from below the bundle of His; PVCs look different; heart rate: 70 (includes both PVCs)

ARTIFACT
unable to determine rhythm or rate

RUN of VENTRICULAR TACHYCARDIA IN A SINUS RHYTHM;
More than 3 PVCs in a row; duration less than 30 seconds; overall heart rate: 110

SINUS BRADYCARDIA
heart rate: 30

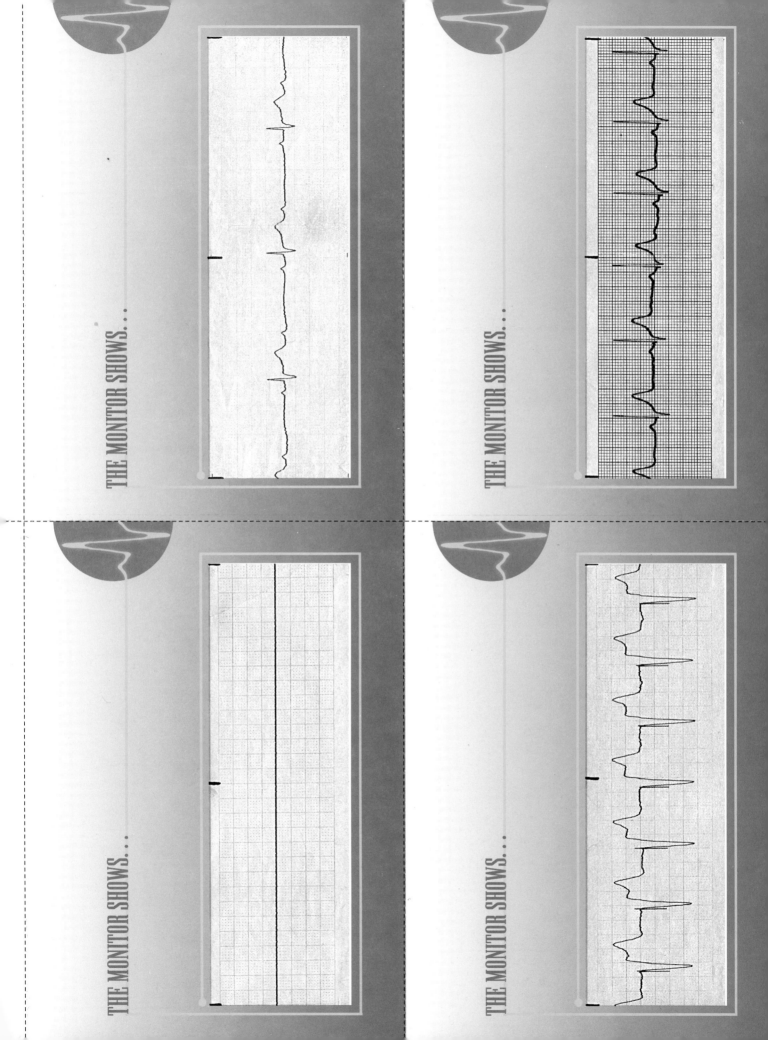

THE MONITOR SHOWS...

THE MONITOR SHOWS...

THE MONITOR SHOWS...

THE MONITOR SHOWS...

RHYTHM IDENTIFICATION

MOBITZ II (Second-Degree, Type II)
in a sinus bradycardia; 2:1 block, 2 P waves for each QRS;
PR intervals do not become progressively longer
heart rate: 30
atrial rate: 70

RHYTHM IDENTIFICATION

ASYSTOLE
heart rate: 0

RHYTHM IDENTIFICATION

NORMAL SINUS RHYTHM
P, PRI, QRS, rate, rhythm are all within normal limits;
heart rate: 60

RHYTHM IDENTIFICATION

PACEMAKER RHYTHM
100% paced; 100% capture;
heart rate: 70

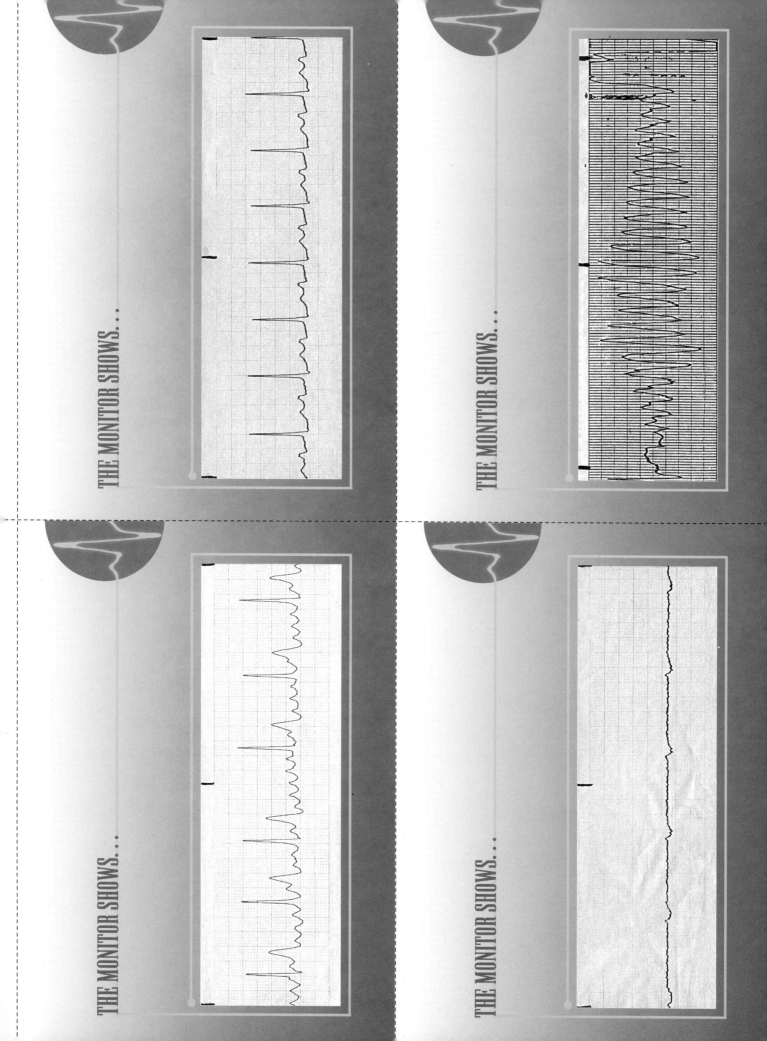

Sinus rhythm with a **FIRST DEGREE BLOCK** prolonged PR interval (greater than 0.20 second); heart rate: 80

ATRIAL FLUTTER with variable ventricular response; sawtooth F waves; ventricular rate: 60; atrial rate: 250-350

TORSADES DE POINTES
QRS increases and decreases in amplitude; heart rate: 270

VENTRICULAR STANDSTILL
no QRS after P wave; ventricular rate: 0; atrial rate: 60

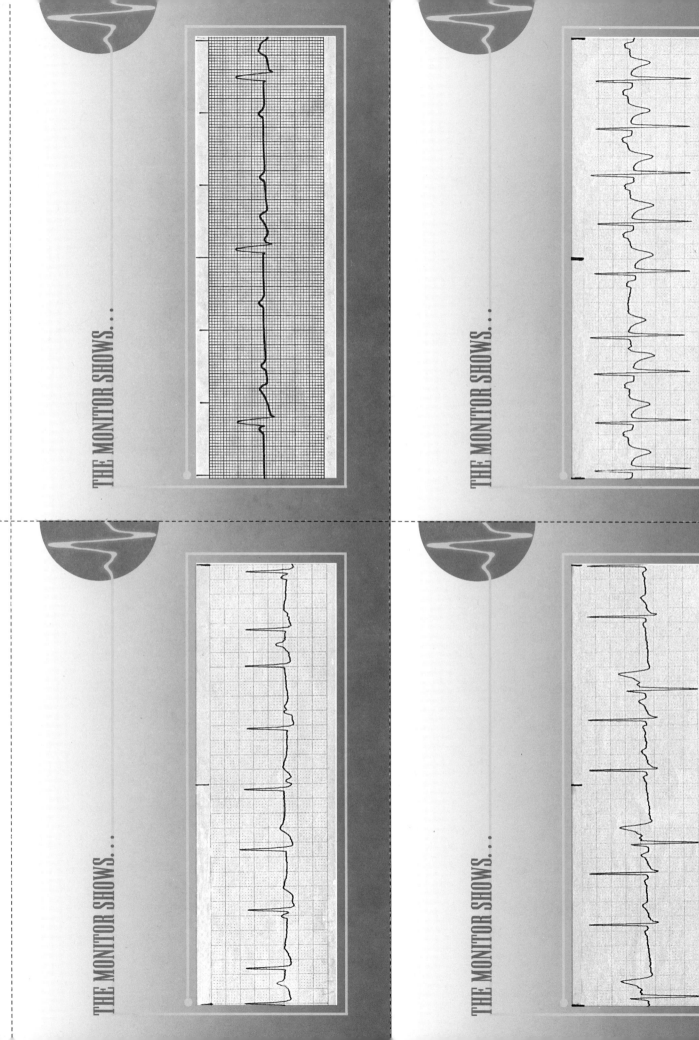

THIRD DEGREE HEART BLOCK

no relationship between P waves and QRS complexes; apparently irregular PR intervals; ventricular rate: 30; atrial rate: 70

PREMATURE ATRIAL CONTRACTION

occurs earlier than expected, originates from atria; heart rate: 90

WANDERING ATRIAL PACEMAKER

complexes originate from at least three sites in SA node, atria, and/or AV junctional area; heart rate: 90

PREMATURE JUNCTIONAL CONTRACTION

occurs earlier than expected; originates from junction; retrograde P wave; narrow QRS in premature complexes; heart rate: 90

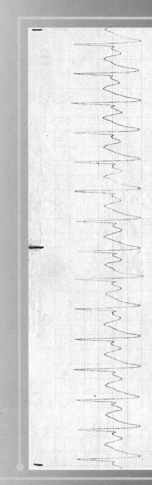

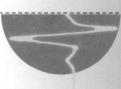

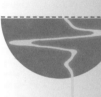

RHYTHM IDENTIFICATION

VENTRICULAR TACHYCARDIA
wide QRS;
no visible P waves;
heart rate: 230-240

RHYTHM IDENTIFICATION

WANDERING JUNCTIONAL PACEMAKER
originates from 3 or more junctional sites;
heart rate: 50

RHYTHM IDENTIFICATION

SINUS TACHYCARDIA
sinus rhythm with heart rate between 101 and 150;
heart rate: 150

RHYTHM IDENTIFICATION

Sinus rhythm with **BUNDLE BRANCH BLOCK**
notched QRS (greater than 0.12 second);
heart rate: 80

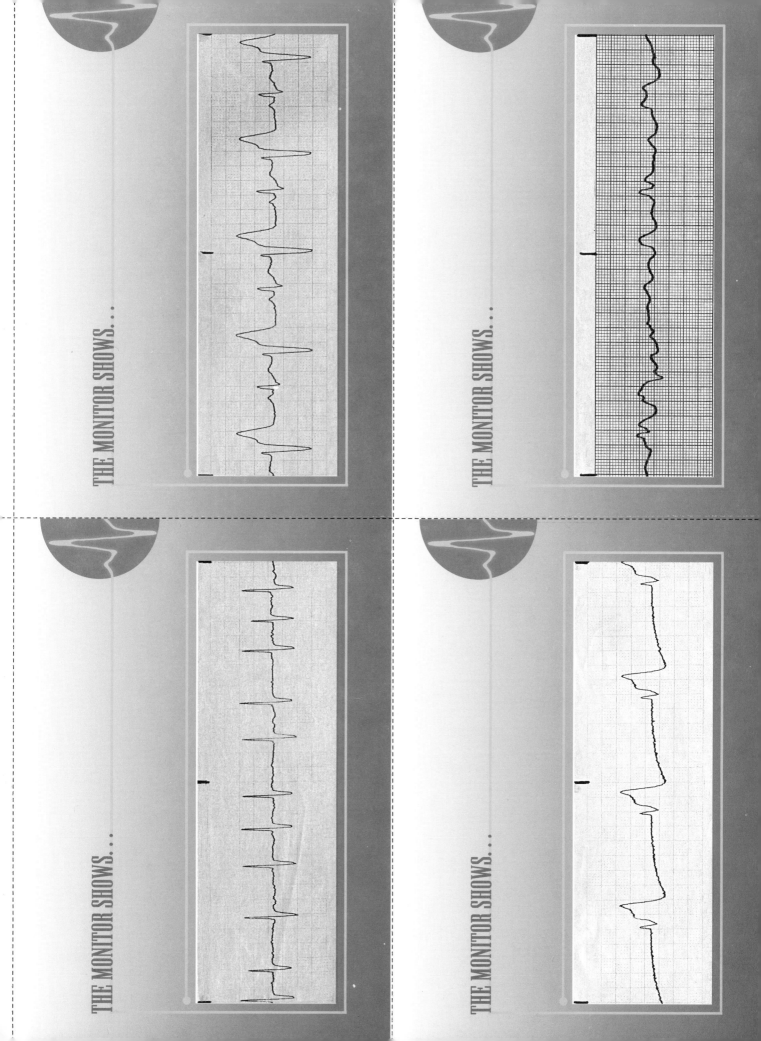

THE MONITOR SHOWS...

THE MONITOR SHOWS...

THE MONITOR SHOWS...

THE MONITOR SHOWS...

RHYTHM IDENTIFICATION

Sinus rhythm with **UNIFOCAL PVCs in BIGEMINY**
every other complex is a PVC;
heart rate: 90

RHYTHM IDENTIFICATION

ATRIAL FIBRILLATION with rapid ventricular response;
irregular rhythm;
no recognizable P wave
heart rate: 110

RHYTHM IDENTIFICATION

VENTRICULAR FIBRILLATION
no P waves;
no QRS complexes;
heart rate: 0

RHYTHM IDENTIFICATION

IDIOVENTRICULAR DYSRHYTHMIA
no P waves;
QRS wide and bizarre;
heart rate between 20 and 40;
heart rate: 40

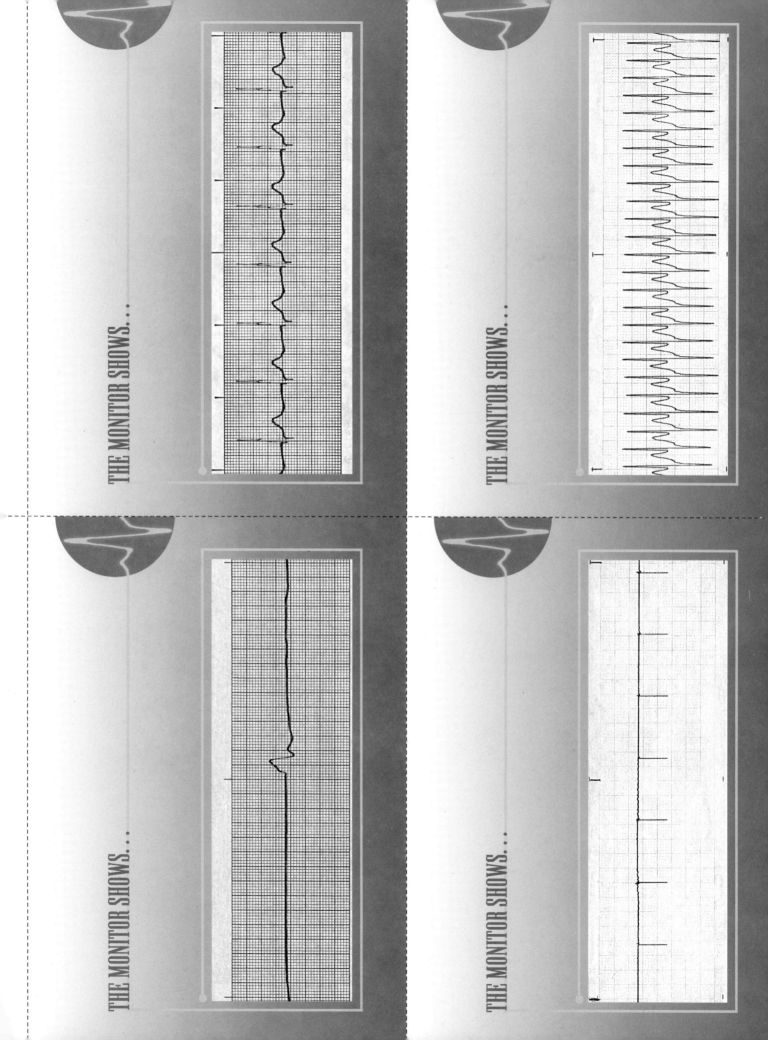

ACCELERATED JUNCTIONAL TACHYCARDIA

junctional rhythm;
rate between 61 and 100;
hidden P waves;
heart rate: 70

SUPRAVENTRICULAR TACHYCARDIA (SVT)

beginning or end of dysrhythmia is not seen;
narrow QRS complexes;
rate greater than 151;
heart rate: 250

AGONAL DYSRHYTHMIA (dying heart)

wide, bizarre complexes;
heart rate less than 20;
usually no pulse;
ventricular rate: 10

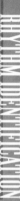

Pacemaker rhythm with **LOSS of CAPTURE**
100% paced;
0% capture; no pulse; no cardiac electrical activity;
pacer rate: 70;
heart rate: 0